Multimedia for Accessible Human Computer Interfaces

Troy McDaniel • Xueliang Liu
Editors

Multimedia for Accessible Human Computer Interfaces

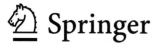 Springer

Editors
Troy McDaniel
Arizona State University
Mesa, AZ, USA

Xueliang Liu
Hefei University of Technology
Hefei, China

ISBN 978-3-030-70718-7   ISBN 978-3-030-70716-3   (eBook)
https://doi.org/10.1007/978-3-030-70716-3

This Springer imprint is published by the registered company Springer Nature Switzerland AG
The registered company address is: Gewerbestrasse 11, 6330 Cham, Switzerland

To my mentor, Dr. Panch, whose curiosity and drive to solve problems that empower individuals with disabilities ignited my own passion for helping people.

Troy McDaniel

Foreword

The field of multimedia, like many other fields in the past few years, has been propelled tremendously by recent developments arising from machine learning, and in particular, deep learning. Indeed, the ability of such extensive models to jointly learn representations and perform prediction/classification through automatic optimization of parameter spaces, directly from training data, has provided a significant boost to solving many problems. Multimedia problems regardless of the modality (audio, speech, images, video, haptic, AR/VR, among others) are no exception to this performance progress.

Accessibility is one of the key usability dimensions for human computer interfaces alongside effectiveness, efficiency, learnability, memorability, and satisfaction. While accessibility refers to the ability of a tool to be used by anyone, it is often perceived as providing similar user experiences for people with disabilities. Anyone within a certain context may require an alternative means of interaction with a device. Take the example of a worker performing repairs on specialized equipment which requires both hands; using a keyboard to find the correct repair step in the manual is not an option, hence speech access or vision-based recognition coupled with content-based retrieval would allow for the pertinent information to be read out or displayed on the worker's augmented reality glasses. In some aspects, accessibility also favors inclusion by allowing for a computer application to be used by diverse people in diverse contexts.

With this book on multimedia for accessible human computer interfaces, the editors, Troy McDaniel and Xueliang Liu, have brought together the multimedia and the HCI community. To the best of my knowledge, this is the very first time a book covers the topic of accessible human computer interface with such breadth, focusing on each modality in turn. Indeed, the manuscript is organized in four parts, each addressing a human sense (vision, auditory, and haptic) with the last part covering multimodal cases.

The book begins by reporting on vision-based accessibility with four chapters. The first chapter, "A Framework for Gaze-contingent Interfaces," details how to track head and eye movement for predicting the next point-of-gaze from depth images. The second chapter, "Sign Language Recognition," proposes a deep neural network solution to the recognition and translation of sign language. The third chapter, "Fusion-based Image Enhancement and its Applications in Mobile Devices," reports a method to produce mixed reality images. The fourth chapter, "Open-domain Textual Question Answering Systems," provides an in-depth look at this hot topic in natural language processing.

Auditory-based accessibility is the topic of the second part of this book, and is comprised of two chapters. The fifth chapter, "Speech Recognition for Individuals with Voice Disorders," introduces and discusses the state-of-the-art in speech recognition technologies for people with voice disorders. The sixth chapter, "Socially Assistive Robots for Storytelling and Other Activities to Support Aging in Place," provides a tour of socially assistive robots aimed at assisting older adults with aging in place.

The third part of this book is composed of two chapters covering haptics for HCI. The part begins with the seventh chapter, "Accessible Smart Coaching Technologies Inspired by Elderly Requisites," which describes how wearable technology can be used for tele-rehabilitation. The eighth chapter, "Haptic Mediators for Remote Interpersonal Communication," provides readers with the state-of-the-art of this emerging field.

The remaining part of the book is concerned with multimodal technologies for accessible human computer interfaces. This part starts with the ninth chapter, "Human-Machine Interfaces for Socially Connected Devices: From Smart Households to Smart Cities," which explores decision systems for evaluating the level of household energy consumption and the type of environmental home. The final chapter, "Enhancing Situational Awareness and Kinesthetic Assistance for Clinicians via Augmented-Reality and Haptic Shared-Control Technologies," details a system leveraging both augmented reality and haptic virtual fixtures to assist surgeons in performing complex surgical tasks.

I strongly believe this book will be of great interest to both academic and industry researchers in the field of HCI and/or multimedia. With such comprehensive and rich content, this book brings state-of-the-art multimedia technologies in the context of accessible HCI to all interested readers regardless of their background and technical level. By pulling together the relevant material, I hope this book will inspire its readers to research and design new and even more accessible human computer interfaces.

Artificial Intelligence & Data Science   Benoit Huet
Director, Median Technologies

Preface

Multimedia for Accessible Human Computer Interfaces is the first resource to provide in-depth coverage of topical areas of multimedia computing (images, video, audio, speech, haptics, and VR/AR) for accessible and inclusive human computer interfaces. Topics are grouped into thematic areas spanning the human senses: vision, hearing, touch, as well as multimodal applications. Each chapter is written by different multimedia researchers to provide complementary and multidisciplinary perspectives. Unlike other related books, which focus on guidelines for designing accessible interfaces, or are dated in their coverage of cutting edge multimedia technologies, *Multimedia for Accessible Human Computer Interfaces* takes an application-oriented approach to present a tour of how the field of multimedia is advancing access to human computer interfaces for individuals with disabilities.

The editors acknowledge the funding support of the National Science Foundation (Grant No. 1828010), Zimin Institute at Arizona State University, the National Major Research Program of China under grant 2018AAA0102002, and in part by the National Natural Science Foundation of China (NSFC) under grant 61976076.

Mesa, AZ, USA   Troy McDaniel

Hefei, China   Xueliang Liu

Contents

About the Editors

Troy McDaniel is an assistant professor of engineering in the Polytechnic School at Arizona State University. He is the director of the Center for Cognitive Ubiquitous Computing and the HAPT-X Laboratory. His research interests span the areas of haptic interfaces, human-robot interaction, human-computer interaction, and smart cities. He is particularly interested in tactile vision sensory substitution and haptic human augmentation. He focuses on applications involving assistive, rehabilitative, and healthcare technologies for individuals with sensory, cognitive, or physical impairments. Within these applications, he explores new haptic interaction paradigms and novel mappings between modalities to convey information in alternative ways. He is also actively exploring challenges related to accessibility and health and well-being within smart city and smart living applications using person- and citizen-centered approaches. He has authored more than 50 peer-reviewed publications and co-edited *Haptic Interfaces for Accessibility, Health, and Enhanced Quality of Life*. He holds a bachelor's and Ph.D. degree in computer science from Arizona State University.

Xueliang Liu is a professor in the School of Computer Science and Information Engineering at Hefei University of Technology, China. His research interests include multimedia retrieval, social media analysis, and object detection. He has authored over 40 journal and conference papers in these areas. He has served as the area chair of ACM Multimedia and is part of technical program committees of numerous multimedia and information retrieval conferences including ACM Multimedia (MM), ACM SIGIR, International Conf. on Multimedia Retrieval (ICMR), and International Conf. on Multimedia and Expo (ICME). Professor Liu has received the outstanding service award at PCM 2018, the best reviewer award at PCM 2013, and the best demo award at ACM MM 2007. He has also been the program chair of the ACM workshop on multimedia for accessible human computer interfaces, and the organizing chair of ICIMCS 2013, MMM 2016, and PCM 2018. Professor Liu received his Ph.D. and M.Sc. from EURECOM France and USTC China in 2013 and 2008, respectively.

Part I
Vision-Based Technologies for Accessible Human Computer Interfaces

A Framework for Gaze-Contingent Interfaces

Yingxuan Zhu, Wenyou Sun, Tim Tingqiu Yuan, and Jian Li

Abstract Mobile devices have become ubiquitous, and most have near infrared cameras. Infrared cameras generate 3D point clouds that can be used as a source of information to create features for better user experiences, especially in gaze-based user interfaces. In this chapter, a system is introduced for using data from mobile devices to detect and predict gaze. The data include 3D point clouds from near infrared cameras and 2D images from visible-light cameras. Because of the hardware setup, 3D reconstruction in these devices has its advantages and challenges. In this work, a variational method is developed to detect the sagittal plane from the data and reconstruct symmetric objects such as faces. Using symmetric face data increases the accuracy of 3D reconstruction and gaze detection. Registration and transformation methods are applied to measure movements of eyes and heads. In order to predict point of gaze, models based on long-short term memory are used to track head and eye movements. Our methods utilize the existing hardware setup and provide features to enhance user experiences. When gaze can be detected and tracked accurately, many gaze-based mobile applications can be developed for users.

Keywords Gaze contingent interface · Gaze detection · Gaze tracking · Variational methods · Long short-term memory

Y. Zhu (✉) · J. Li
Futurewei Technologies, Framingham, MA, USA
e-mail: yingxuan.zhu@futurewei.com; jian.li@futurewei.com

W. Sun
Huawei Technologies, Xi'an, China
e-mail: sunwenyou@huawei.com

T. T. Yuan
Huawei Technologies, Shenzhen, China
e-mail: tqy@huawei.com

3

1   Introduction

A gaze-contingent interface (GCI) assists people with motion difficulties to navigate devices and help improve mobility. Infrared camera-equipped mobile devices bring new features to GCIs and can significantly improve user experiences.

1.1   Gaze-Contingent Interface

A GCI is a human-computer interface (HCI) that changes display and screen content based on what the viewer is looking at [35]. In terms of convenience and user friendliness, GCIs have advantages. Compared to voice-based interfaces, the performance of GCIs will not change significantly in a noisy environment; and compared to hand-based or gesture-based interfaces, GCIs are convenient to use among people with physical impairments.

GCIs have a wide range of applications and can improve user experiences in computer assisted driving, gaming, marketing, medicine, among other areas [20, 27, 33, 39]. After a device detects the point of gaze (POG), or point of regard, a user's attention is detected. For instance, after a GCI detects that the POG of a user has been on a screen button for a specific amount of time, which can be regarded as the user selecting that button, the device will proceed with the function(s) of the button. GCIs can also adjust the resolution of a screen according to the user's focus, or remove objects that are beyond the user's attention to maintain user focus [16]. Garcia-Barrios et al. [8] proposed a framework of real-time eye tracking and content tracking for e-learning, and concluded that the framework had multiple benefits: improved knowledge of users' behavior, developed correction and adaptation mechanisms, and identified problematic areas in content flow or structuring. Li et al. [31] introduced an eye gaze-contingent ultrasound interface for a surgical system, which helped surgeons control the ultrasound system without using their hands during operations. Recently, GCIs have been widely embedded into augmented and virtual reality (AR/VR) applications, such as gaming.

Utaminingrum et al. [42] proposed a framework to recognize and detect eye movement for handling position, which used Haar Cascade to observe the area of the eyes, applied thresholding to the image using morphology to obtain the focus of the eyes, and utilized Hough Circle Transform with several rules to decide the handling position of eye movement. Raymond et al. [37] introduced a gaze-based wheelchair control interface that combined eye tracking with a 3D depth camera system to investigate identifiable patterns between eye movement and driving intentions. The gaze-based wheelchair control interface showed that a GCI was sufficient in restoring mobility by wheel chair and to increase participation in daily life. Subramanian et al. [41] further investigated gaze-based wheelchair interfaces, and developed a "Zero UI" driving platform that allowed users to control the visual scene via gaze and provided a destination to the wheelchair for autonomous driving.

Using gaze as a form of input, GCIs have unique benefits and problems. Compared to other input resources, vision provides fast and high bandwidth information to guide actions, requires no training, and is directly relative to the user's attention. On the other hand, GCI developers should pay attention to eye movement noise, accuracy, and Midas Touch problems [28]. Midas Touch is a situation where the detected gaze or eye movement does not reflect the user's attention because a user can look at an object while thinking about something unrelated. In addition, GCIs require fixed head movement to some extent [46].

1.2 Eye Tracking and Gaze Detection

GCIs rely on eye tracking and gaze detection techniques. Eye gaze tracking is a useful technique in vision-based HCI, and a critical component of GCIs [24, 25]. The techniques to find POGs can be categorized into three groups: eye-attaching tracking, optical tracking, and electric potential measurement [7, 13, 15, 34, 36]. Among these techniques, optical tracking with video recording is prevalent. This method does not require any attachments to the eyes nor placement of electrodes around the eyes. In our proposed method, optical tracking techniques are used. Note that some of the optical tracking devices are embedded in glasses, but even these are not attached to the eyes directly.

In terms of camera location, eye tracking systems include head-mounted systems and remote systems [21]. Head-mounted systems have better tolerance for head movement, but usually need to be attached to users' heads, which lack comfort and convenience. In addition, head-mounted systems usually block part of users' visual fields, which affect vision. Remote systems refer to eye tracking systems that are not attached to users' heads. These systems are usually less intrusive but require stabilization of the head. Aleem et al. [2] described a laser eye tracking system that scanned a laser light over the eyes to detect diffuse reflections of the laser light with one or more photodetector(s). This approach was based on reduction in reflection intensity due to transmission of laser light through the pupil and/or increased diffusivity of reflections from the cornea relative to reflections from the sclera.

POG is determined by the positions of both head and eyeballs. In order to have precise tracking results, single-camera-and-single-light (SCSL) methods usually require head stabilization or perfect device attachment to the head [19]. For example, Bulling et al. showed multiple models of eye trackers in [10], including the first generation of video-based eye trackers from Mobile Eye and iView X HED, the first eye tracker integrated into a glasses frame from Tobii Glasses, and wearable electrooculography (EOG) goggles from Swiss Federal Institute of Technology (ETH) Zurich [11]. However, it is not practical nor comfortable for users to maintain the same position so that the SCSL methods can work well. Thus, methods using multiple cameras and multiple lights (MCML) were introduced to address the trade-off between comfort and performance [45]. In MCML methods, multiple cameras acquire both a large field of view and a limited field of view. The acquisition of a large field of view allows head motion, and obtaining a limited field of view captures high resolution eye images for gaze estimation. However, adding multiple cameras and multiple lights for GCIs increases the cost of mobile devices. Moreover, MCML methods have the problems of stereo such as point matching, occlusion, and large data to process [23].

In addition to the methods summarized in [23], Bae et al. [6] proposed an iris recognition device using reflection from near infrared light to detect the iris, and the authors used the plurality of reference signals in different phases to remove the offset of the reflected light signal. Berkner-Cieslicki et al. [9] proposed an eye tracking system for detecting positions and movements of users' eyes in a head-mounted display (HMD). This eye tracking system emits near infrared light at users' eyes and tracks position and motion using cameras at each side of the face. The gaze tracker [29] was used to collect gaze information for depth estimation of gazed object and to construct sparse depth maps of augmented reality spaces for controlling visual information displayed to the viewer. Cao et al. [12] presented a cascade learning-based method that alternatively optimized both eye detection and gaze estimation. A convolutional neural network (CNN) model with minimal computational requirements was proposed for efficient appearance-based gaze estimation in low-quality consumer imaging systems [30].

1.3 Gaze-Contingent Interface Based on Near Infrared Camera of Mobile Device

Infrared cameras or depth cameras, coupled with time-of-flight techniques, have brought great features to mobile, AR/VR, and gaming devices. For example, the infrared camera of the Apple® iPhone® X can generate a point cloud of more than 30,000 dots for the function of Face ID® [17]. These kinds of point clouds are so sophisticated that the subtle differences between faces can be captured, enabling features such as biometric signature to unlock personal devices. Kinect® uses a depth camera to support scene reconstruction [3]. Infrared cameras bring new applications to mobile devices in AR/VR, multiexperiences, computer assisted driving, gaming, healthcare, among a myriad of other application areas.

In this chapter, the term infrared refers to near infrared with a wavelength of 700–900 nm. Near infrared does not distract users and has been approved by the Food and Drug Administration (FDA) to be used in a variety of medical devices. Methods of video-based eye tracking are mostly based on infrared. The performance of infrared-based cameras is consistent under variable illumination, which make gaze detection methods robust to indoor lighting conditions. Corneal reflection (bright pupil, dark pupil, or both) is commonly used to detect gaze. As an example, Zhu et al. presented an algorithm for gaze estimation without calibration under a large amount of head movement, based on corneal reflection and generalized regression neural networks [26].

However, there are challenges in using data from infrared cameras of mobile devices. Light travels straight, and a camera cannot see through obstacles. In addition, it is not practical to ask users to always maintain the best position for cameras to perform well. In reality, data caught by cameras usually only have partial faces, i.e., symmetric objects in unsymmetrical shapes. For example, if a camera is placed perfectly in front of a user but he or she is looking to the left, part of the left side of the face will be missing in the data because light can only reach the right side of the face. In addition, also because light travels straight, the part of the face that is more perpendicular to the light beams receives more light points and has higher density in the point cloud. Thus, it is very possible that point density is not even in the data of the point cloud. Moreover, most current methods in GCIs need the positions of both head and eyes to decide POGs to develop applications and enhance user experiences. Object symmetry is an important factor in perception problems [18] and has been applied to detect faces and face features in [32, 38]. Reconstruction of symmetric objects from imperfect data improves shape representation, geometric deep learning, and detection of geometric features.

In this chapter, we share a method for using data (point clouds and RGB images) from mobile devices to detect gaze and predict POG. A variational method [14, 40, 43, 44] is developed to reconstruct symmetric face data from imperfect camera data, and the reconstructed data are applied to a long short-term memory (LSTM) network for gaze prediction. Specifically, the variational method finds a sagittal plane that can map the face data from the left side to the right side, and vice versa, to regenerate a symmetric face. Compared to an unsymmetrical face, a symmetrical face improves registration results and reduces processing time; thus, finding the sagittal plane eventually helps detect the subtle movements of the head and eyes. After detection, a sequence of positions of faces and eyes are inputted to the LSTM network for prediction of the next possible movement and POG.

The proposed method takes advantage of symmetric objects to increase accuracy and to reduce the time needed for reconstruction and registration. In some scenarios, reconstruction and registration can be achieved directly by using UseR Standard Data (URSD) and a sagittal plane, which dramatically reduces the time in finding positions. Our methods rely on the assumption that the object in question is symmetric, which is generally true for the human head. In addition, symmetric and rigid objects, such as heads, have better accuracy than symmetric but nonrigid objects, such as the human body. For example, it is hard to detect the sagittal plane when a person is in an asymmetrical pose. However, the proposed method can be used to detect part of the human body, and can work with other 3D reconstruction and recognition methods, such as those in [1, 22].

The methods proposed in this chapter belong to a research project on future mobile devices, which were first introduced in [47]. Our methods use two kinds of facial data: 3D point clouds and 2D images. A 3D point cloud is a set of 3D data points that show the structure of an object, such as a face. The point clouds from infrared cameras do not have color and usually have depth information. Depending on the hardware setup, 2D images include images with bright pupils, dark pupils, eye color images, or any combination of these. Because 2D images are mostly used for detection of eyes in our methods, we also refer to these images as eye images, even though 2D images include faces and other objects. The movements of heads and eyes can be subtle in gaze detection. Theoretically, when the distance between a camera and an object becomes larger, the object becomes smaller in the photo. Thus, the further the distance between the user and the camera, the more subtle the changes and less a camera can capture. Combining information from both 3D point clouds and eye images provides more detail for gaze detection and leads to better results. When captured using cameras, 3D point clouds and eye images are not in the same coordinate system. Because camera locations in a device are mostly fixed after manufacture, the parameters to transform between one coordinate system and another can be obtained during calibration. The movements of heads and eyes are measured by position differences obtained from registration and transformation.

2 Methods

To utilize infrared cameras in mobile devices and add new functions for better user experiences, we propose methods to use data from infrared cameras for GCIs of mobile device. Our methods can be easily adjusted to improve accessibility. In our methods, we assume that there is no cover attention, i.e., what a user is looking at is what the user is paying attention to.

2.1 Framework

The framework of our method is shown in Fig. 1. The user standard data are obtained during calibration. During the first use of a device, cameras are calibrated to obtain parameters and standard information of each user. After the data of 3D point clouds and eye images are captured, these data are fused into the same coordinate system using parameters from calibration. Faces and eyes are detected by image registration methods using URSD as references. A variational method is used to find the sagittal plane from facial data and to reconstruct the face by the sagittal plane. POGs are calculated based on reconstructed facial data. Finally, the LSTM network is applied to predict the next POG after learning a sequence of POGs.

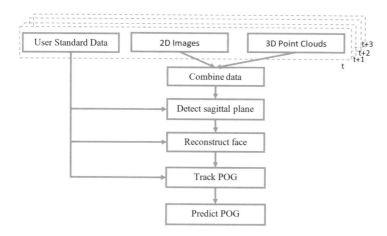

Fig. 1 Framework for gaze detection and prediction

2.2 Calibration and Standard Acquisition

After manufacture, a device's hardware components, including infrared light emitters and cameras, are set. Each user has his or her unique facial structure. Data acquired in calibration are important references and are used as standards for comparison and registration. As described earlier, these data are called UseR Standard Data, or URSD, in our methods. URSD include, but are not limited to, user's data with facial information, parameters to transfer data from one domain to another, positions and movements of faces and eyes when a user looks at different given points on the screen. There are different ways to calibrate; generally, the more calibration points there are, the better the result will be.

The 9-point calibration method is used in our experiments, see Fig. 2. Specifically, let $P_S = \{(x_{S_q}, y_{S_q}, z_{S_q}) | q = 1, \ldots, n\}$ be the given standard POGs on the screen, S be a set of 3D point clouds with one for each POG, and C be the corresponding eye images, where n is the number of POGs. A user will first look at the given POGs on a screen at the farthest distance d_1 in normal use. When the user is looking at a given POG, he or she can send a command to record and save the corresponding URSD. Methods of sending a command include, but are not limited to, pressing a button on the remote of the device, pressing a button on the device, and/or sending a voice command. Calibration is done at two distances. After recording the parameters obtained from distance d_1, the user moves to distance d_2 to perform the above steps again to obtain a second set of URSD.

3D point clouds from infrared cameras and eye images from visible-light cameras are in different coordinate systems. Because camera locations are fixed, parameters to transform data from one domain to another can be obtained during calibration, such as parameters to transform between the point cloud domain and the eye color

Fig. 2 Illustration of POGs
in calibration

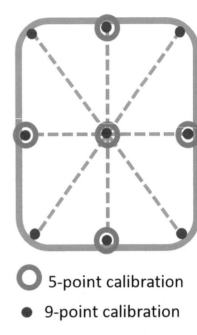

○ 5-point calibration

● 9-point calibration

image domain. Let G be the function that fuses the 3D point cloud S and eye image C using parameters ω to obtain data $\mathcal{V}$, then

$$\mathcal{V} = G(S, C, \omega). \tag{1}$$

Some parameters of ω are obtained during manufacturing calibration.

The data captured by cameras might include multiple faces including those of bystanders. The URSD obtained during calibration are also used as references to identify authorized users. During system setup, the number of users for one device can be specified and the corresponding URSD of each user will be recorded. When a device is in regular use, URSD are used as reference and computer vision methods (such as registration and transformation) are applied to detect faces and eyes.

2.3 Determination of Sagittal Plane

The positions of both heads and eyes are required in most of the current methods to decide POGs. However, as described in Sect. 1.3, real-time data of heads and eyes may not be in optimal shapes because light travels straight and cannot go through objects. In addition, a user usually looks at the screen instead of looking at the camera, i.e., cameras of a device usually cannot capture the user's whole face. Thus, only part of a user's face will be recorded in the data.

The sagittal plane symmetrically separates a human body into its left and right sides. Because heads and faces are mostly symmetric, knowing one side of the face and the sagittal plane, a whole face can be reconstructed. Lighting conditions may lead to the left and right sides of a face being in very different colors. However, the structure of the left and right sides of a face are mostly the same, simply because the face is symmetric. Furthermore, a user's eyes will usually look in the same direction and focus on the same object. Based on the aforementioned problems and observations, a method based on variational functions is proposed to find the sagittal plane and reconstruct the face.

Let $p = (x, y, z) \in \mathbb{R}^3$ be a point in point cloud Ω. Let f with $f(p) = 0$ to present sagittal plane.

$$\begin{cases} \text{Saggital plane}: f(x, y, z) = 0\} \\ \text{Left}: f(x, y, z) > 0\} \\ \text{Right}: f(x, y, z) < 0\}. \end{cases} \tag{2}$$

Now, let p' be symmetric to p with respect to the sagittal plane, that is, the line formed by p and p' is perpendicular to f. Because of symmetry, the distance D of p to f should be equal to the distance of p' to f, that is, their difference in distance should be 0. The cost function $\mathcal{F}(f)$ presents the above ideas in a mathematical way. When the sagittal plane f is found, $\mathcal{F}(f)$ is minimized.

$$\mathcal{F}(f) = \int_\Omega \lambda_1 (D(p)H(f(x, y, z)) - D(p')(1 - H(f(x, y, z))))^2 \\ + \lambda_2 (D(p)(1 - H(f(x, y, z))) - D(p')H(f(x, y, z)))^2 dxdydz \tag{3}$$

where λ_1 and λ_2 are parameters, and $H(f)$ is a Heaviside Function.

$$H(f) = \begin{cases} 1, & \text{if } f \geq 0 \\ 0, & \text{if } f < 0 \end{cases} \tag{4}$$

For the purpose of simplicity, (3) is written as

$$\begin{aligned} \mathcal{F}(f) &= \int_\Omega \lambda_1 (DH - D'(1 - H))^2 \\ &\quad + \lambda_2 (D(1 - H) - D'H)^2 dxdydz \\ &= \int_\Omega \lambda_1 (DH - D' + D'H)^2 \\ &\quad + \lambda_2 (D - DH - D'H)^2 dxdydz \\ &= \int_\Omega \lambda_1 (D^2 H^2 + D'^2 \\ &\quad + D'^2 H^2 - 2DD'H \\ &\quad + 2DD'H^2 - 2D'^2 H) \\ &\quad + \lambda_2 (D^2 + D^2 H^2 \\ &\quad + D'^2 H^2 - 2D^2 H \\ &\quad - 2DD'H + 2DD'H^2)dxdydz \end{aligned} \tag{5}$$

where D, D', and H represent $D(p)$, $D(p')$ and $H(f(x, y, z))$ in (3), respectively. If $\lambda_1 = \lambda_2$, (5) can be simplified as

$$\mathcal{F}(f) = \int_\Omega D^2 + D'^2 + 2(D + D')^2(H^2 - H)dxdydz \tag{6}$$

Let $E = D^2 + D'^2 + 2(D + D')^2(H^2 - H)$, keep D and D' fixed, and deduce the associate Euler-Lagrange equation for f.

Solve for f, and parameterize with step size t:

$$\frac{\partial f}{\partial t} = 2\delta(f(x, y, z))((D + D')^2(2H - 1), \tag{7}$$

or

$$f^{(n)} = f^{(n-1)} + 2\Delta t\delta(f(x, y, z))((D + D')^2(2H - 1), \tag{8}$$

where $\delta(f(x, y, z)) = \frac{d}{df}H(f)$ and Δt is a step size. The initial plane can be a plane perpendicular to the line between two eyes, which can be approximately detected from digital photos. In experiments, the step size is set to 1, and the Heaviside Function is

$$H(z) = \frac{1}{2}\left(1 + \frac{2}{\pi}\arctan\left(\frac{z}{\epsilon}\right)\right). \tag{9}$$

where π and ϵ are parameters of the Heaviside Function.

Because light from the device emitter lands on a person's face at different locations, the density of points is not even in the point cloud. Locations that are closer to the light source and more perpendicular to light beams have larger density than those that are not. Thus, the number of points on the right side may not be the same as the number of points on the left side, and vice versa, i.e., there may not be a p' for each p. Given that not every point p has a symmetric point p' that can form a line perpendicular to f, we loosen the definition of p' to the closest ideal point of p' within distance d, where d is a parameter. If there is no p' within distance d, p will not be included in the calculation.

In addition, using the points on $f(x, y, z)$, the sagittal plane is obtained by a Support Vector Machine (SVM), and $f(x, y, z) = Ax + By + Cz + K$, where A, B, C, K are parameters. Thus, the distance $L(p)$ between p and f can be obtained by

$$L(p) = \frac{Ax + By + Cz + K}{\sqrt{A^2 + B^2 + C^2}}. \tag{10}$$

Once the sagittal plane is determined, data from one side of the face are mapped to the other side and a mainly symmetric user face is reconstructed.

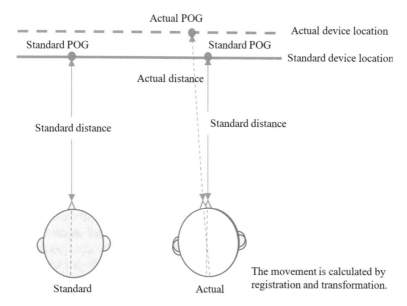

Fig. 3 Illustration of standard POG and actual POG

2.4 Calculation of POG with Head Adjustment

A user can look at different locations by moving only the eyes while keeping his or her head motionless, and vice versa. Thus, movements of heads and eyes need to be determined together to calculate actual POG. Registration and transformation are used to measure movements of heads and eyes. Figure 3 shows the locations of a standard POG in URSD and an actual POG.

POG is computed from both head and eyeball positions. To obtain accurate POG, the head movement needs to be compensated for using the approach in [4].

$$d_t - d_S = \alpha(d_{G_t} - d_S) \tag{11}$$

where d_S, d_t, and d_{G_t} are reference directions—the directions of head and gaze at time t, respectively. α is a parameter depending on head pose.

The calculation of POG with head adjustment is based on the methods in [15] and [5]. Specifically, let $P_{G_t} = \{(x_{G_t}, y_{G_t}, z_{G_t})\}$ be the POG at time t, a be the distance between the plane of standard POGs and the actual plane of the device, and b be the distance between the eyes. If $P_{L_t} = \{(x_{L_t}, y_{L_t}, z_{L_t})\}$ and $P_{R_t} = \{(x_{R_t}, y_{R_t}, z_{R_t})\}$ are the view points of standard device location for the left and right eyeballs at time t, then P_{G_t} can be calculated as

$$x_{G_t} = (1 - \frac{b}{x_{L_t} - x_{R_t} + b})x_h + (\frac{b}{x_{L_t} - x_{R_t} + b})(\frac{x_{L_t} + x_{R_t}}{2}) \tag{12}$$

$$y_{G_t} = (1 - \frac{b}{x_{L_t} - x_{R_t} + b})y_h + (\frac{b}{x_{L_t} - x_{R_t} + b})(\frac{y_{L_t} + y_{R_t}}{2}) \qquad (13)$$

$$z_{G_t} = (1 - \frac{b}{x_{L_t} - x_{R_t} + b})z_h + (\frac{b}{x_{L_t} - x_{R_t} + b})a. \qquad (14)$$

2.5 Gaze Prediction by LSTM

If a device can predict the next POG for the user, it can proactively provide relevant options and improve user experiences. To predict how a user moves his or her head and eyes, the changes in position of the head and eyes over a time interval need to be known, which can be measured using registration and transformation methods. LSTM is a machine learning method that can detect changes in data sequences. The LSTM network is applied in our methods to capture the changes in head and eye movements to predict the next possible POG(s). Even though 1 second is used as the step size in our methods, the time unit can be any time interval and is not necessarily 1 second. The LSTM model of our method is shown in Fig. 4.

In our system, registration and transformation methods are embedded into LSTM cells. The registration and transformation applied to data are discussed in Sect. 2.6. Specifically, the LSTM parameters and formulas in an LSTM cell, Fig. 5, are defined below.

- $\mathbf{X}_t$: input data of an LSTM cell at time t, including 3D point clouds and eye images.
- $\mathbf{H}_t \in \mathbb{R}^h$, and $\mathbf{H}_t = \{S, \mathbf{h}_t\}$: the hidden variable of an LSTM unit, including the standard face data S and the aligned data at t. $\mathbf{h}_t$ is the fused 3D face data (3D point cloud with intensity values), and can be obtained by registration and transformation (combining the registration result and new point of gaze). $\mathbf{H}_t$ is

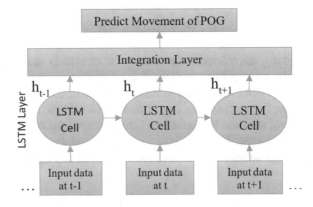

Fig. 4 Illustration of LSTM model

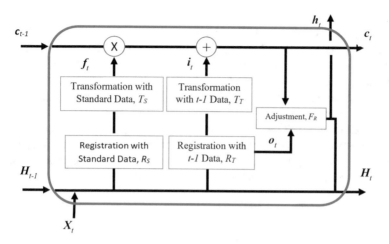

Fig. 5 Design of LSTM cell in our method

passed from one LSTM cell to another. The superscript h refers to the number of hidden units.

- $\mathbf{f}_t$: forget gate's activation function applied to registration result of S and $\mathbf{X}_t$. $\mathbf{f}_t$ indicates whether the current input data match URSD, i.e., whether the detected face belongs to the authorized user(s). If it belongs to the user, $\mathbf{f}_t$ is 1, otherwise it is 0, i.e., the current input data should not be processed if it does not belong to an authorized user.
- $\mathbf{i}_t$: input gate's result from registration and transformation of $\mathbf{X}_t$ and $\mathbf{H}_{t-1}$. $\mathbf{i}_t$ represents the difference between $\mathbf{X}_t$ and $\mathbf{H}_{t-1}$, i.e., the movement of eyes between the current and previous POGs. It is one of the components deciding the current point of gaze.
- $\mathbf{o}_t$: output gate's result obtained from registration. $\mathbf{o}_t$ represents pairs of corresponding points in data $\mathbf{X}_t$ and data $\mathbf{h}_{t-1}$.
- $\mathbf{c}_t \in \mathbb{R}^2$, and $\mathbf{c}_t = \{P_S, P_t\}$: cell state vector, or POG, including standard POG P_S and current POG P_t at time t. P_t indicates where the user is looking at on the screen, which is obtained by combining the previous point of gaze and the movement. $\mathbf{c}_t$ as a whole can be presented as a 2 by 2 matrix, where each row represents a point in x and y on the screen.

$$\mathbf{f}_t = \sigma_f(W_f T_S(R_S(\mathbf{X}_t, \mathbf{H}_{t-1}))) \tag{15}$$

$$\mathbf{i}_t = \tanh(W_i T_T(R_T(\mathbf{X}_t, \mathbf{H}_{t-1})) \tag{16}$$

$$\mathbf{o}_t = W_o R_T(\mathbf{X}_t, \mathbf{H}_{t-1}) \tag{17}$$

$$\mathbf{c}_t = \mathbf{f}_t \circ \mathbf{c}_{t-1} + \mathbf{i}_t \tag{18}$$

$$\mathbf{h}_t = F_R(\mathbf{o_t}, \mathbf{c_t}) \tag{19}$$

where

- R_S: registration of S and $\mathbf{X}_t$, which represents pairs of corresponding points between standard data S and current input data $\mathbf{X}_t$. Note that S is included in $\mathbf{H}_{t-1}$ and passed to the next LSTM cell by $\mathbf{H}_t$; specifically, the active component of $\mathbf{H}_{t-1}$ in R_S is S, which can be set by the parameters.
- T_S: transformation of $\mathbf{H}_{t-1}$ (only S) and $\mathbf{X}_t$, which represents the movement between these two data.
- R_T: registration of $\mathbf{X}_t$ and $\mathbf{h}_{t-1}$, which represents pairs of corresponding points of these two datasets. Note that $\mathbf{h}_{t-1}$ is included in $\mathbf{H}_{t-1}$ with S; specifically, only $\mathbf{h}_{t-1}$ of $\mathbf{H}_{t-1}$ is active in R_T, which can be set up by the parameters.
- T_T: transformation of $\mathbf{X}_t$ and $\mathbf{h}_{t-1}$, which indicates the eye movement from $\mathbf{h}_{t-1}$ to $\mathbf{X}_t$.
- F_R: based on $\mathbf{c}_t$, for each pair of corresponding points in $\mathbf{X}_t$ and $\mathbf{h}_{t-1}$, refines the point in $\mathbf{X}_t$ to remove small inconsistencies.
- σ_f: heaviside function, or sigmoid function.
- W_f, W_i, and W_o are weight matrices, and ∘ denotes element-wise product.

It is worth mentioning that solving an LSTM model with back propagation requires variable differentiability between LSTM cells. Generally, a human face remains the same over a short period of time. If a user's face changes significantly, this user will be decided by the device as an unauthorized user and the data will not be processed. Thus, it is reasonable to assume that the registration of face data from two different time points is rigid and linear, i.e., there is no significant changes in face structure, but only changes in coordinate systems of two datasets. Therefore, the registration of face data can be seen as mapping the coordinate system of one dataset to another. A linear function is generally differentiable. Based on linearity and differentiability, registration and transformation results can be used to directly calculate movements of heads and eyes between LSTM cells.

2.6 Measurement of Head and Eye Movements

Registration and transformation are used to measure movements of heads and eyes against references in URSD, and to decide POGs. In addition, in order to predict what a user will be looking at, the head and eye movements of the user should be measured and recorded. The URSD obtained in calibration are used as references in registration to measure how the head and eyes move by comparing the current position and the position recorded in the URSD. Registrations in our methods include registration of heads and faces, and registration of eyes. Face registration also helps decide if the detected face belongs to an authorized user, and to determine where the eyes are in the current data. Eye registration is to learn how the eyes move and the location of the current POG. Registration also includes registration against previous data to determine how faces and eyes move. Note that in some literature, registration includes transformation. In our method, the goal of

Table 1 Registration in LSTM cells

Registration	Standard, R_S	$t - 1$, R_T
Face	Output corresponding pairs of points to T_S; found the closest point of gaze in standard data	Output corresponding pairs of points to T_T
Eye	Output corresponding pairs of points to T_S; found the closest point of gaze in standard data	Output corresponding pairs of points to T_T

Table 2 Transformation in LSTM cells

Registration	Standard, T_S	$t - 1$, T_T
Face	Measure and decide if it is the face of authorized user(s); estimate face moving distance	Determine the movement of face, and approximate movement of point of gaze
Eye	Detect the range for point of gaze approximately, based on standard face data	Determine the movement of eyes, and thus, the movement of point of gaze

registration is to match two datasets, and find the corresponding pairs of points. A variety of registration methods can be used. Transformation is to quantify the movement. Tables 1 and 2 show the registrations (R_S, R_T) and transformations (T_S, T_T) embedded into LSTM cells.

3 Use Cases

The use of infrared cameras in mobile devices creates much potential for GCIs. Compared with bulky headsets, which may require users to sit in front of cameras, mobile devices are usually compact and convenient to use. The detection of POG can be a function of the mobile device, and users can enable and disable the feature. In this section, two examples of GCIs are discussed below.

3.1 Use Case #1: Select an Option on Screen

In a GCI, the device can provide options on the screen for the user to choose by using POGs. There are more than one way to confirm a user selection, including the duration a user looks at the option (length of gaze), a pop-up confirmation dialog, and voice command. Depending on the design of a GCI, the selections are not necessary to be at fixed locations on the screen, but can be near or even at the locations of POGs. Such a design can reduce the time that a user has to move his or her head and eyes and refocus, which creates a better user experience. In addition, because a user does not have to move his or her head and eyes to make

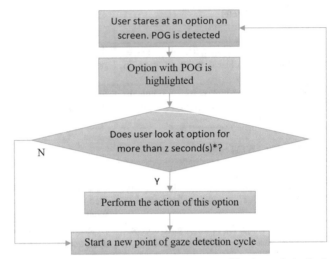

Fig. 6 A workflow of using POG to select an option on screen

every selection, it will reduce time and increase smoothness in using GCIs. Figure 6 shows a workflow where the user selects and confirms a selection by the length of time that he or she focuses on the screen location (the duration of a POG).

The orange dot in (a) of Fig. 7 shows the detected POG. Because the POG is in the region of an option, that option is highlighted, Fig. 7b. If the user looks at that region for a predefined amount of time, the option is selected.

3.2 Use Case #2: Auto Screen Scrolling

When the user is reading an ebook, his or her head and eyes will move consistently on the screen. The proposed LSTM method can capture this consistency and anticipate that the user may want to read the next lines of the ebook. In this case, we show an example of navigating content on the screen using POGs. The content here can be PDF files such as a paper or a book, a website, an email, etc. Let l_s be the height of a screen, the top left corner of the screen $(0, 0)$ be the screen origin, and (x, y) be the detected POG in the screen coordinate system, where x is the row on the screen and y is the column. If y is not in the range of $[l_s/3, 2l_s/3]$, the device will move the content automatically:

$$\begin{cases} \text{When } y < l_s/3, \text{ scroll the screen down for } l_s/3, \\ \text{When } y > 2l_s/3, \text{ scroll the screen up for } l_s/3. \end{cases} \tag{20}$$

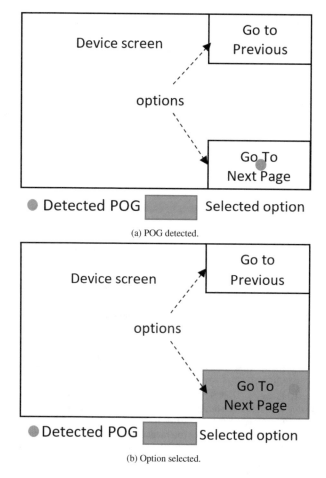

(a) POG detected.

(b) Option selected.

Fig. 7 Select an option on screen. (**a**) POG detected. (**b**) Option selected

The design above includes scrolling the screen up. It is possible a user will search back for something that he or she desires to read, maybe line-by-line instead of word-by-word. The LSTM method should also be able to predict the next POGs for this type of behavior.

4 Future Work

Near infrared cameras bring new functions to mobile devices, and provide opportunities in assistive computing to improve user experiences. In this chapter, we proposed a framework to use data from mobile devices (3D point clouds from infrared cameras and photos from visible-light cameras) to detect and track POGs for GCIs. Our methods include reconstructing symmetric objects from imperfect 3D point cloud data, measuring movement against references using registration methods, detecting and predicting POGs using an LSTM network. In addition to assistive computing, these methods can be used in a variety of devices, including autonomous driving, AR/VR, multiexperiences, among others. The use of 3D infrared cameras is still new to mobile devices, but we believe this feature will be utilized in more and more applications to provide better user experiences.

References

1. Achlioptas, P., Diamanti, O., Mitliagkas, I., Guibas, L.: Learning representations and generative models for 3d point clouds. In: Proceedings of the 35th International Conference on Machine Learning (ICML) (2018)
2. Aleem, I.S., Chapeskie, M.V.J.: Systems, devices, and methods for laser eye tracking (2016). https://patents.google.com/patent/US9904051B2/en. Patent No. US9904051B2, Filed October 21st., 2016
3. Azure kinect DK depth camera. https://docs.microsoft.com/en-us/azure/kinect-dk/depth-camera
4. Ba, S.O., Odobez, J.: Recognizing visual focus of attention from head pose in natural meetings. IEEE Trans. Syst. Man Cybern. **39**(1), 16–33 (2009). https://doi.org/10.1109/TSMCB.2008.927274
5. Ba, S.O., Odobez, J.: Multiperson visual focus of attention from head pose and meeting contextual cues. IEEE Trans. Pattern Anal. Mach. Intell. **33**(1), 101–116 (2011). https://doi.org/10.1109/TPAMI.2010.69
6. Bae, K., Kim, T., Jeong, S., Cho, S.: Iris recognition device and mobile device having the same (2014). https://patents.google.com/patent/US9418306B2/en?oq=US9418306B2. Patent No. US9418306B2, Filed November 11th., 2014, Issued Aug. 16th., 2016
7. Bajaj, D.: Gaze-contingent displays for interactive text enhancement. Master's thesis (2017)
8. Barrios, V.G., Gütl, C., Preis, A.M., Andrews, K., Pivec, M., Mödritscher, F., Trummer, C.: Adele: A framework for adaptive e-learning through eye tracking. In: Proceedings of I-Know'04, pp. 609–616 (2004)
9. Berkner-Cieslicki, K., Motta, R.J., LIM, S.H., Kim, M., Saito, K., Petljanski, B., Sauers, J.C., Shinohara, Y.: Eye tracking system (2017). https://patents.google.com/patent/US20180113508A1/en. Patent No. US20180113508A1, Filed October 19th., 2017
10. Bulling, A., Gellersen, H.: Toward mobile eye-based human-computer interaction. In: IEEE Pervasive Computing, vol. 9, pp. 8–12 (2010)
11. Bulling, A., Roggen, D., Tröster, G.: It's in your eyes: towards context-awareness and mobile HCI using wearable EOG goggles. In: Proceedings of the Tenth International Conference on Ubiquitous Computing (2008). https://doi.org/10.1145/1409635.1409647
12. Cao, L., Gou, C., Wang, K., Xiong, G., Wang, F.Y.: Gaze-aided eye detection via appearance learning. In: Proceedings of the 24th International Conference on Pattern Recognition (ICPR), pp. 1965–1970. IEEE, Piscataway (2018). https://doi.org/10.1109/ICPR.2018.8545635
13. Chennamma, H., Yuan, X.: A survey on eye-gaze tracking techniques. Indian J. Comput. Sci. Eng. **4**(5), 388–393 (2013)
14. Cremers, D., Soatto, S.: Motion competition: a variational approach to piecewise parametric motion segmentation. Int. J. Comput. Vis. **62**, 249–265 (2005). https://doi.org/10.1007/s11263-005-4882-4
15. Duchowski, A.T.: Eye Tracking Methodology, 3rd. edn. Springer, New York (2017)

16. Duchowski, A.T., Cournia, N., Murphyi, H.: Gaze-contingent displays: A review. CyberPsychol. Behav. **7**(6), 621–634 (2004). https://doi.org/10.1089/cpb.2004.7.621
17. Face ID your face is your password. https://www.apple.com/iphone-xs/face-id/
18. Gesù, V.D., Valenti, C.: Symmetry operators in computer vision. Vistas Astron. **40**(4), 461–468 (1996). https://doi.org/10.1016/S0083-6656(96)00030-X
19. Gneo, M., Schmid, M., Conforto, S., DAlessio, T.: A free geometry model-independent neural eye-gaze tracking system. J. NeuroEng. Rehab. **9**(82) (2012). https://doi.org/10.1186/1743-0003-9-82
20. Goldberg, J.H., Schryver, J.C.: Eye-gaze-contingent control of the computer interface: Methodology and example for zoom detection. Behav. Res. Methods Instrum. Comput. **27**(3), 338–350 (1995)
21. Goldberg, J.H., Wichansky, A.M.: Eye tracking in usability evaluation: a practitioner's guide. In: The Mind's Eye: Cognitive and Applied Aspects of Eye Movement Research, chap. 23, pp. 493–516. Elsevier Science (2003). https://doi.org/10.1016/B978-044451020-4/50027-X
22. Güler, R.A., Kokkinos, I.: Holopose: Holistic 3d human reconstruction in-the-wild. In: Proceedings of IEEE Conf. on Computer Vision and Pattern Recognition (CVPR), pp. 10884–10894. IEEE, Piscataway (2019). https://doi.org/10.1109/ICPR.2018.8545635
23. Hansen, D.W., Ji, Q.: In the eye of the beholder: A survey of models for eyes and gaze. IEEE Trans. Pattern Anal. Mach. Intell. **32**(3), 478–500 (2010). https://doi.org/10.1109/TPAMI.2009.30
24. Jacob, R.J.: The use of eye movements in human-computer interaction techniques: what you look at is what you get. ACM Trans. Inf. Syst. **9**(3), 152–169 (1991)
25. Jacob, R.J.: Eye tracking in advanced interface design. In: Barfield, W., Furness, T.A. (eds.) Virtual Environments and Advanced Interface Design, pp. 258–288. Oxford University Press, New York (1995)
26. Ji, Q., Zhu, Z.: Eye and gaze tracking for interactive graphic display. Mach. Vis. Appl. **15**(3), 139–148 (2004). https://doi.org/10.1007/s00138-004-0139-4
27. Kar, A., Corcoran, P.: A review and analysis of eye-gaze estimation systems, algorithms and performance evaluation methods in consumer platforms. IEEE Access **5** (2017). https://doi.org/10.1109/ACCESS.2017.2735633
28. Kumar, M.: Gaze-enhanced user interface design. Ph.D. thesis, Stanford University, Palo Alto, CA (2007)
29. Kuo, T.S., Shih, K.T., Chung, S.L., Chen, H.H.: Depth from gaze. In: Proceedings of the 25th IEEE International Conference on Image Processing (ICIP), pp. 2910–2914. IEEE, Piscataway (2018). https://doi.org/10.1109/ICIP.2018.8451156
30. Lemley, J., Kar, A., Drimbarean, A., Corcoran, P.: Convolutional neural network implementation for eye-gaze estimation on low-quality consumer imaging systems. IEEE Trans. Consum. Electron. **65**(2), 179–187 (2019). https://doi.org/10.1109/TCE.2019.2899869
31. Li, Z., Tong, I., Salcudean, S.E.: Eye gaze contingent ultrasound interfaces for the da Vinci® surgical system. In: Proceedings of the 2017 International Conference on Intelligent Robots and Systems (IROS), Shared Platforms Workshop. IEEE, Piscataway (2017)
32. Loy, G., Zelinsky, A.: Fast radial symmetry for detecting points of interest. IEEE Trans. Pattern Anal. Mach. Intell. **25**(8), 959–973 (2003). https://doi.org/10.1109/TPAMI.2003.1217601
33. Lupu, R.G., Ungureanu, F.: A survey of eye tracking methods and application Buletinul Institutului Politehnic din Iasi, Automatic Control and Computer Science Section, (2014). https://scholar.google.com/citations?user=66PuewoAAAAJ&hl=da https://silo.tips/download/a-survey-of-eye-tracking-methods-and-applications
34. Majaranta, P., Bulling, A.: Eye tracking and eye-based human – computer interaction. In: Fairclough, S.H., Gilleade, K. (eds.) Advances in Physiological Computing, Human–Computer Interaction Series, chap. 3, pp. 39–65. Springer, London (2014)
35. Majaranta, P., Aoki, H., Donegan, M., Hansen, D.W., Hansen, J.P.: Gaze Interaction and Applications of Eye Tracking: Advances in Assistive Technologies, 1st. edn. IGI Global, Hershey (2011). https://doi.org/10.4018/978-1-61350-098-9. https://doi.org/10.1007/3-540-09237-4

36. Morimoto, C.H., Mimica, M.R.M.: Eye gaze tracking techniques for interactive applications. Comput. Vis. Image Understanding **98**(1), 4–24 (2005). https://doi.org/10.1016/j.cviu.2004. 07.010
37. Raymond, L.A., Piccini, M., Subramanian, M., Pavel, O., Faisal, A.: Natural gaze data driven wheelchair. In: Proceedings of the 11th IAPR International Conference on Pattern Recognition (2018). Preprint. https://doi.org/10.1101/252684
38. Reisfeld, D., Yeshurun, Y.: Robust detection of facial features by generalized symmetry. In: Proceedings of the 11th IAPR International Conference on Pattern Recognition, pp. 117–120. IEEE, Piscataway (1992). https://doi.org/10.1109/ICPR.1992.201521
39. Richardson, D.C., Spivey, M.J.: Eye-tracking: Research areas and applications. In: Bowlin, G.L., Gary, E.W. (eds.) Encyclopedia of Biomaterials and Biomedical Engineering. CRC Press (2008). https://doi.org/10.1201/b18990-101
40. Spencer, J.A.: Variational methods for image segmentation. Ph.D. thesis, University of Liverpool, Liverpool (2016)
41. Subramanian, M., Songur, N., Adjei, D., Orlov, P., Faisal, A.A.: A.eye drive: Gaze-based semi-autonomous wheelchair interface. In: Proceedings of the 2019 41st Annual International Conference of the IEEE Engineering in Medicine and Biology Society (EMBC). IEEE, Piscataway (2019). https://doi.org/10.1109/EMBC.2019.8856608
42. Utaminingrum, F., Fauzi, M.A., Sari, Y.A., Primaswara, R., Adinugroho, S.: Eye movement as navigator for restricted disabled person in handling position. In: Proceedings of the 2016 International Conference on Communication and Information Systems, pp. 1–5. ACM (2016). https://doi.org/10.1145/3023924.3023926
43. Vese, L.A., Guyader, C.L.: Variational Methods in Image Processing, 1st. edn. Chapman and Hall/CRC, Boca Raton (2015)
44. Wainwright, M.J., Jordan, M.I.: Graphical models, exponential families, and variational inference. Found. Trends Mach. Learn. **1**, 1–305 (2008). https://doi.org/10.1561/2200000001
45. Yoo, D.H., Chung, M.J.: A novel non-intrusive eye gaze estimation using cross-ratio under large head motion. Comput. Vis. Image Understanding **98**(1), 25–51 (2005). https://doi.org/10.1016/j.cviu.2004.07.011
46. Zhang, X., MacKenzie, I.S.: Evaluating eye tracking with iso 9241 - part 9. In: International Conference on Human-Computer Interaction, vol. 4552, pp. 779–788. Springer, Berlin (2007)
47. Zhu, Y., Sun, W., Yuan, T.T., Li, J.: Gaze detection and prediction using data from infrared cameras. In: Proceedings of the 2nd Workshop on Multimedia for Accessible Human Computer, ACM Multimedia 2019, pp. 41–46 (2019). https://doi.org/10.1145/3347319. 3356838

Sign Language Recognition

Dan Guo, Shengeng Tang, Richang Hong, and Meng Wang

Abstract This chapter covers several research works on sign language recognition (SLR), including isolated word recognition and continuous sentence translation. To solve isolated SLR, an Adaptive-HMM (hidden Markov model) framework (Guo et al., TOMCCAP 14(1):1–18, 2017) is proposed. The method explores the intrinsic properties and complementary relationship among different modalities. Continuous sentence sign translation (SLT) suffers from sequential variations of visual representations without any word alignment clue. To exploit spatiotemporal clues for identifying signs, a hierarchical recurrent neural network (RNN) is adopted to encode visual contents at different visual granularities (Guo et al., AAAI, pp 6845–6852, 2018; Guo et al., ACM TIP 29:1575–1590, 2020). In the encoding stage, key segments in the temporal stream are adaptively captured. Not only RNNs are used for sequential learning; convolutional neural networks (CNNs) can be used (Wang et al., ACM MM, pp 1483–1491, 2018). The proposed DenseTCN model encodes temporal cues of continuous gestures by using CNN operations (Guo et al., IJCAI, pp 744–750, 2019). As SLT is a weakly supervised task, due to the gesture variation without word alignment annotation, the pseudo-supervised learning mechanism contributes to solving the word alignment issue (Guo et al., IJCAI, pp 751–757, 2019).

Keywords Sign language recognition · Sign language translation · Sequence-to-sequence learning · Connectionist temporal decoding · Pseudo-supervised optimization

---

D. Guo (✉) · S. Tang · R. Hong · M. Wang
Hefei University of Technology, University of Hefei, Hefei, China
e-mail: guodan@hfut.edu.cn; tsg1995@mail.hfut.edu.cn

© The Author(s), under exclusive license to Springer Nature Switzerland AG 2021
T. McDaniel, X. Liu (eds.), *Multimedia for Accessible Human Computer Interfaces*,
https://doi.org/10.1007/978-3-030-70716-3_2

1 Online Early-Late Fusion Based on Adaptive HMM for Sign Language Recognition

1.1 Introduction

For sign language recognition (SLR) based on multi-modal data, a sign word can be represented by various features with existing complementary relationships among them. To investigate these complementary relationships, we present an online early-late fusion model based on an adaptive hidden Markov model (HMM) [8]. Inherent latent patterns of signs are not only associated to key gestures and body poses, but also related to the relationships among them. The proposed adaptive-HMM is designed to acquire the hidden state number of each sign through affinity propagation clustering. For complementary learning, we suggest an online early-late fusion scheme. The early fusion (feature fusion) is used to exploit the joint feature learning to achieve higher complementary scores while the late fusion (score fusion) uncovers and aggregates various scores in a weighting paradigm. This fusion is query-adaptive. Experiments verify viability on signer-independent SLR tasks with a large vocabulary. The proposed adaptive-HMM demonstrates consistent robustness in terms of performance on different dataset sizes and SLR models.

In this section, the remarkable GMM (Gaussian mixture model)-HMM model is chosen as a basic framework to tackle the isolated SLR problem. Given N signs' training data, each sign n has its own HMM $\lambda_n (1 \leq n \leq N)$, thus we have N signs' HMMs: $\{\lambda_1, \lambda_2, \ldots, \lambda_N\}$. We use the public toolkit[1] to learn $\{\lambda_n\}$. The recognition process is implemented using the Viterbi algorithm, and the most likely sign class λ^* of observation sequence O is found by Eq. 1.

$$\lambda^* = \underset{\{\lambda_1, \lambda_2, \ldots, \lambda_n, \ldots, \lambda_N\}}{argmax} P(\lambda_n | O). \tag{1}$$

where $P(\lambda_n | O)$, learned by the model $\lambda_n (n = 1, \ldots, N)$, indicates the relevance probability of query O related to the n-th sign. To be specific, HMM-states adaptation and early-late fusion are elaborated in Sects. 1.2 and 1.3.

1.2 Adaptive HMMs

The HMM model is sensitive to its inherent latent states. To obtain a superior sign recognizer, we attempt to learn appropriate latent states for each sign word. Here, we propose HMM-state adaptation to decide the individual state number $Q_n (1 \leq n \leq N)$ for each sign model. Before learning the HMM λ_n, we split all

---

[1]HMM package: http://www.cs.ubc.ca/~murphyk/Software/HMM/hmm/html. Parameters Q and M are discussed, whereas A, B and π can be handled by this code package.

the data samples of sign n into reasonable clusters and ensure an appropriate sort number for gesture variation. We adopt affinity propagation (AP) clustering [6] to adaptively acquire the centroid number of the training data. For sign n, we embed the distance measurement in the AP approach to build a frame-similarity net. The net is used to calculate the mutual responsibility and accessibility log-probability ratios between any two frames f_i and f_j. We explore the similarity function in AP to iteratively locate the best frame as exemplar f_k, which has larger responsibility weight than all other frames, until no more new exemplars appear. Thus, these best exemplars $\{f_k\}$ are taken as the centroid and we can naturally obtain the centroid number k_n (Fig. 1).

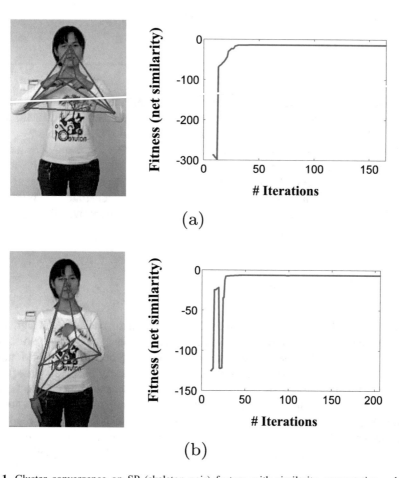

Fig. 1 Cluster convergence on SP (skeleton pair) feature with similarity computation, where "fitness" is a metric [6]. While fitness is closer to 0, clustering convergence is vastly improved. (**a**) Sign "*people*". (**b**) Sign "*I*"

Algorithm 1 Early-late fusion based on adaptive GMM−HMM (adaptive-HMM)

Require: N signs' training sample sets; Query O
Ensure: the sign class of query O
    Training:
 1: **for** sign $n(1 \leq n \leq N)$ under feature $i(1 \leq i \leq m)$ **do**
 2:    Extract feature set $F_n^{(i)}$ from sign n's training set $Set\ O_n$;
 3:    Compute the number of clusters $k_n^{(i)}$ on $F_n^{(i)}$ by AP clustering;[2]
 4:    $Q_n^{(i)} = k_n^{(i)}/M$;
 5:    Learn the GMM-HMM model $\lambda_n^{(i)} = (A, B, \pi)$ with $Set\ O_n$ and $Q_n^{(i)}$;
 6: **end for**
    Testing:
 7: Feature selection: e.g. remove "bad" HOG feature in the work;
 8: Obtain O's remaining m' score lists $\{s_O^{(i)}\}$ by SLR models $\{\lambda_n^{(i)}\}$;
 9: Calculate the fused score list s_O^* by Eq. 2∼ Eq. 5;
10: $n^* = \arg\max_{n^* \in N} s_O^*$;

In the Adaptive-HMM, M denotes the cluster number of data distribution in the GMM stage and Q represents the number of latent states in the HMM stage. Classical SLR methods set M as a constant value, and typically set $M = 3$; we follow this usage. We take the hidden state number $Q_n(1 \leq n \leq N)$ as a to-be-learned factor, which reflects the characterization of key gestures. With a fixed M-component in the GMM stage of the model, the state number Q_n is set to be proportional to the number of clusters k_n, where k_n demonstrates the number of centroids of the gesture sample sequence. The proposed Adaptive-HMM is shown in step $1 \sim 5$ of Algorithm 1.

1.3 Early-Late Fusion

The adaptive-HMM can be applied to model the hidden states of each sign under multi-modalities, e.g., RGB images and skeletal coordinate data that are discussed in this subsection. We then discuss the complementarity of different HMM models under various feature types through the exploitation of early fusion and late fusion. The early fusion is straightforwardly implemented by concatenating various features into a combined feature as elaborated in Sect. 1.4.1. To explore the score fusion, we build the score list (a score vector) of query O within each feature type (including the combined feature). For multiple feature types $F^{(i)}(i = 1, \ldots, m)$, we obtain the **score list** set of query O by N signs' adaptive HMMs $\{\lambda_1^{(i)}, \lambda_2^{(i)}, \ldots, \lambda_N^{(i)}\}$ in Eq. 2:

$$s_O^{(i)} = [P(\lambda_1^{(i)}|O), P(\lambda_2^{(i)}|O), \ldots, P(\lambda_N^{(i)}|O)] \tag{2}$$

---

[2]As in [6], here we set similarity preference to media similarity in AP.

where $P(\lambda_n^{(i)}|O)$ represents the relevance of query O related to the n-th sign within feature $F^{(i)}$, $(n = 1, \ldots, N)$; it is derived from the Viterbi algorithm on $\lambda_n^{(i)}$. Thus, we obtain score lists $\{s_O^{(1)}, s_O^{(2)}, \ldots, s_O^{(m)}\}$ of query O under m feature types.

1.3.1 Feature Selection

Given that a "bad" feature can pull down the overall fusion performance, we propose a feature selection paradigm; namely, if the performance of a combined feature is superior to its single component, we abandon the "bad" component feature whose performance is worse than the combined feature. Therefore, the complementary relationship in the combined feature is maintained while filtering the redundant, "bad" information. We take the average variance of score lists on the training data as the feature selection criterion. Given a score list (a score vector), its variance means the deviation degree from its own mean value. A smaller variance means that different signs have similar scores in the list, and thus, cannot be distinguished. In contrast, a larger variance represents good discrimination power. As illustrated in Fig. 2, we build a LOO (leave-one-out) cross-validation experiment on a partial small size dataset: the 50-sign CSL dataset. Under various features, variances and average variances of score lists of a total of 1000 training samples are separately illustrated in Fig. 2a and b. The performance of variance on the feature HOG of RGB images is not as good compared to the combined feature SP (skeletal pair coordinate)-HOG. Thus, we eliminate HOG, and select SP and SP-HOG as to-be-fused features.

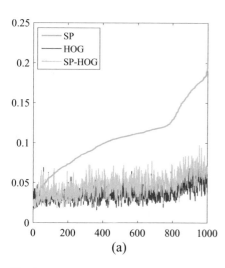
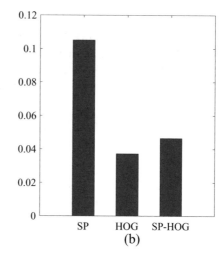

Fig. 2 Variance curves and average variances of score lists of the training samples under different features. Feature SP is superior, followed by SP-HOG and HOG. (**a**) Variance comparison with an arranged sample order sorted on the SP feature. (**b**) Average variance

1.3.2 Query-Adaptive Weighting

After feature selection, we weight the remaining m' score lists $\{s_O^{(i)}\}$. The fusion weight is inversely relative to the area of normalized sorted score curve. This is because a better $s_O^{(i)}$ is assigned a larger weight, while having a higher score on the right word label, and a much lower score on other irrelevant labels. In other words, if the arranged score list has a much sharper curve, the score list with its feature is much more discriminative and helpful. To be more explicit, we sort $s_O^{(i)}$ in decreasing order and apply min-max normalization. We denote it as $s_O'^{(i)}$ and weight on $s_O'^{(i)}$ ($1 \le i \le m'$) as follows:

$$
\begin{cases}
s_O'^{(i)} = \dfrac{s_O'^{(i)} - min s_O'^{(i)}}{max s_O'^{(i)} - min s_O'^{(i)}} \\[3mm]
w_O^{(i)} = \dfrac{1/A_{s_O'^{(i)}}}{\sum\limits_{1 \le i \le n} 1/A_{s_O'^{(i)}}}
\end{cases}
\tag{3}
$$

where $A_{s_O'^{(i)}}$ denotes the curve area of the i-th score list $s_O'^{(i)}$ under feature $F^{(i)}$ ($1 \le i \le m'$). It represents that the weighting paradigm is conditioned on $s_O'^{(i)}$, i.e., the query Q itself. The weighting stage is query-adaptive and unsupervised.

1.3.3 Score Fusion

We then fuse m' score lists. The product rule typically results in better performance than other rules in biometric multi-modality fusion [15, 35]. The fusion formula is shown in Eq. 4 and a deformation in Eq. 5. Using the publicly available MATLAB package in footnote 1, we directly implement Eq. 5 in a sum format.

$$
s_O^* = \left[\prod_{i=1}^{n} (s_O'^{(i)})^{w_O^{(i)}} \right], \quad s.t. \sum_{i=1}^{n} w_O^{(i)} = 1
\tag{4}
$$

$$
s_O^* = \left[\sum_{i=1}^{n} w_O^{(i)} \cdot \log(s_O'^{(i)}) \right], \quad s.t. \sum_{i=1}^{n} w_O^{(i)} = 1
\tag{5}
$$

The predicted sign class of query O corresponds to the maximum value in s_O^*.

$$
n^* = \arg\max_{n^* \in N} s_O^* = \arg\max_{n^* \in N} [s_{O,n}^*]
\tag{6}
$$

Table 1 The details of 370-sign CSL dataset

Signs	Dataset	Signer number	Repetition time	Sample number
370	Training	4	5	20×370
	Testing	1	5	5×370

where s_O^* denotes an N-dim classification vector. Its n^*-th component $s_{O,n}^*$ represents the probability of query O related to the n^*-th sign under feature $F^{(i)}$.

1.4 Experiments

1.4.1 Experiments Setup

Dataset We conducted experiments on the CSL (Chinese sign language) dataset, which is an RGB-D dataset collected using a Kinect sensor [30]. As shown in Table 1, the dataset consists of 370 signs performed 5 times by 5 signers including both men and women. The heights and gesture habits of signers are completely different. To guarantee the signer-independent test, we use the leave-one-out (LOO) cross-validation strategy to test SLR models in the experiments.

Feature Extraction This RGB-D SLR dataset contains color (RGB images) and depth (skeletal coordinates) modalities. We aim to learn the complementarity of these two modalities. In this work, we take the skeleton pair feature (D: 10-dimensional SP feature), hand feature (RGB: 51-dimensional HOG feature by PCA dimensionality reduction) and SP-HOG (RGB-D: 61-dimensional fused feature) as the basic features for each sign word.

- **Hand-crafted feature (RGB images)**: The HOG feature F_{HOG} is derived from the area of the two hands in the images by using an adaptive skin model and depth constraint as in [30].[3] Due to the high dimensionality of the original HOG feature, Principal Component Analysis (PCA) is adopted. We hold about 80% of the information energy of the dataset through PCA and obtain the 51-dimensional HOG feature. The PCA transformation matrix is acquired on the training data, and applied to the test samples.
- **Skeleton pair feature (Depth Data)**: For depth data, we first extract mutual distances of five skeleton points (head, left elbow, right elbow, left hand, and right hand), then convert them to a 10-dimensional SP distance feature F_{SP} [29]. Every signer has a different body shape. In order to unify the gesture postures of different signers, we normalize each SP vector by its maximum value. We then

---

[3]In this work, HOG features were extracted through OpenCV with basic parameters [30] and further optimized, e.g., some invalid frames are deleted.

obtain the SP feature sequence F_{SP} of each sign video sample. The characteristic of SP features is invariant to rotation, scaling, and translation.

- **Combined feature (RGB-D Data)**: We concatenate the F_{HOG} and F_{SP} features to create the SP-HOG feature (61-dimensional combined feature). The SP-HOG feature is considered to be early (feature) fusion.

Data Augmentation on Feature SP In the following experiments, we enhance our restricted training data with data augmentation [3]. To avoid overfitting, we investigate random Gaussian perturbation on the skeleton coordinates to enrich additional gesture positions. Given the 3D-depth skeleton point (x, y, z) extracted by the Kinect sensor, we take the coordinate x as an example to clarify Gaussian disturbance, and both y and z coordinates are tackled similarly. First, we calculate the range of x in all training samples within each sign n: $[x_{max}^n, x_{min}^n]$. Let $\Delta x^n = x_{max}^n - x_{min}^n$. Then, we set a Gaussian random variable $X \sim N(0, (\eta \Delta x^n)^2)$, where η is the disturbance parameter. We set the empirical parameter to $\eta = 0.01$. Under sign n, an additional combination of (x', y', z') coordinates of the skeleton point is generated, as shown below. By implementing data augmentation once, the original dataset is expanded to twice the original size.

$$\begin{cases} x' = & x + N(0, (\eta \Delta x^n)^2) \\ y' = & y + N(0, (\eta \Delta y^n)^2) \\ z' = & z + N(0, (\eta \Delta z^n)^2) \end{cases} \tag{7}$$

Compared Approaches We compare the proposed approach with other SLR methods, e.g., DTW [2, 25], GMM-HMM (HMMs) and Light-HMM [30]. In addition, we also compare the early-later fusion strategy with other fusion approaches, for example, early fusion for SLR [30] and late fusion [35].

- GMM-HMM [30]: For the classical GMM-HMM, a better parameter setting is $Q = M = 3$, where Q denotes the number of states in the HMM and M denotes the number of mixture models in the GMM.
- Light-HMM [30]: In order to trade off accuracy and run time, the Light-HMM determines key frames and chooses Q adaptively. Here $M = 3$ and Q is adaptive. In order to acquire excellent performance, we set Light-HMM's threshold ε_0 to 0.001 and threshold λ to the average value of the RSS score curve of parameter ε.
- DTW [2, 25]: Different from HMM calculating the probability score of query O under each sign class, DTW searches its nearest neighbor among the entire training samples and regards the sign class of the nearest neighbor as its class. In the late fusion testing of this work, the DTW score list is set as the reciprocal of the distances from all training samples.

1.4.2   Experiment with HMM-States Adaptation

We evaluate the Adaptive-HMM. The adaptation is set to HMM(Q) with adaptive Q and $M = 3$. We also evaluate adaptation HMM(M), in which M is adaptive and $Q = 3$. As shown in Table 2, compared with various HMMs, DTW is significantly more time-consuming as it compares all training samples to the to-be-identified sample, while the HMM merely learns the hidden states. Light-HMM performs worse than Adaptive-HMM due to dropping a few key frames. In the proposed adaptive HMM, the parameter Q has considerably more influence than M. Q indicates status changes, while M simulates data distribution. Due to rare samples and chaos characteristic of Gaussian simulation, the impact of M is not exceptionally clear on the CSL SLR dataset. Thus, we adopt the Adaptive-HMM(Q) as our adaptation paradigm.

1.4.3   Comparison on Different Fusion Steps

Table 3 lists different fusion strategies. In Table 4, under Recall@R=1, the precision with the SP feature is 34.82% and HOG feature just reaches 21.52%. The performance of Fusion I (early fusion) is lower than that of a single SP feature; HOG features have a negative influence. Both Fusion II, Fusion III and our early-late fusion acquire obvious improvements. These fusions, involving late (score) fusion, have learned the positive effect of complementary features. As shown in Fig. 3, the performance of Fusion II and Fusion III are close, but our fusion performance is superior. Compared with Fusion II and Fusion III, our fusion further reduces the negative impact of "bad" single feature HOG.

Table 2 Performance comparison with the single SP feature

Methods	Top 1	Top 5	Top 10	Testing time (ms/sign)
DTW	0.3159	0.5284	0.6245	1730
GMM-HMM	0.2751	0.5384	0.6583	159
LightHMM	0.2196	0.4529	0.6322	128
Adaptive-HMM (M)	0.2810	0.5404	0.6662	82
Adaptive-HMM (Q)	**0.3482**	**0.6129**	**0.7080**	88

Table 3 Setting details of different fusion strategies

Fusion I	Fusion II	Fusion III	Early-late fusion
Early fusion	Late fusion	Early-late fusion	Feature selection + Early-late fusion
SP-HOG	SP ⊗ HOG	SP ⊗ HOG ⊗ SP-HOG	SP ⊗ SP-HOG
Feature fusion	Score fusion	(feature + score) fusion	(feature + score) fusion

Table 4 Performance comparison with different fusion types

	Recall@R		
Feature	$R = 1$	$R = 3$	$R = 5$
SP	0.3482	0.5326	0.6129
HOG	0.2152	0.3403	0.3989
Fusion I [30]	0.3202	0.4571	0.5192
Fusion II [35]	0.4121	0.5627	0.6275
Fusion III	0.4140	0.5674	0.6299
Early-late fusion	**0.4532**	**0.6075**	**0.6734**

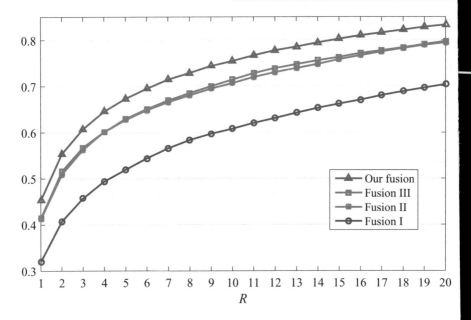

Fig. 3 Recall@R on the 370-sign CSL dataset

1.4.4 Comparison on Different Dataset Sizes

In this section, we test the Adaptive-HMM with different dataset sizes. We sample several of 370 sign words as subsets (e.g., the top 50, 100, and 200 words). As illustrated in Fig. 4a, with the increase of Recall@R, the precision improves; when the number of sign word increases, the performance drops. The differences between our fusion and other fusions are shown in Fig. 4b. Our fusion has obviously better precision and stability.

1.4.5 Comparison on Different SLR Models

As shown in Tables 5 and 6, the HOG feature achieves poor performance, and DTW still performs with the worst precision. Due to HOG delivering poor performance,

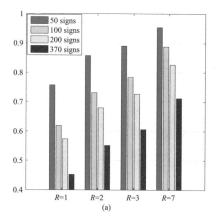
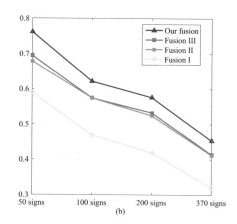

Fig. 4 (a) Precision comparison of our fusion with different dataset sizes. (b) Precision differences of our fusion to Fusions I, II and III at Recall@ $R=1$

the performance of Fusion I (early fusion) on the 50-sign dataset is very poor. What is interesting is that Fusion II (late fusion) effectively utilizes HOG. Our fusion further improves the accuracy. To summarize, our method provides the best performance by exploiting the advantages of early and late fusion as well as complementarity. The time costs of different SLR models are shown in Table 7. Compared with other HMMs, DTW takes much more time. The time costs of various HMMs are close to each other. GMM-HMM has a stable time cost when Q is fixed with 3. Under a few key frames, the time cost of Light-HMM is higher than GMM-HMM, as its average adaptive Q is nearly $4 \sim 5$ times of GMM-HMM's Q. Compared with GMM-HMM, it has a higher computational complexity of adaptive state transitions, so the Adaptive-HMM also has a variable Q. In any case, the score fusion time is insignificant compared with the query time under different SLR models. Fusion computation is effective for online fusion.

2 Hierarchical LSTM for Sign Language Translation

2.1 Introduction

Sign Language sentence Translation (SLT) is challenging due to the specific linguistics under continuously changing gestures. To address this issue, a hierarchical LSTM (HLSTM) based encoder-decoder model is proposed [12]. It tackles different visual clues of frames, clips, and sub-sign units. As shown in Fig. 5, firstly, a 3D CNN is used to learn the temporal and spatial clues of video clips, and then the online adaptive variable length key clip mining method is used to pack sub-sign units. Afterward, we realize a temporal attention mechanism to balance the

Table 5 Fusion comparison on different SLR models with 50 signs

	DTW		GMM-HMM		Light-HMM [30]		Our adaptive HMM	
	Recall@1	Recall@4	Recall@1	Recall@4	Recall@1	Recall@4	Recall@1	Recall@4
SP	61.84%	82.08%	61.60%	88.96%	55.44%	82.00%	71.68%	93.60%
HOG	20.24%	39.68%	44.64%	68.64%	29.12%	55.92%	46.88%	68.24%
Fusion I [30]	22.88%	43.44%	58.40%	81.36%	50.40%	74.64%	58.96%	79.20%
Fusion II [35]	63.12%	82.96%	66.08%	84.96%	49.92%	75.76%	67.84%	87.12%
Fusion III	63.96%	83.76%	66.16%	86.88%	57.68%	80.08%	69.44%	87.36%
Our fusion	63.04%	83.04%	72.64%	90.40%	61.92%	83.52%	76.16%	91.84%

Table 6 Fusion comparison on different SLR models with 370 signs

	GMM-HMM			Light-HMM			Our adaptive HMM		
	Recall@1	Recall@3	Recall@5	Recall@1	Recall@3	Recall@5	Recall@1	Recall@3	Recall@5
SP	27.51%	45.56%	53.84%	21.96%	37.41%	45.29%	34.82%	53.26%	61.29%
HOG	21.38%	33.51%	39.61%	10.50%	19.29%	24.93%	21.52%	34.03%	39.89%
Fusion I [30]	32.00%	46.13%	52.63%	24.50%	38.49%	45.28%	32.02%	45.71%	51.92%
Fusion II [35]	37.46%	52.95%	59.39%	22.22%	36.23%	43.57%	41.21%	56.27%	62.75%
Fusion III	38.93%	54.42%	60.79%	29.04%	44.41%	51.72%	41.40%	56.75%	62.99%
Our fusion	**41.50%**	**57.36%**	**63.91%**	**33.88%**	**49.64%**	**56.67%**	**45.32%**	**60.75%**	**67.34%**

Table 7 Time comparison on 50 signs. Fusion time in this table merely indicates time of fusion computation

Avg. testing time (s)	DTW	GMM-HMM	Light-HMM	Our adaptive HMM
SP	1.730	0.088	0.128	0.159
HOG	8.495	0.123	0.399	0.179
Fusion I	9.025	0.124	0.217	0.156
Fusion II	**0.014**	**0.011**	**0.011**	**0.011**
Fusion III	**0.015**	**0.011**	**0.011**	**0.011**
Our fusion	**0.014**	**0.011**	**0.011**	**0.011**

Fig. 5 The overall framework of HLSTM

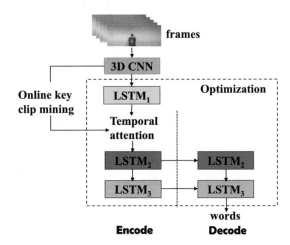

relationship among sub-sign locations. Finally, two LSTM layers are used to recurse sub-sign semantics. After condensing the original visual features extracted by the 3D CNN and top LSTM layer, the bottom two LSTM layers have less computational complexity.

2.2 Online Key Clip Mining

Discriminative motion patterns sparsely occur throughout video, such as sign speed, habits of signers, and special characteristics of sign words. In this work, we attempt to automatically obtain the variable-length key clips, rather than fixed interval for key frames or volumes segmentation [31, 36]. We employ a low-rank approximation method [30] to calculate the linear correlation of the frame sequence, which is implemented by calculating the residual sum of square (RSS) of feature ε between the previous frame and the current frame.

Given feature sequence $F = [f_1, f_2, \cdots, f_n]$ of a video, we model a correlation matrix M to compute the residual error ε_c of feature f_c at time step c. Based on the subset $F_c = [f_1, f_2, \cdots, f_c]$, ε_c and M are initialized as $\varepsilon_1 = 0$

and $M = (f_1^T f_1)^{-1}$. The correlation coefficient π_c and residual error ε_c at time step c $(2 \leq c \leq n)$ are learned by:

$$\begin{cases} \pi_c = MF_{c-1}^T f_c \\ \varepsilon_c = (f_c - F_{c-1}\pi_c)^T (f_c - F_{c-1}\pi_c) = \left\| f_c - F_{c-1}MF_{c-1}^T f_c \right\|^2 \end{cases} \tag{8}$$

Then, the matrix M is updated as follows:

$$M = \begin{bmatrix} M + \pi_c^T \pi_c \varepsilon_c & -\pi_c/\varepsilon_c \\ -\pi_c^T \varepsilon_c & 1/\varepsilon_c \end{bmatrix} \tag{9}$$

where M indicates the inherent linear correlation of F_c, π_c builds the relevance of F_{c-1} to f_c, and $F_{c-1}\pi_c$ is the approximate reconstruction of f_c by using F_{c-1} at time step c. Thus, we acquire $\varepsilon = [\varepsilon_1, \cdots, \varepsilon_c, \cdots, \varepsilon_n]$.

Previous works captured optimal subsets by selecting discrete frames; however, as shown in Fig. 6, the RSS curve tackles the continuous key and non-key variable-length clips (e.g., invalid segments for word-to-word conversion). Each peak on the RSS variable curve represents the local maximum gain of continuous variations. We keep the monotonously increasing part of ε curve as profit—a **key clip**, because the residual error increases, it cannot be replaced by the previous frame. Thereafter, the ε gradually decreases along the monotonically decreasing portion of the curve, where the monotonically increasing parts are denoted as **non-key clips**. This indicates that the reduced portion can be linearly reconstructed from the

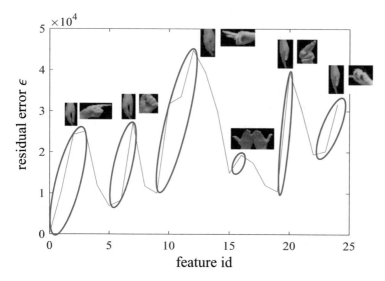

Fig. 6 Curve of ε of a video. Each peak corresponds to a sign's discriminative gesture

previous frame's downward error. To summarize, we avoid over-learning of non-key fragments in videos.

2.3   Hierarchical LSTM Encoder

The HLSTM model is a three-tier LSTM encoder architecture. The top $LSTM_1$ is responsible for extracting the recurrent representation based on the 3D spatio-temporal features $F = [f_1, f_2, \ldots, f_n]$ obtained by the well-known C3D [27]. And then, with the use of pooling and attention-based weighting, we condense the length of $LSTM_1$ features into n'' for $LSTM_2$ and $LSTM_3$. Finally, $LSTM_2$ is mainly used for visual embedding during the encoding stage, and $LSTM_3$ is used for modeling word embedding during the decoding stage and for sequence learning. $LSTM_2$ and $LSTM_3$ are both used in the encoding and decoding phases. Their parameters are shared in these two phases.

2.3.1   Hierarchical Encoder

The input video frames $(f_1, \cdots, f_N)$ are encoded by using both CNN and LSTM modules. A visual embedded representation V is learned by:

$$
\begin{aligned}
V &= \theta_{lstms}[\mathcal{G}(\theta_{cnn}(f_1, \cdots, f_N))] \\
&= \theta_{lstms}[\mathcal{G}(f_1, f_1, \cdots, f_n)] \\
&= \theta_{LSTM_3, LSTM_2, LSTM_1}[(f'_1, \cdots, f'_{n'})] \\
&= \theta_{LSTM_3, LSTM_2}(\widetilde{h}_1, \cdots, \widetilde{h}_{n''}) \\
&= (v_1, \cdots, v_{n''})
\end{aligned}
\tag{10}
$$

where $\mathcal{G}(\cdot)$ represents the key clip mining operation. As shown in Table 8, N, n and n' are of variable length. We set $n'' = l_{ave}$, where l_{ave} is the average of features for all training videos. $\{\widetilde{h}_1, \cdots, \widetilde{h}_{n''}\}$ is the inputs for $LSTM_2$, which is described in detail in the following section about polling and attention-based weighting. $\{v_1, \cdots, v_{n''}\}$ is the hidden states of $LSTM_3$ during the encoding phase.

Table 8 Parameter description

Symbol	Description
N	The number of original frames of a video
n	The number of extracted features
n'	The number of selected features by $\mathcal{G}(\cdot)$
n''	The number of encoding time steps of $LSTM_2$

2.3.2 Pooling Strategy

To condense less important clips, the outputs $\{h_t\}$ $(t \in [1, n])$ of $LSTM_1$ are compressed for $LSTM_2$. As shown in Fig. 7, h_t is taken as an independent sub-sign vector if it belongs to key clips, and we perform pooling on the non-key block if h_t belongs to non-key clips. Each non-key block includes consecutive, less important clips and the first frame of the next adjacent key clip. The pooled feature block is defined as $\{h_t\}$ $(t \in [t_1^*, t_{T_c}^*])$, where T_c is the length of the pooling block. Three pooling schemes can be applied as follows:

- **Key-pooling:** The last time stamp of the block $h'_t = h_{key}$ is directly fed into $LSTM_2$. This eliminates the effect of the non-key clips.

- **Mean-pooling:** Take the average vector of the block along the time dimension as $h'_t = h_{mean}$, which balances the recurrent output of each block.

- **Max-pooling:** The maximization of the block $h'_t = h_{max}$ highlights the block's salient response.

After pooling, we fix the recurrent sequence $\{h'_t\}$ $(t \in [1, n'])$ with variable n' for different video samples into the same length n''. There are two processes: if $n' < n''$, the sequence is filled with zero-padding vectors; if $n' \geq n''$, $\{h'_t\}$ is evenly sampled to n''.

2.3.3 Attention-Based Weighting

Figure 8 describes the weighting mechanism which shows the impact of each source position on the time dimension. The learnable attention vector $W \in \mathbb{R}^{T_e}$ is modelled by end-to-end training $\widetilde{h}_t = w_t \cdot h'_t$, where h'_t is the pooled vector, and $T_e = n''$. We denote the proposed HLSTM with or without this attention module as HLST and HLSTM-attn, respectively.

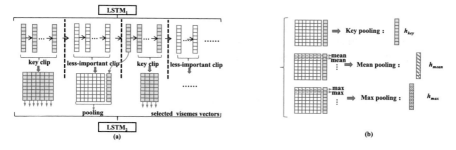

Fig. 7 Illustration of pooling strategy on non-key clips. (**a**) The pooling process. (**b**) Different pooling strategies

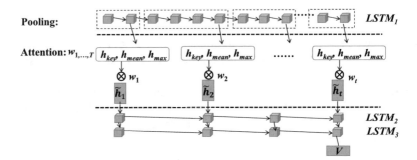

Fig. 8 Attention-based weighting mechanism

2.4 Sentence Generation

For the decoding stage, we apply $LSTM_2$ and $LSTM_3$ for sentence generation, where $LSTM_3$ recurrently outputs the generated sentences. With V obtained in the encoding stage, the decoder outputs the conditional probability of the generated sentence $(y_1, \cdots, y_m)$ as follows:

$$p(y_1, \cdots, y_m | V) = \prod_{t=1}^{m} p(y_t | v_{n''+t-1}, y_{t-1}) \tag{11}$$

We take zero-padding vectors as visual input of $LSTM_2$. $LSTM_3$ starts with $<BOS>$, and then inputs the previous word. During training, $LSTM_3$ is fed with the previous ground-truth word at each step. During the test, we select the current word (y_t) with the highest probability from the output (z_t) of $LSTM_3$ in Eq. 12, and its word embedding is the input at the next time step.

$$p(y_t | z_t) = \frac{exp(W_y z_t)}{\sum_{z'_t = V} exp(W_y z'_t)} \tag{12}$$

We utilize the entropy of the generated sentences to learn the model parameters θ. Loss optimization is performed during the decoding phase.

$$\theta^* = \underset{\theta}{\operatorname{argmax}} \sum_{t=1}^{m} p(y_t | v_{n''+t-1}, y_{t-1}; \theta) \log p(y_t | v_{n''+t-1}, y_{t-1}; \theta) \tag{13}$$

Table 9 Details of the
USTC-CSL dataset

		Signers	Sentences	Samples
Split I	Train	40	100	$40 \times 100 = 4000$
	Test	10	100	$10 \times 100 = 1000$
Split II	Train	50	94	$50 \times 94 = 4700$
	Test	50	6	$50 \times 6 = 300$

2.5 Experiment

2.5.1 Experiment Setup

Dataset The USTC-CSL dataset consists of sign videos that cover 100 daily sentences in Chinese sign language (CSL).[1] There are 50 signers to play each sentence, resulting in 5000 videos. And each sentence comprises 4 ~ 8 (average 5) sign words (phrases). The vocabulary size is 179. As shown in Table 9, the dataset is split as follows: **Split I—signer independent test:** Videos played by 40 signers are taken as the training set, and videos played by the remaining 10 signers are taken as the test set. In other words, the training and test sets have the same sentences but are played by different signers. **Split II—unseen sentences test:** 6 sentences are selected in which words separately appeared in the remaining 94 sentences so that a word appears in different sentences with different occurrence orders and usages.

Evaluation Metrics **Precision** reflects the ratio of correct sentences. **Acc-w** calculates the mean ratio of the correct word to the reference word in a sentence. Word error rate (**WER**) [4] is used to measure the minimum number of operations to change a generated sentence to reference. Semantic evaluation metrics widely used in NLP, NMT and image captioning are also reported, such as **BLEU**, **METEOR**, **ROUGE-L** and **CIDEr**.

2.5.2 Model Validation

We set the LSTM hidden state to $n_{hid} = 1000$. Features are extracted by C3D, which crops from every 16 frames with 8 frames overlapping [27].

Evaluation on Pooling Strategies The results in Table 10 demonstrate the properties of the pooling schemes. Key-pooling maintains the recurrent character on the time dimension, mean-pooling averages the recurrent output, and max-pooling emphasizes the significant responses. For Split I, mean-pooling is superior, whereas max-pooling performs better for Split II. Thus, we set mean-pooling and max-pooling for Split I and Split II, respectively.

---

[1]http://mccipc.ustc.edu.cn/mediawiki/index.php/SLR_Dataset.

Table 10 Comparison on different pooling strategies

Pooling strategy	Precision on Split I	*Acc-w* on Split II
Key-pooling	0.920	0.479
Mean-pooling	**0.924**	0.458
Max-pooling	0.912	**0.482**

Table 11 Comparison on different encoder frameworks

Model	Precision
S2VT ($n = 21$)	0.897
S2VT ($n = 66$)	0.850
S2VT (3-layer, $n = 21$)	0.903
S2VT (3-layer, $n = 66$)	0.854
HLSTM (SYS sampling)	0.910
HLSTM	**0.924**
HLSTM-attn	**0.929**

Evaluation on n'' Settings In the experiments, 66 is the maximum length of video C3D features of all training samples, and 21 is the average length. Note that N, n and n' are variable length for different videos. When $n'' = 66$, it recursively leads to all the sequence representations; if $n'' = 21$, compression features provide an average length. As shown in Table 11, $n'' = 21$ performs better compared to $n'' = 66$. When $n'' = 66$, there is little benefit in adding useless padding vectors to the $LSTM_2$ and $LSTM_3$ layers.

Evaluation on Encoder Frameworks Table 11 lists five similar but different encoding methods. Observing Table 11, encoders with fixed LSTM length have lower performance, such as S2VT and S2VT (3-layer). We extend S2VT to S2VT (3-layer) and make further comparisons. The S2VT (3-layer) encoder is a 3-layer LSTM of equal length, while the 2-layer decoder as our own. The hierarchical recurrent encoder performs better. In addition, the settings of the 3-layer encoder is better than the 2-layer as it combines the recurring features by the top layer LSTM. The system sampling is inferior to variable length key clip mining, and HLSTM-attn is superior with temporal attention.

2.5.3 Comparison to Existing Methods

Summary on Seen Sentences We compare the proposed approach with the following methods: **LSTM&CTC** model,[2] **S2VT** [28], **LSTM-E** [22], **LSTM-Attention** [33] and **LSTM-global-Attention** [21]. In the following experiments, if not explicitly stated, our HLSTM used only C3D features without temporary attention. HLSTM selects the mean pooling for Split I and the max pooling for Split II. As for extensions, HLSTM (SYS Sampling) has removed the selection of

---

[2]https://github.com/baidu-research/warp-ctc

key clips and directly inputs the outputs of $LSTM_1$ into $LSTM_2$ through system sampling in HLSTM. HLSTM-attn introduces temporal attention into HLSTM. The HLSTM models perform better than the others. Among different settings, HLSTM-attn performs the best (Table 12).

Experiment on Unseen Sentences Unseen sentences give a new challenge for SLT than seen sentences. In the test Split II, the words appear in different videos. Various variants of HLSTM are still better than other methods at identifying more meaningful words, as shown in Table 13.

3 Dense Temporal Convolution Network for Sign Language Translation

3.1 Introduction

Due to the lack of precise mapping annotation between visual actions and text words, sign language sentence translation (SLT) is a weakly supervised task. Aligning sign actions and the corresponding words is the goal of this work; thus, Dense Temporal Convolutional Network (DenseTCN) is proposed to capture actions in a hierarchical view [11]. The overview of DenseTCN is shown in Fig. 9; a temporal convolution (TC) unit is used to learn the short-term correlation between adjacent features, and is further expanded into a dense hierarchical structure. Finally, the output sets of all the previous layers will be integrated together at the kth TC layer. The merits of DenseNet consist of: (1) the deeper TC layer captures longer-term temporal context through hierarchical content aggregation, and (2) leveraging short-term and extended long-term sequential learning is useful to address the sequential alignment in the SLT task. The CTC loss and a fusion strategy are used to refine the predicted sentences.

3.2 DenseTCN

Different from classical RNN cells, TC is a convolutional operation to tackle short-term temporal calculation. DenseNet captures long-term temporal context through hierarchical TC layers. Taking the $k-$th TC layer as an example, the technical details of TC are shown in Fig. 10; using TC on the input feature matrix $H_k = \{h_i\}_{i=1}^{M} \in \mathbb{R}^{k \times M \times d'}$, it is transformed into the output feature matrix $\{h_i'\}_{i=1}^{M} \in \mathbb{R}^{M \times d'}$, where M is the length of the feature sequence and d' is the feature dimension. Specifically, each TC layer embeds all the outputs of previous TC layers into a new compact representation. The parameters of the kth$(k > 0)$ TC layer are defined as [number of filters, k, n, the input feature dimension, $padding, stride$]. As shown in Fig. 10,

Table 12 Evaluation under Split I for seen sentence recognition

	Precision	CIDEr	BLEU-4	BLEU-3	BLEU-2	BLEU-1	ROUGE-L	METEOR
LSTM&CTC	0.858	8.632	0.899	0.907	0.918	0.936	0.940	0.646
S2VT	0.897	8.512	0.874	0.879	0.886	0.902	0.904	0.642
S2VT (3-layer)	0.903	8.592	0.884	0.889	0.896	0.911	0.911	0.648
HLSTM (SYS)	0.910	8.907	0.911	0.916	0.922	0.935	0.938	0.683
HLSTM	**0.924**	**9.019**	**0.922**	**0.927**	**0.932**	**0.942**	**0.944**	**0.699**
HLSTM-attn	**0.929**	**9.084**	**0.928**	**0.933**	**0.938**	**0.948**	**0.951**	**0.703**

Table 13 Evaluation under Split II for unseen sentence translation

	Acc-w	CIDEr	BLEU-3	BLEU-2	BLEU-1	ROUGE-L	METEOR	WER
LSTM&CTC	0.332	0.241	0.039	0.124	0.343	0.362	0.111	0.757
S2VT	0.457	0.479	0.135	0.258	0.466	0.461	0.189	0.670
S2VT (3-layer)	0.461	0.477	0.145	0.265	0.475	0.465	0.186	0.652
HLSTM (SYS)	0.459	0.476	0.185	0.293	0.463	0.462	0.173	**0.630**
HLSTM	**0.482**	**0.561**	**0.195**	**0.315**	**0.487**	**0.481**	**0.193**	0.662
HLSTM-attn	**0.506**	**0.605**	**0.207**	**0.330**	**0.508**	**0.503**	**0.205**	0.641

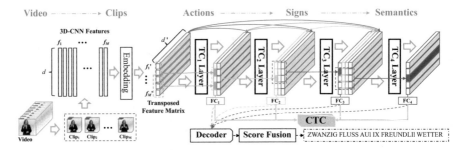

Fig. 9 The overview of DenseTCN with $K = 4$ layers for SLT

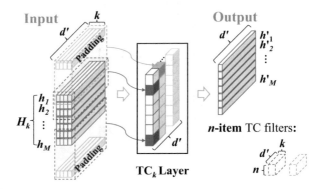

Fig. 10 Detailed operations of the TC_k layer (e.g. $k = 4, n = 3$)

we set the parameters to $[d', k, 3, d', 1, 1]$, where $n = 3$ indicates associating three adjacent features to realize short-term awareness. H_k and O_k represent the input and output of the kth TC layer, respectively. The calculation of the TC layer is formulated as follows:

$$
\begin{cases}
H_0 = \mathcal{F} \in \mathbb{R}^{M \times d}, & if \ k = 0 \\
H_k = [O_{k-1}, O_{k-2}, \ldots, O_0] \in \mathbb{R}^{k \times M \times d'}, & else; \\
O_0 = \Phi(H_0) \in \mathbb{R}^{M \times d'}, & if \ k = 0 \\
O_k = TC_k(H_k) \in \mathbb{R}^{M \times d'}, & else;
\end{cases}
\tag{14}
$$

where $H_0 = \mathcal{F}$ denotes the original features and function Φ denotes a FC layer that transforms the d-dimension features to d'. After each TC layer, we employ activation functions and Dropout [20] to avoid over-fitting. By cascading the outputs of all previous calculation layers, DenseNet expands the temporal receptive fields in the hierarchical design.

3.3 Sentence Learning

3.3.1 CTC Decoder

Each TC layer is followed by a fully connected (FC) layer, which converts each densely encoded feature into a word vocabulary to predict consecutive possible words. Voc is a set of all the words in the training set. and we add a blank word '_' to the vocabulary Voc to build a new vocabulary $Voc'=Voc \cup \{'\_'\}$.

$$p_k = FC_k(O_k) = O_k \cdot W_k + b_k , \tag{15}$$

where $p_k \in \mathbb{R}^{M \times w} = \{p_k^i\}_{i=1}^M$ is a predicted score matrix of the kth TC layer and w is the size of the vocabulary Voc'.

CTC [7] is adopted as the objective function to decode sentences. CTC applies a many-to-one mapping operation $\mathcal{B}$, which deletes the blank words and repeated words in π_k, e.g. $\mathcal{B}(\_a\,a\,\_\_pencil) = \{a\,pencil\}$, to convert π_k into a variable sentence $\mathcal{Y} = \{apencil\}$. Therefore, the probability of a labeling $\mathcal{Y} = (y_1, y_2, \ldots, y_L)$ containing L words is the sum of the probability that all words are aligned as follows:

$$Pr(\mathcal{Y}|p_k) = \sum_{\pi_k \in \mathcal{B}^{-1}(\mathcal{Y})} Pr(\pi_k|p_k) \tag{16}$$

where $\mathcal{B}^{-1}(\mathcal{Y}) = \{\pi_k|\mathcal{B}(\pi_k) = \mathcal{Y}\}$ involves all possible paths $\{\pi_k\}$. And the probability of a path π_k is defined as follow:

$$Pr(\pi_k|p_k) = \prod_{j=1}^M Pr(\pi_{k,j}|p_k), \forall \pi_{k,j} \in Voc' \tag{17}$$

where $\pi_{k,j}$ is the jth element of π_k.

A hierarchical CTC optimization is the novelty of this work. Let $P = \{p_k\}_{k=1}^K$ be the input of all the CTC decoders, where K is the depth of the DenseTCN, and the total CTC loss is defined as follows:

$$\mathcal{L}_{CTC} = -\log Pr(\mathcal{Y}|P) = -\sum_{k=1}^K \log Pr(\mathcal{Y}|p_k) \tag{18}$$

3.3.2 Score Fusion and Translation

Until now, we obtain a probability score set $P = \{p_k\}_{k=1}^K$, where $p_k \in \mathbb{R}^{M \times w}$ and w is the size of vocabulary. We choose the *softmax* operation to normalize each probability p_k, and further sum all the normalized variables of $\{p_k\}$.

$$p^i_{fusion,j} = \frac{1}{K}\sum_{k=1}^{K}\frac{e^{p^i_{k,j}}}{\sum_{j'=1}^{w}e^{p^i_{k,j'}}} \tag{19}$$

Next, we use the function *argmax* on p^i_{fusion} and output the ith word classification label with the maximum value. At last, we have to delete the blank '_' and reduplicate words by the above-mentioned two-stage greedy strategy, and output the final generated sentence.

3.4 Experiments

3.4.1 Datasets

We evaluated our method on the German sign language dataset (PHOENIX),[3] which involves daily news and weather forecasts in German sign language. As shown in Table 14, it consists of 6841 videos executed by 9 signers.

3.4.2 Evaluation Metrics

Word error rate (WER) is a widely used metric to measure the similarity of two sentences. The distance from a generated sentence to the ground-truth is required to be the minimal operations of substitution (S), deletion (D), and insertion (I). We use G to indicate the number of words in the ground truth, and WER is formulated as follows:

$$\text{WER} = (S + D + I)/G \times 100\% \tag{20}$$

When WER is lower and accuracy is higher, the model is better. Further, auxiliary evaluations *del* and *ins* represent the ratio of delete and insert operations as follows:

$$del = D/G \times 100\%, \quad ins = I/G \times 100\% \tag{21}$$

Table 14 Details of PHOENIX dataset

	Signers	Sentences	Videos	Words
TRAIN	9	5672	5672	1231
VAL	9	540	540	461
TEST	9	629	629	497

---

[3] https://www-i6.informatik.rwth-aachen.de/$\sim$koller/RWTH-PHOENIX/.

3.4.3 Implementation Details

For data processing, each video is divided into clips with 8 frames and an overlapping 4 frames to get 190,536 clips of the TRAIN subset, 17,908 clips of the VAL subset and 21,349 clips of the TEST subset of the PHOENIX dataset. We extract clip features with a dimension of 512 through an 18-layer 3D-ResNet [13] pre-trained on the SLR dataset [34]. The linear function Φ transforms d-dimensional features to d'. Here, d=512. The parameters of the kth$(k > 0)$ TC layer are defined as [number of filters, k, n, the input feature dimension, $padding$, $stride$]. As mentioned earlier, the parameters of the kth TC are set to $[d', k, 3, d', 1, 1]$. We discuss d' in the latter Sect. 3.4.4. For the PHOENIX dataset, the input feature dimension size is 512, and the size of vocabulary is 1232. The activation function ReLU [20] is adopted after each TC layer. We train the DenseNet model with ADAM optimizer and dropout ratio $\rho = 0.5$ on each TC layer. The initialized learning rate is 10^{-4} and the weight attenuation is 10^{-5}. After 30 training epochs, the learning rate changes to be 0.9 times of the original. The training is constrained to stop while the learning rate is lower than 10^{-6}. Dropout is not considered during the testing phase.

3.4.4 Depth Discussion

In the experiments, the minimum network depth K is 1 and the maximum is 16. We test different depths in the two cases with or without (w/o) dropout. As shown in Fig. 11, the experimental results demonstrate that on the PHOENIX VAL dataset, the performance with dropout and a deeper dense network is better. Observing the experimental results, we set the empirical parameter K to 10, and embedding size d' to 512 for the PHOENIX dataset.

3.4.5 Comparison

As shown in Table 15, the symbol ▲ marks the models that introduce other features, such as "face image"; △ indicates that additional offline optimizations are used, e.g., multiple EM iterations are used for weak supervision in the hybrid CNN-HMM (CNN-Hybrid) model [19]. We analyze the differences between the models in Table 15. HMM-based models include HOG-3D and CMLLR, which employ hand-crafted features [16]. Based on deep features, Cui et al. developed a three-steps training optimization named staged-Opt [5]. 1M-Hands [17] and SubuNets [1] consider more visual clues, i.e., both hands and global images. LS-HAN solves the SLT task by an attention mechanism [14]. Through the offline EM optimization, [24] Dilated-CNN was trained five times. CTF-SLT [32] applies BGRU and TCOV to tackle long-term and short-term sequential learning respectively. Dense TC operation and the hierarchical CTC optimization are the main contributions of this work. Our proposed approach is superior to other methods. Figure 12 shows

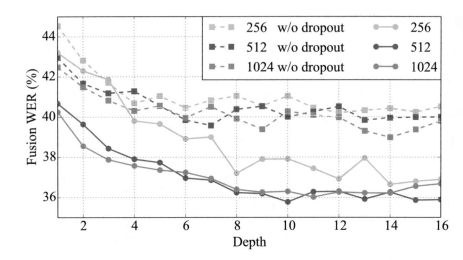

Fig. 11 Performance of DenseTCN with different depths on PHOENIX VAL set

Table 15 Evaluations under PHOENIX

Methods	VAL del/ins	WER	TEST del/ins	WER
HOG-3D ▲	25.8/4.2	60.9	23.2/4.1	58.1
CMLLR ▲	21.8/3.9	55.0	20.3/4.5	53.0
1M-Hands ▲ △	16.3/4.6	47.1	15.2/4.6	45.1
CNN-Hybrid ▲ △	12.6/5.1	38.3	11.1/5.7	38.8
Staged-Opt ▲ △	13.7/7.3	39.4	12.2/7.5	38.7
SubuNets ▲	14.6/4.0	40.8	14.3/4.0	40.7
Dilated-CNN △	8.3/4.8	38.0	7.6/4.8	37.3
LS-HAN	–	–	–	38.3
CTF-SLT	12.8/5.2	37.9	11.9/5.6	37.8
DenseNet*	–	49.7	–	49.2
Our DenseTCN	10.7/5.1	**35.9**	10.5/5.5	**36.5**

▲: Other modality, △: Extra supervision

the translation process in DenseTCN with $K = 10$ layers. With reference to the "ground-truth", the WER value of the translated sentence of each TC layer is in the range of 50% to 8%. As a result, the deletion (D) words ("MOEGLICH" and "VERSCHIEDEN"), the insertion (I) word ("UNTERSCHIED"), and the substitution (S) words ("WIND" and "loc-REGION") are modified with all the TC layers.

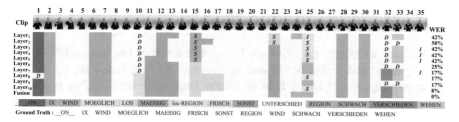

Fig. 12 The prediction results of the DenseTCN with depth $K = 10$

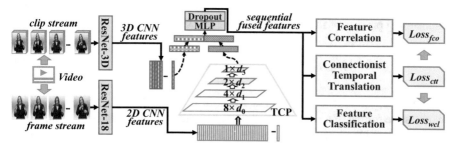

Fig. 13 The framework of the proposed CTM method for online SLT. Except for the Temporal Convolution Pyramid (TCP) module for feature extraction, the CTTR (Connectionist Temporal TRanslation) module is designed to generate sequential words that are further taken as supervision to optimize FCLS (Feature CLaSsification) and FCOR (Feature CORrelation) modules. Thus, the entire CTM method is learned in a pseudo-supervised mode

4 Joint Optimization for Translation and Sign Labeling

4.1 Introduction

Online sign translation faces challenges of hybrid semantic learning, such as visual representation, textual grammar, and sign linguistics. A Connectionist Temporal Modeling (CTM) framework is proposed for sentence translation and sign labeling [10]. As shown in Fig. 13, in order to obtain short-range temporal correlations, we designed a Temporal Convolution Pyramid (TCP) module to convert 2D CNN features to pseudo 3D' features. After feature fusion of 2D and pseudo 3D' features, the fused features are fed into three optimization modules in the CTM framework, i.e., Connectionist Temporal TRanslation (CTTR), Feature CLaSsification (FCLS), and Feature CORrelation (FCOR) for long-range sequential learning. Besides, dynamic programming is embedded into the decoding process, which maps sequential features to sign labels and generates sentences. During the connectionist decoding process, we regard the classification labels of clips as pseudo-labels, which are used as pseudo-supervised hints in the end-to-end framework. To be specific, we designed a joint objective function combining $\mathcal{L}_{fcor}$, $\mathcal{L}_{cttr}$, and $\mathcal{L}_{fcls}$ to optimize the decoding phase.

4.2   Clip Feature Learning in Videos

In this part, we clarify the clip-level feature extraction of two-stream CNNs, i.e., the alignment and fusion of 2D and 3D features. At first, motivated by the Δt-gram language model in the field of natural language processing, we propose a Temporal Convolution Pyramid (TCP) module to obtain contiguous features. The TCP gradually condenses temporal cues via multi-layer convolution operations with contiguous Δt-items. We use an l-layer TCP to transform the original 2D frame features $\{f_{2d}\} \in \mathbb{R}^{d_0 \times \mathcal{N}}$ into pseudo clip-level features $\{f'_{3d}\} \in \mathbb{R}^{d_l \times \frac{\mathcal{N}}{\Pi_{i=1}^{l}(s_i)}}$. The embedding process of features in TCP is expressed as Eq. 22.

$$\{f'^{n}_{3d}\}_{n=1}^{N} = TCL_{\Phi_l}\left\{ \cdots \left[TCL_{\Phi_1}(f^{n}_{2d}|_{n=1}^{\mathcal{N}}) \right] \right\} \tag{22}$$

where Φ_i represents the parameter of TCL_i in TCP, and $\Phi_i = (ch_i, d_i, \Delta t_i, s_i, pad_i)$ denotes the format of a convolutional parameter (number of channels, height, width, stride, and padding). $d_i \times \Delta t_i$ denotes the convolutional kernel size, and s_i is the temporal sliding window. Here, $d_{i+1} = ch_i$, i.e., the kernel size for the $(i+1)$-th layer, is set to the output dimension of the i-th layer. In other words, TCP is a combination of 2D spatial and 1D temporal convolution to compact a 2D clip into a 3D feature. We deem this operation as pseudo 3D' features, rather than real 3D CNN operations.

As shown in Fig. 14, a three-layer TCP is realized with ($\Delta t_i = 2$)-gram and as non-overlapping ($s_i = 2$); the frame-level 2D features are transformed into a short clip-level 3D feature. After that, we fuse the f'_{3d} and f_{3d} by the MLP, which can be formulated as Eq. 23.

$$F_{fus} = \{f_n\}_{n=1}^{N} = MLP(f'_{3d} \oplus f_{3d}) \tag{23}$$

where $\oplus$ is the concatenation operation for feature vectors.

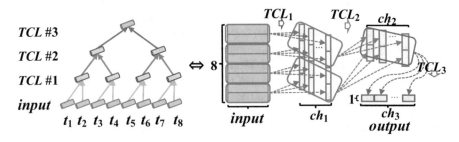

Fig. 14   TCP module for pseudo 3D' feature extraction

4.3 Joint Loss Optimization

After feature fusion, we tackle long-range sequential learning. First, we discuss the CTTR module which generates the predicted sentence $\pi = \{\pi_n\}_{n=1}^{N}$. In order to further improve the temporal correlation and classification accuracy of features, we construct a pseudo-supervised learning framework. Here, $\pi = \{\pi_n\}_{n=1}^{N}$ is regarded as pseudo-labels of words for alignment learning of sequential features. According to the pseudo-labels, the FCLS module and the FCOR module respectively calculate the entropy of feature classification and the similarity of feature samples with the same or different labels. Both of the above two modules prevent the CTTR module from overfitting the training data. We combine the three loss functions $\mathcal{L}_{fcor}$, $\mathcal{L}_{cttr}$, and $\mathcal{L}_{fcls}$ to jointly optimize the model. The entire loss function is expressed as Eq. 24.

$$\mathcal{L} = \frac{1}{|\mathcal{S}|} \sum \mathcal{L}_{cttr} + \frac{1}{|\mathcal{M}|} \sum \mathcal{L}_{fcls} + \frac{1}{|\mathcal{T}|} \sum \mathcal{L}_{fcor} \qquad (24)$$

where $\mathcal{S}$, $\mathcal{M}$ and $\mathcal{T}$ respectively represent the set of training samples, the set of clip-level features and the set of all pseudo triplets. $\mathcal{L}_{cttr}$ is expressed in Eq. 25, while $\mathcal{L}_{fcls}$ and $\mathcal{L}_{fcor}$ will be given in Eqs. 26 and 28.

4.3.1 CTC Loss for CTTR Module

The CTTR module is composed of a BGRU and CTC-decoder. BGRU is adopted to encode long-term temporal hints of visual features. Then, a fully connected layer embeds the embedding sequential features into non-normalized categorical probabilities $\{p_n\}$. Following the same operations as Eqs. 16 ~ 18 in Sect. 3.3.1 of DenseTCN, we take the CTC loss as the objective function of the CTTR module, as shown in Eq. 25.

$$\mathcal{L}_{cttr} = -\sum_{\pi \in \mathcal{B}^{-1}(\mathcal{Y})} \sum_{n \in N} log(p_n^{\pi_n}) \qquad (25)$$

where $\mathcal{B}^{-1}(\mathcal{Y})$ represents the set of alignments from the decoding path π to the target sentence $\mathcal{Y}$. Note that the CTC decoder selects the word label with the maximum value in each probability vector p_n to compose the generated sentence, which are regarded as pseudo-labels for the loss calculation in the following FCLS and FCOR modules.

4.3.2   Cross-Entropy Loss for FCLS Module

We use an FC layer with batch normalization and softmax to realize the FCLS module. This module obtains the predicted probability of each clip-level feature from the fusion feature $\{f_n\}$. Based on the assumption that the pseudo-label is reliable, the optimization goal of the network is to make the new predicted probabilities trend toward the pseudo-labels. We calculate the cross-entropy loss to evaluate the distance between the predictions and the pseudo labels as Eq. 26.

$$\mathcal{L}_{fcls}(\mathcal{M}) = -\sum_{m\in\mathcal{M}}\sum_{k\in K} y_m^k \log(p_m^k) \tag{26}$$

where p_m^k represents the predicted probability of the sample m calculated by the FCLS module. y_m^k is a boolean value indicating whether the label of the sample m is π_m according to the output of CTTR.

4.3.3   Triplet Loss for FCOR Module

We design a triplet loss to promote the features with the same label to gather in the embedding space, while the features with different labels are far away from each other. In the FCOR module, FC with batch normalization is used to model features into the embedding space to obtain new features $\{f_n\}$.

According to the word decoding path π with the maximum probability of P_{max}^π, the embedding features are divided into different groups. Specifically, clip features with the same label are classified as positive pairs, denoted as (e_+, e_+); while clip features with different labels are regarded as negative pairs, denoted as (e_+, e_-) and (e_-, e_+). Thus, the set of all sample pairs can be represented as $\mathcal{T} = \{(e_+, e_+), (e_+, e_-), (e_-, e_+)\}$. Taking the video shown in Fig. 15 as an example, e_1 and e_6 are (e_+, e_+), while e_1 and e_2 are (e_+, e_-) or (e_-, e_+). We use colored squares and gray squares in the matrix to represent positive and negative pairs, respectively. Here, we ignore self-pairs (along the diagonal) and pairs with blank label samples (squares with snowflake dots). The constraint of the distance of positive and negative pairs is formulated in Eq. 27.

$$\begin{cases} s(e_+, e_+) > s(e_+, e_-) + \alpha \\ s(e_+, e_+) > s(e_-, e_+) + \alpha \\ s.t. \quad s(a,b) = \frac{a^T b}{\|a\|\|b\|} = L_2(a)^T \cdot L_2(b) \end{cases} \tag{27}$$

where $s(a,b)$ represents the similarity function with samples a and b, and L_2 denotes L_2-normalization. We use parameter α to control similarity intensity during the training process.

Then, we implement the measurement of triplet loss. For each batch, we randomly select the same number of negative pairs as positive pairs, and perform the triplet loss calculation as follows:

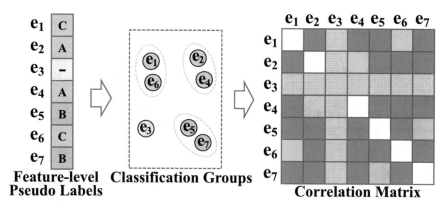

Fig. 15 Calculation of triplet loss with different labels. e_3 indicates the blank label

$$\mathcal{L}_{fcor}(\mathcal{T}) = \sum_{t \in \mathcal{T}} max(s(t_{neg}) - s(t_{pos}) + \alpha, 0)$$

$$= \sum_{t \in \mathcal{T}} max(s(t_{neg}) - \beta, 0) + \sum_{t \in \mathcal{T}} max(\beta - s(t_{pos}), 0)$$

(28)

where β controls similarity intensity in the training process.

4.4 Experiment

4.4.1 Experiment Setup

Dataset and Evaluation We conduct experiments on RWTH-PHOENIX-Weather (PHOENIX) [16] and USTC-CSL—Split II [14] datasets for unseen sentences test. We adopt Word Error Rate (**WER**) [18] as the evaluation metric, which measures the minimal cost of insertion, deletion, and replacement operations during sequence conversion. For a sequence of length $|L|$, the proportions of inserted and deleted words are recorded as **ins** and **del**, respectively.

Implementation The resolutions of sign videos in the PHOENIX and USCT-CSL datasets are 210×260 pixels and 1280×720 pixels, respectively. We crop out the area covering the human body from the original frames and resize them to 224×224 pixels. We extract features with four-frames overlapping, and parameter setting of the TCP module are shown in Table 16, where the parameter $d_0 = d_1 = d_2 = d_3 = 512$-dim. We adopt the ADAM optimizer with batch size 40, and set the initial learning rate to 1×10^{-4}. The learning rate is reduced by $1/10$ every 20 epochs until the learning rate becomes 1×10^{-6}. ReLU and Dropout operations are adopted after each TCL layer, and the Dropout parameter is set to 0.2.

Table 16 Parameter setting of the TCP module

Input size	Layer	Kernel, channel, stride	Output size
$t \times d_0$	TCL_1	$2 \times d_0,\ d_1,\ 2$	$(t/2) \times d_1$
	TCL_2	$2 \times d_1,\ d_2,\ 2$	$(t/4) \times d_2$
	TCL_3	$2 \times d_2,\ d_3,\ 2$	$(t/8) \times d_3$

Table 17 Performance comparison on the PHOENIX dataset with different features and $\mathcal{L}_{cttr}$ loss

Features	VAL(%) del/ins/WER	TEST (%) del/ins/WER
f_{2d}	55.1/1.5/69.4	53.6/1.8/68.3
f_{3d}'	27.5/5.8/63.6	26.8/6.1/62.2
f_{3d}	21.0/5.1/45.1	20.0/5.5/45.4
$f_{3d}' + f_{3d}$	10.5/7.3/42.2	10.8/7.8/42.2
$Fusion_{\{f_{3d}', f_{3d}\}}$	10.6/6.9/**41.0**	10.1/7.9/**41.3**

Table 18 Performance comparison using different losses on PHOENIX dataset

Loss	VAL (%) del/ins/WER	TEST (%) del/ins/WER
$\mathcal{L}_{cttr}$	10.6/6.9/41.0	10.1/7.9/41.3
$\mathcal{L}_{cttr}+\mathcal{L}_{fcls}$	10.2/6.7/39.9	10.3/7.7/40.2
$\mathcal{L}_{cttr}+\mathcal{L}_{fcor}$	11.3/6.7/39.8	10.9/6.9/40.0
$\mathcal{L}_{cttr}+\mathcal{L}_{fcls}+\mathcal{L}_{fcor}$	11.8/5.9/**38.9**	10.6/6.1/**38.7**

4.4.2 Model Validation

To verify the TCP module, we conducted experiments with different features. As shown in Table 17, the **del** value of f_{2d} is 55.1%, which is much worse. TCP improves the performance with 27.5%. Compared to direct addition of f_{3d}' and f_{3d}, MLP fusion has better performance, and the WER value is reduced from 42.2% to 41.3% on the TEST set. We test the effectiveness of the pseudo-supervised learning framework. As shown in Table 18, the introduction of $\mathcal{L}_{fcls}$ improves the performance by 1.1% on both VAL and TEST sets. With the auxiliary of $\mathcal{L}_{fcor}$, the model learns the similarities and differences between clip-level representations, thereby further reducing the WER on the VAL and TEST sets by 1.0% and 1.5%. When using $\mathcal{L}_{cttr}$, $\mathcal{L}_{fcls}$, and $\mathcal{L}_{fcor}$ simultaneously, CTM can achieve the best results (Fig. 16).

4.4.3 Main Comparison

Here, the proposed model is compared to the state-of-the-art. We observe two obvious conclusions from Table 19. (1) The previous work always introduces extra visual hints to improve the performance, such as using visual representations of face or hands, and pose trajectory. In addition, the pre-trained sign language vocabulary is utilized in 1M-Hands [18], while CNN-Hybrid [17] introduces additional supervision. In contrast, our method has no extra hints and additional supervision. (2) Most methods use offline iterations, such as 1-M-H, CNN-Hybrid, Staged-Opt [5], and DCNN [24]. Without offline optimizations, our CTM achieves

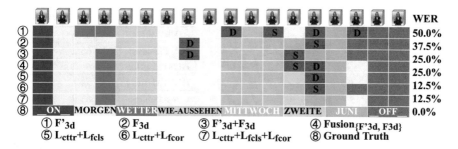

① F'₃d   ② F₃d   ③ F'₃d+F₃d   ④ Fusion{F'₃d, F₃d}
⑤ L_cttr+L_fcls   ⑥ L_cttr+L_fcor   ⑦ L_cttr+L_fcls+L_fcor   ⑧ Ground Truth

Fig. 16 Sentence decoding results using different setting of features and losses. "S" and "D" represent substitution and deletion operations

Table 19 Comparison with the state-of-the-art on the PHOENIX dataset

Methods	Off-line Iterations	Extra Augmentation	VAL (%) des/ins/WER	TEST (%) des/ins/WER
HOG-3D [16]	–	√	25.8/4.2/60.9	23.2/4.1/58.1
CMLLR [16]	–	√	21.8/3.9/55.0	20.3/4.5/53.0
1-M-H [18]	3	√	19.1/4.1/51.6	17.5/4.5/50.2
1-M-H+CMLLR [18]	3	√	16.3/4.6/47.1	15.2/4.6/45.1
CNN-Hybrid [17]	3	√	12.6/5.1/38.3	11.1/5.7/38.8
Staged-Opt-init [5]	–	√	16.3/6.7/46.2	15.1/7.4/46.9
Staged-Opt [5]	3	√	13.7/7.3/39.4	12.2/7.5/38.7
SubUNets [1]	–	√	14.6/4.0/40.8	14.3/4.0/40.7
DCNN-init [24]	–		18.5/2.6/60.3	18.1/2.8/59.7
DCNN [24]	5		**8.3/4.8/38.0**	**7.6/4.8/37.3**
Our Method	–		**11.6/6.3/38.9**	**10.9/6.4/38.7**

"Extra Augmentation" refers to the date of face, hand or trajectory. "Off-line Iterations" represents the number of iterations during offline optimization, and "-" indicates the framework was trained in an end-to-end manner

better performance than HOG-3D [16], CMLLR [16], SubUNets [1], Staged-Opt-init and DCNN-init. It is worth noting that Staged-opt and DCNN obtain good performance through offline iterative optimization. Their initial results of WER reduce rapidly to 46.9% and 59.7% on the test dataset, which are much lower than the values obtained by our approach. Note that offline iteration requires repeated training. The optimization process is time-consuming. Our CTM model does not suffer from this limitation and achieves comparable performance to these offline iterative models.

From the results of Table 20, the proposed CTM achieves the best performance on the USTC-CSL dataset with performance improvements of 2.2~5.1% compared with other models. Different from S2VT and HLSTM based on the encoder-decoder framework, CTM directly utilizes connectionist temporal modeling along the temporal dimension, which is also more flexible for online SLT.

Table 20 Comparison with
the state-of-the-art on the
USTC-CSL dataset

Methods	TEST WER (%)
S2VT [28]	67.0
S2VT(3-layer) [33]	65.2
HLSTM [9]	66.2
HLSTM-attn [9]	64.1
Our method	**61.9**

Acknowledgments This work is supported in part by the State Key Development Program under Grant 2018YFC0830103, in part by the National Natural Science Foundation of China (NSFC) under Grant 61876058, and in part by the Fundamental Research Funds for the Central Universities.

References

1. Camgoz, N.C., Hadfield, S., Koller, O., Bowden, R.: Subunets: End-to-end hand shape and continuous sign language recognition. In: Proceedings of the IEEE international conference on computer vision (ICCV), pp. 3075–3084 (2017)
2. Celebi, S., Aydin, A.S., Temiz, T.T., Arici, T.: Gesture recognition using skeleton data with weighted dynamic time warping. In: VISAPP, pp. 620–625 (2013)
3. Chatfield, K., Simonyan, K., Vedaldi, A., Zisserman, A.: Return of the devil in the details: Delving deep into convolutional nets (2014). Preprint. arXiv:14053531
4. Cui, R., Liu, H., Zhang, C.: Recurrent convolutional neural networks for continuous sign language recognition by staged optimization. In: CVPR, pp. 7361–7369 (2017)
5. Cui, R., Liu, H., Zhang, C.: Recurrent convolutional neural networks for continuous sign language recognition by staged optimization. In: Proceedings of the IEEE Conference on Computer Vision and Pattern Recognition (CVPR), pp. 1610–1618 (2017)
6. Frey, B.J., Dueck, D.: Clustering by passing messages between data points. Science **315**(5814), 972–976 (2007)
7. Graves, A., Fernández, S., Gomez, F., Schmidhuber, J.: Connectionist temporal classification: labelling unsegmented sequence data with recurrent neural networks. In: International Conference on Machine Learning (ICML), pp. 369–376 (2006)
8. Guo, D., Zhou, W., Li, H., Wang, M.: Online early-late fusion based on adaptive HMM for sign language recognition. TOMCCAP **14**(1), 1–18 (2017)
9. Guo, D., Zhou, W., Li, H., Wang, M.: Hierarchical LSTM for sign language translation. In: AAAI, pp. 6845–6852 (2018)
10. Guo, D., Tang, S., Wang, M.: Connectionist temporal modeling of video and language: a joint model for translation and sign labeling. In: IJCAI, pp. 751–757 (2019)
11. Guo, D., Wang, S., Tian, Q., Wang, M.: Dense temporal convolution network for sign language translation. In: IJCAI, pp. 744–750 (2019)
12. Guo, D., Zhou, W., Li, A., Li, H., Wang, M.: Hierarchical recurrent deep fusion using adaptive clip summarization for sign language translation. ACM TIP **29**, 1575–1590 (2020)
13. Hara, K., Kataoka, H., Satoh, Y.: Learning spatio-temporal features with 3d residual networks for action recognition. In: ICCV Workshop on Action, Gesture, and Emotion Recognition, vol. 2, p. 4 (2017)
14. Huang, J., Zhou, W., Zhang, Q., Li, H., Li, W.: Video-based sign language recognition without temporal segmentation (2018). Preprint. arXiv:180110111
15. Kittler, J., Hatef, M., Duin, R.P., Matas, J.: On combining classifiers. IEEE Trans. Pattern Anal. Mach. Intell. **20**(3), 226–239 (1998)

16. Koller, O., Forster, J., Ney, H.: Continuous sign language recognition: towards large vocabulary statistical recognition systems handling multiple signers. Comput. Vision Image Understanding **141**, 108–125 (2015)
17. Koller, O., Ney, H., Bowden, R.: Deep hand: How to train a cnn on 1 million hand images when your data is continuous and weakly labelled. In: Proceedings of the IEEE Conference on Computer Vision and Pattern Recognition (CVPR), pp. 3793–3802 (2016)
18. Koller, O., Ney, H., Bowden, R.: Deep hand: How to train a cnn on 1 million hand images when your data is continuous and weakly labelled. In: CVPR, pp. 3793–3802 (2016)
19. Koller, O., Zargaran, O., Ney, H., Bowden, R.: Deep sign: hybrid cnn-hmm for continuous sign language recognition. In: British Machine Vision Conference (BMVC), p. 12 (2016)
20. Krizhevsky, A., Sutskever, I., Hinton, G.E.: Imagenet classification with deep convolutional neural networks. In: Advances in Neural Information Processing Systems (NIPS), pp. 1097–1105 (2012)
21. Luong, M.T., Pham, H., Manning, C.D.: Effective approaches to attention-based neural machine translation. In: EMNLP, pp. 1412–1421 (2015)
22. Pan, Y., Mei, T., Yao, T., Li, H., Rui, Y.: Jointly modeling embedding and translation to bridge video and language. In: Proceedings of the IEEE Conference on Computer Vision and Pattern Recognition (CVPR), pp. 4594–4602 (2016)
23. Pei, X., Guo, D., Zhao, Y.: Continuous sign language recognition based on pseudo-supervised learning. In: MAHCI, pp. 33–39 (2019)
24. Pu, J., Zhou, W., Li, H.: Dilated convolutional network with iterative optimization for coutinuous sign language recognition. In: International Joint Conference on Artificial Intelligence (IJCAI), pp. 885–891 (2018)
25. Salvador, S., Chan, P.: Toward accurate dynamic time warping in linear time and space. Intell. Data Anal. **11**(5), 561–580 (2007)
26. Song, P., Guo, D., Zhou, W., Wang, M., Li, H.: Parallel temporal encoder for sign language translation. In: ICIP, pp. 1915–1919 (2019)
27. Tran, D., Bourdev, L., Fergus, R., Torresani, L., Paluri, M.: Learning spatiotemporal features with 3d convolutional networks. In: Proceedings of the IEEE international conference on computer vision (ICCV), pp. 4489–4497 (2015)
28. Venugopalan, S., Rohrbach, M., Donahue, J., Mooney, R., Darrell, T., Saenko, K.: Sequence to sequence-video to text. In: Proceedings of the IEEE International Conference on Computer Vision (ICCV), pp. 4534–4542 (2015)
29. Wang, J., Liu, Z., Wu, Y., Yuan, J.: Mining actionlet ensemble for action recognition with depth cameras. In: IEEE Conference on Computer Vision and Pattern Recognition, pp. 1290–1297 (2012)
30. Wang, H., Chai, X., Zhou, Y., Chen, X.: Fast sign language recognition benefited from low rank approximation. In: Automatic Face and Gesture Recognition (FG), vol. 1, pp. 1–6 (2015)
31. Wang, L., Xiong, Y., Wang, Z., Qiao, Y., Lin, D., Tang, X., Van Gool, L.: Temporal segment networks: towards good practices for deep action recognition. In: ECCV, pp. 20–36 (2016)
32. Wang, S., Guo, D., Zhou, W., Zha, Z., Wang, M.: Connectionist temporal fusion for sign language translation. In: ACM MM, pp. 1483–1491 (2018)
33. Yao, L., Torabi, A., Cho, K., Ballas, N., Pal, C., Larochelle, H., Courville, A.: Describing videos by exploiting temporal structure. In: Proceedings of the IEEE International Conference on Computer Vision (ICCV), pp. 4507–4515 (2015)
34. Zhang, J., Zhou, W., Xie, C., Pu, J., Li, H.: Chinese sign language recognition with adaptive HMM. In: International Conference on Multimedia and Expo (ICME), pp. 1–6 (2016)
35. Zheng, L., Wang, S., Tian, L., He, F., Liu, Z., Tian, Q.: Query-adaptive late fusion for image search and person re-identification. In: IEEE Conference on Computer Vision and Pattern Recognition, pp. 1741–1750 (2015)
36. Zhu, W., Hu, J., Sun, G., Cao, X., Qiao, Y.: A key volume mining deep framework for action recognition. In: CVPR, pp. 1991–1999 (2016)

Fusion-Based Image Enhancement and Its Applications in Mobile Devices

Shijie Hao, Xu Han, Yuanhang Wu, and Lei Xu

Abstract In this chapter, we introduce a general framework for fusion-based image enhancement to produce photorealistic or non-photorealistic enhancement effects from natural images. For example, based on the contrast adjustment technique, we can produce the naturalness-preserving low-light enhancement effect for dark or back-light images. Also, based on the pencil drawing stylization and the semantic segmentation technique, we can convert a natural image into the mixed reality-virtuality effect. In these applications, we adopt a simple-but-effective method to construct a pixel-wise fusion map, aiming to guarantee the fusion-based enhancement effects. Furthermore, we have realized the techniques in mobile devices. For better user experiences, we use Fast Fourier Transform (FFT) to accelerate some computationally expensive steps. In addition, we introduce GrabCut to allow users to extract any interested regions for generating the mixed reality-virtuality effect. Demo APPs for Android phones are available for downloading.

Keywords Image enhancement · Image stylization · Image fusion

1 Introduction

With the rapid development of mobile phones, it has become convenient to take pictures of what we see at any time. Despite the great progress, it is still not easy to obtain a visually appealing image. On one hand, only a small percentage of the population have photography expertise. On the other hand, various interference factors exist in real-world photography, such as imperfect lightness conditions. Furthermore, beyond photorealistic visual effects, people are also interested in obtaining various non-photorealistic visual effects. In this context, it is useful

S. Hao (✉) · X. Han · Y. Wu
Hefei University of Technology, Hefei, China

L. Xu
Shanghai Polytechnic University, Shanghai, China

© The Author(s), under exclusive license to Springer Nature Switzerland AG 2021
T. McDaniel, X. Liu (eds.), *Multimedia for Accessible Human Computer Interfaces*,
https://doi.org/10.1007/978-3-030-70716-3_3

61

to develop image enhancement techniques that efficiently generate high-quality photorealistic images and diversified non-photorealistic images.

In this chapter, we aim to develop a general fusion-based framework for image enhancement. According to the enhancement tasks, the framework can be specified into different enhancing models to generate photorealistic and non-photorealistic effects from a given image. Specifically, we can fuse an input low-light image and a partially over-enhanced image to produce a naturalness-preserving low-light enhancement effect. Also, we can fuse a photorealistic image and its pencil drawing stylization to produce a mixed reality-virtuality effect. Among these applications, the key requirement is the seamless fusion, which is satisfied based on a simple-but-effective fusion weight map.

To make the framework more applicable in our daily life, we implement the model in mobile devices. To optimize the user experience, we apply the Fast Fourier Transform (FFT) to accelerate the filtering process needed in both photorealistic and non-photorealistic enhancements. Second, we adopt the interactive segmentation technique to give users control over the process of mixed reality-virtuality effect generation.

The rest of the chapter is organized as follows. Section 2 surveys related work. In Sect. 3, we describe the general fusion model and two specific applications. In Sect. 4, we introduce the technical details of acceleration and user interaction, and present some experimental results. Section 5 summarizes the chapter and discusses challenges worth further exploring.

2   Related Works

In this section, we introduce related work on the topics of low-light enhancement, pencil drawing generation, and semantic segmentation.

Fusion-based methods are commonly used in low-light image enhancement. Kou et al. [1] proposed a multi-exposure image fusion framework by designing a novel edge-preserving filter. Ma et al. [2] proposed a robust multi-exposure image fusion method in which the multi-exposure image blocks are decomposed jointly into structural elements. Despite the success, the problem we often face is that there is only one image at hand, which is often encountered in downloading an image from the Internet. A feasible strategy is to generate one or more reliable fusion sources from a single image. Fu et al. [3] generated three images of different contrasts from a single input, and then used the pyramid model to multi-scale fuse these three images to achieve good results. Feng et al. [4] used a simplified Retinex model to generate fusion sources similar to multi-exposure images, and then used multi-exposure image fusion methods to fuse these generated images. Hao et al. [5] used a simplified Retinex model to generate an initial enhanced image and designed a light-and structure-aware guidance matrix, which was used to fuse the original image with the initial enhanced image. In this chapter, we use the fusion framework proposed in [5]. Furthermore, we extend the application of this framework to support non-photorealistic enhancement.

Pencil drawing generation is an example of a non-photorealistic stylization technique. Lu et al. [6] proposed a subtle framework for generating pencil drawings in which the line sketches and the shadings are separately produced. The pencil drawing is finally obtained by combining the line sketches and the pencil shadings. Many proposed approaches follow this route, trying to improve the framework from multiple aspects. For example, Hao et al. [7] used the multi-scale filtering technique to enhance sketch lines. Qiu et al. [8] optimize computational efficiency by introducing parallel computation based on GPUs. Following the framework in [6], Li et al. [9] designed convolutional neural networks (CNNs) to produce lines and shadings. In our application, we also follow [6] to initially produce the fusion source. Specifically, we introduce the FFT technique to lift computational efficiency. We then fuse the pencil drawing with the original image, producing the mixed reality-virtuality effect, such as a photorealistic person standing in a pencil-drawn sketch.

Image segmentation aims at associating each pixel with a semantic label [10]. Despite the current success of supervised semantic segmentation methods, collecting sufficient training data with full supervision is not a trivial task. Further, the large size and FLOPs of trained networks are expensive for mobile applications with limited hardware resources. In this context, traditional interactive segmentation techniques are still attractive. The Intelligent Scissors [11] model uses live-wire boundary detection to obtain the optimal boundaries for image segmentation and composition. Boykov et al. [12] proposed a general interactive segmentation method for N-dimensional images called GraphCut. Users can manually marks certain pixels as "object" or "background" to provide hard constraints for segmentation. Through the promotion of graph cut theory, the GrabCut [13] method achieves better segmentation effects through iterative optimization and less user interaction. These method are flexible enough to extract arbitrary objects under human interaction. Recently, interactive segmentation methods based on deep learning have been developed. For example, Zhang et al. [14] proposed an Inside-Outside Guidance (IOG) approach to extract object segmentation masks with minimized user interaction.

3 Fusion-Based Enhancement Models

In this section, we first introduce a general linear fusion model framework. We then present two specific applications, i.e., the naturalness-preserving low-light enhancement, and the mixed pencil drawing generation.

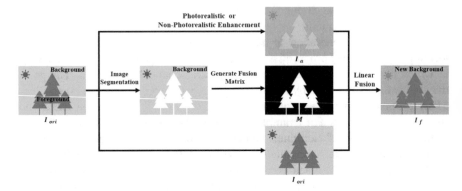

Fig. 1 A general framework for the linear fusion model

3.1 A General Framework of Linear Fusion

The framework introduced in this section is essentially a linear two-source fusion model, as shown in Fig. 1. Specifically, the model has two key elements: the fusion map and the fusion sources. Based on semantic segmentation terminology, for an input image I_{ori}, we term the region of interest as "object", and the rest as "background". Through a certain image segmentation technology, "object" and "background" can be separated. This binary partition can be used as the fusion matrix, denoted as M, in which the binary pixel values are taken as the fusion weights. For the fusion sources, the choice is open. In our application, we choose one fusion source as the input image I_{ori}. The other one I_a is the initial enhancement at any form according to the specific application. As for the low-light enhancement task, I_a can be an initial low-light enhancement. As for the mixed pencil drawing generation, I_a can be the pure pencil drawing image, converted from I_{ori}. The fusion can be formulated as:

$$I_f = I_{ori} \cdot M + I_a \cdot (1 - M), \qquad (1)$$

where $\cdot$ means element-wise multiplication. From Eq. 1, we can see that the fused image I_f simply combines I_{ori} and I_a under the guidance of M. In the following applications, the technical details of producing I_a and M are presented.

3.2 Naturalness-Preserving Low-Light Enhancement

Despite the rapid development of mobile devices, it is still difficult to take a satisfying photo in a complex lighting environment. Low light and back light usually cause weak and imbalanced lightness distribution. The images taken under these situations

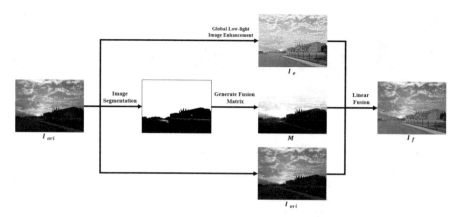

Fig. 2 Low-light image enhancement framework based on fusion model

have low visual quality, and many image details are hidden in darkness. Many low-light enhancement algorithms have been proposed to solve this problem, such as histogram-base methods [15], Retinex-based methods [16], or deep-learning-based methods [17]. A common limitation, namely, over-enhancement, still exists in these methods. The reason for this is that well-illuminated regions usually exist in low-light images, which need no enhancement. However, most current methods do not know which regions should be preserved during processing, and therefore, these algorithms over-enhance the well-illuminated regions. Based on this observation, we introduce a fusion-based low-light enhancement model. Aiming at preserving naturalness, the model enhances low-light regions while retaining well-illuminated regions of the original image, as shown in Fig. 2.

As a specific case of Eq. 1, this model can be represented as:

$$I_f = I_{ori} \cdot M + I_e \cdot (1 - M), \tag{2}$$

where I_f is the final fusion image, I_{ori} is the input low-light image, I_e is an initially enhanced image, and M is the fusion matrix. As shown in Fig. 2, M distinguishes the areas that need to be enhanced, and preserves the originally-bright sky region in I_{ori}. Therefore, the key in this model is the construction of M in which two demands are expected to be satisfied. First, M should be aware of the lightness distribution. Second, M should be aware of the image content structure. In the following, we present the details of the construction of M.

We first obtain the max-RGB channel of I_{ori}:

$$T_0(p) = \max_{c \in \{R,G,B\}} I_{ori}^c(p). \tag{3}$$

To make the fusion map aware of lightness, a straightforward threshold segmentation is used to partition T_0 into dark regions and bright regions. Here, we can simply

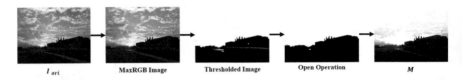

I_{ori} MaxRGB Image   Thresholded Image   Open Operation M

Fig. 3 The pipeline of generating M

set the threshold as $t = 0.2$ on T_0. However, the simple binarization is still far
from being structure-aware, which may cause many incorrect instances of fusion.
We further conduct the following refinement steps. First, we use the morphological
open operation to remove small outlier regions. We then use the guided filter [18]
to refine the fusion matrix at the pixel level. Here, the guidance image is chosen
as T_0. The output of the joint filter is used as our fusion matrix M. An example
of the above process is shown in Fig. 3. From the example, we have the following
observations. First, M clearly indicates which part of the image is dark, allowing
the preservation of the originally-bright regions in I_{ori} based on Eq. 2. Second,
compared with the binary image, M is consistent with the image structures in T_0. In
addition, the relaxed fusion weights facilitate seamless combination of I_{ori} and I_e.

We now introduce how to obtain I_e based on the Retinex model. The Retinex
theory assumes an observed image I_{ori} is the element-wise product of a reflectance
map R and an illumination map T:

$$I_{ori} = R \cdot T. \qquad (4)$$

In this application, we simplify the Retinex model solution by directly taking
the reflectance map R as the initial enhancement I_e. Based on this assumption, we
can directly obtain R by element-wise division $R = I_{ori}/T$, where T_0 is the initial
estimation of T, and ε is a small positive number to avoid numerical instability and
control the enhancing strength:

$$R = I_{ori}/(T_0 + \varepsilon). \qquad (5)$$

To obtain a better initial enhancement, T_s, as in [19], a common approach is to
further refine T_0 with an edge-preserving filter. Therefore, I_e can be obtained by:

$$I_e = I_{ori}/(T_s + \varepsilon). \qquad (6)$$

Compared with the low-light enhancement technique based on Eq. 4, the model
based on Eq. 6 can be seen as a simplified Retinex model, as it fully decouples
the inter-dependency between R and T. The enhanced image I_e can be directly
obtained based on T_s and a pre-defined ε. Typically, I_e has good performance on
lightening the dark regions in I_{ori}, but it usually contains over-enhanced regions.
Therefore, aiming at preserving the naturalness of the enhanced result, we use the

fusion model in Eq. 2, which subtly combines the enhanced dark regions in I_e and the originally-bright regions in I_{ori}.

3.3 Mixed Pencil Drawing Generation

It has become attractive to automatically transfer a natural image into a non-photorealistic form to create diversified visual effects. The fusion model of Eq. 1 can be used to generate non-photorealistic effects. A mixed reality-virtuality effect is depicted in Fig. 4, where a photorealistic person is shown standing in a non-photorealistic pencil drawing.

It is important to obtain the fusion matrix M to combine I_a and I_{ori}. Take Fig. 4 as an example: after the person is selected as the foreground, the interactive segmentation technique [11–13] is adopted to obtain the binary mask. Similar to the application in the previous section, the mask is further refined by the guided filter, aiming to avoid obvious discontinuity in the fusion.

Any artistic medium may be used, but for demonstrative purposes, we will continue to use a pencil drawing as the artistic image I_a in this chapter. The framework is as follows. The input image I_{ori} is first converted to the HSV color space where only the V channel (also known as the intensity channel) I is used for further processing. The pencil drawing generation can be divided into two stages.

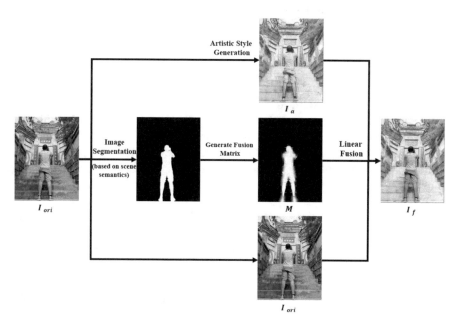

Fig. 4 Artistic image generation framework based on the fusion model

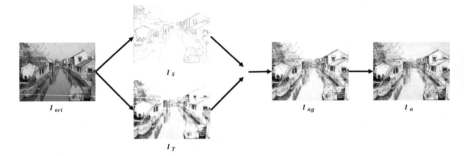

Fig. 5 Grayscale and color pencil drawing composite framework

The first stage aims to generate a structure-aware sketch layer I_S, while the second stage aims to generate the tone layer I_T. By multiplying I_S and I_T, we can obtain the pencil drawing I_{ag} in grayscale. Furthermore, combined with the unchanged H and S channels, we take I_{ag} as the new V channel, and convert back to RGB space, producing the color pencil drawing I_a. An example is shown in Fig. 5.

To make I_S structure-aware, we produce multiple filtered images $\{I_{Bi}\}$ based on an edge-preserving filter. By imposing different filtering strengths, $\{I_{Bi}\}$ is a set of smoothed images under different scales. Based on [6], we then use the 8-direction $(0, \pi/4, \ldots, 7\pi/4)$ convolution for $\{I_{Bi}\}$ to generate the sub-sketch-layers $\{I_{Si}\}$, making the lines in the pencil drawing resemble the line patterns in human sketches. We then fuse all the sub-layers $\{I_{Si}\}$ to obtain the sketch layer I_S via pixel-wise multiplication:

$$I_S = \prod_i I_{Si}. \tag{7}$$

The process is depicted in Fig. 6.

To obtain I_T, the tone mapping is first applied using histogram matching in which the histogram of I is reshaped to resemble the intensity distribution of pencil drawings. Then, the texture pattern t is transferred onto the tone mapped image I_H. Following [6], the transferring model is chosen as a pixel-wise exponential mapping function:

$$I_H(p) \approx t(p)^\beta, \tag{8}$$

where β is the transferring matrix. It is estimated via solving the following optimization problem:

$$\beta^* = \min_\beta \|\beta \ln t - \ln I_H\|_2^2 + \lambda \|\nabla \beta\|_2^2, \tag{9}$$

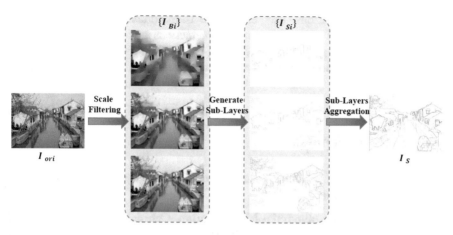

Fig. 6 Multi-scale sub-sketch-layer generation framework

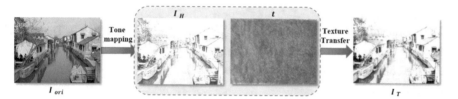

Fig. 7 Tone layer generation framework

where λ is the weight (we empirically set it as 0.2 as in [6]). The tone layer I_T can finally be obtained by Eq. 10. A typical example of the above process is shown in Fig. 7.

$$I_T(p) = t(p)^{\beta^*}. \tag{10}$$

4   Applications in Mobile Devices

To validate the effectiveness of our proposed enhancing models introduced in Sect. 3, we developed two prototype Android APPs in which all computations are carried out on mobile devices. This enables users to generate high-quality photorealistic images or diversified non-photorealistic images at any time and any place. Free downloads of the installation packages are available.[1,2]

---

[1]https://drive.google.com/file/d/1n2ABS-MyldIFvMxFWdEiJjfTuE0pfh1M/view?usp=sharing.
[2]https://drive.google.com/file/d/1bnxzygK4yfZr5uDLUb4icPZ1RBa8PEj7/view?usp=sharing.

For mobile applications, user experience is important. For example, a fast implementation speed and convenient user interactions are always appreciated. We first introduce FFT to accelerate the filtering process. We then adopt an interactive segmentation algorithm to allow users to extract the semantic regions according to their interests.

4.1 FFT Acceleration

We first introduce the preliminary steps for using FFT to speed up the solution of polynomial multiplication.

Using FFT to Solve Polynomial Multiplication Calculate the multiplication of two polynomials, for example $A \times B$, where $A = a_0 x_0 + a_1 x_1 + \ldots + a_{n-1} x_{n-1}$, $B = b_0 x_0 + b_1 x_1 + \ldots + b_{n-1} x_{n-1}$. We assume the product is C.

a. Direct Calculation
The coefficient of C can be expressed as: $\sum_{k=0}^{j} a_k b_{j-k}, 0 \leq j \leq 2n - 2$. Therefore, the polynomial C can be expressed as: $C = \sum_{j=0}^{2n-2} \sum_{k=0}^{j} a_k b_{j-k} x^j$. We can see that the complexity of direct calculation is $O(n^2)$.

b. Fast Calculation
Based on concepts in digital signal processing, the above multiplication is actually a convolution of two sequences. Here, the coefficients a_j and b_j of the polynomials A and B can be regarded as vectors; then the coefficients c_j of the polynomial C can be regarded as the convolution of a_j and b_j. As we have the important property that the time (or spatial) domain convolution corresponds to the frequency domain multiplication, the fast calculation can be designed as follows:

1. Obtain the frequency domain expression of A and B respectively via FFT, of which the complexity is $O(n \log(n))$.
2. Point-wise multiply the frequency domain expressions of A and B, of which the complexity is $O(n)$.
3. Convert the multiplied sequence back to the spatial domain via IFFT, of which the complexity is $O(n \log(n))$.

The above process can be expressed as $C = A \times B = \mathscr{F}^{-1}(\mathscr{F}(A) \cdot \mathscr{F}(B))$, where $\cdot$ means element-wise multiplication. In this way, the polynomial multiplication with complexity $O(n^2)$ is reduced to $O(n \log(n))$. As n becomes very large, the saved implementation time can be dramatically increased.

Based on the above acceleration ideas, we introduce FFT as the accelerator of the filtering process used in the proposed applications. Using the mixed pencil drawing as an example, we produce multiple images $\{I_{Bi}\}$, which are obtained by applying a TV-based edge-preserving filter:

$$arg\min_{I_{Bi}} \|I_{Bi} - I\|_2^2 + \lambda \left(\mathbb{R}_x + \mathbb{R}_y\right), \tag{11}$$

$$\begin{cases} \mathbb{R}_x = \left\| \dfrac{\nabla_x I_{Bi}}{(\overline{\nabla_x L})^\gamma} \right\|_1 \\ \mathbb{R}_y = \left\| \dfrac{\nabla_y I_{Bi}}{(\overline{\nabla_y L})^\gamma} \right\|_1, \end{cases} \tag{12}$$

where $L = log(I_{Bi})$, $\overline{\nabla_{x,y}L} = \frac{1}{\Omega}\sum_\Omega \nabla_{x,y}L$, Ω is a local patch with the size of 3×3, and γ is a scale parameter.

First, the gradient descent method is used to solve Eq. 11 directly. For the regularization term $\mathbb{R}$, the following approximation can be made:

$$\mathbb{R} = \left\| \frac{\nabla I_{Bi}}{(\overline{\nabla L})^\gamma} \right\|_1 \approx \omega \|\nabla I_{Bi}\|_2^2, \omega = \frac{1}{\max(|\nabla I_{Bi}|, \epsilon)(\overline{\nabla L})^\gamma}. \tag{13}$$

Equation 11 can be converted into:

$$\underset{I_{Bi}}{\operatorname{argmin}} \|I_{Bi} - I\|_2^2 + \lambda(\omega_x \|\nabla_x I_{Bi}\|_2^2 + \omega_y \|\nabla_y I_{Bi}\|_2^2). \tag{14}$$

We further convert Eq. 14 into the matrix form:

$$\underset{\mathbf{I}_{Bi}}{\operatorname{argmin}}(\mathbf{I}_{Bi} - \mathbf{I})^{\mathrm{T}}(\mathbf{I}_{Bi} - \mathbf{I}) + \lambda(\mathbf{I}_{Bi}^{\mathrm{T}}\mathbf{D}_x^{\mathrm{T}}\mathbf{W}_x\mathbf{D}_x\mathbf{I}_{Bi} + \mathbf{I}_{Bi}^{\mathrm{T}}\mathbf{D}_y^{\mathrm{T}}\mathbf{W}_y\mathbf{D}_y\mathbf{I}_{Bi}). \tag{15}$$

$\mathbf{I}_{Bi}$ and $\mathbf{I}$ are the matrix representations of I_{Bi} and I, respectively. $\mathbf{D}_x$ and $\mathbf{D}_y$ are the Toeplitz matrices composed of forward-difference discrete gradient operators. The diagonal matrices $\mathbf{W}_x$ and $\mathbf{W}_y$ are formed by the weights ω_x and ω_x. Equation 15 can be solved via setting its derivative to 0:

$$\mathbf{I}_{Bi} = (\mathbf{1} + \lambda\mathbf{Q})^{-1}\mathbf{I}, \tag{16}$$

where $\mathbf{1}$ is the identity matrix, and $\mathbf{Q} = \mathbf{D}_x^{\mathrm{T}}\mathbf{W}_x\mathbf{D}_x + \mathbf{D}_y^{\mathrm{T}}\mathbf{W}_y\mathbf{D}_y$ is a sparse five-point definite Laplacian matrix [20]. To obtain a piecewise smoothing result, we can further gradually refine $\mathbf{I}_{Bi}^k$ in an iterative way:

$$\mathbf{I}_{Bi}^k = (\mathbf{1} + \lambda\mathbf{Q}^{k-1})^{-1}\mathbf{I}. \tag{17}$$

However, directly calculating the inverse of $(\mathbf{1} + \lambda\mathbf{Q}^{k-1})^{-1}$ in Eq. 17 is not suitable for mobile devices due to the expensive computation, especially when the image size is large. To address this limitation, we use FFT to speed up the solution of Eq. 11.

For Eq. 11, we have:

$$\underset{I_{Bi}}{\text{argmin}} \|I_{Bi} - I\|_2^2 + \lambda \|W \cdot \nabla I_{Bi}\|_1, \ W = \frac{1}{(\nabla L)^\gamma}. \tag{18}$$

Equation 18 can be solved by the Alternating Direction Minimization (ADMM) technique in which $\nabla I_{Bi} = X$ is used as the constraint term. Therefore, we aim to solve the following optimization problem:

$$\underset{I_{Bi}}{\text{argmin}} \|I_{Bi} - I\|_2^2 + \lambda \|W \cdot X\|_1 \qquad s.t. \qquad X = \nabla I_{Bi}. \tag{19}$$

We convert the symbols in Eq. 19 into matrix form, and the augmented Lagrangian function can be shaped as follows:

$$\mathscr{L} = \|\mathbf{I}_{Bi} - \mathbf{I}\|_2^2 + \lambda \|\mathbf{W} \cdot \mathbf{X}\|_1 + \frac{\rho}{2} \|\nabla \mathbf{I}_{Bi} - \mathbf{X}\|_2^2 + \langle \mathbf{Y}, \nabla \mathbf{I}_{Bi} - \mathbf{X} \rangle. \tag{20}$$

In Eq. 20, $\langle \cdot, \cdot \rangle$ is the matrix inner product, ρ is a positive penalty scalar, and $\mathbf{Y}$ is the Lagrangian multiplier. Equation 20 can be solved via the alternative optimization strategy in which three sub-problems are solved in turn.

(1) $\mathbf{I}_{Bi}$ Sub-Problem

$$\mathbf{I}_{Bi}^k = \underset{\mathbf{I}_{Bi}}{\text{argmin}} \|\mathbf{I}_{Bi} - \mathbf{I}\|_2^2 + \frac{\rho^{k-1}}{2} \left\| \nabla \mathbf{I}_{Bi} - \mathbf{X}^{k-1} \right\|_2^2 + \left\langle \mathbf{Y}^{k-1}, \nabla \mathbf{I}_{Bi} - \mathbf{X}^{k-1} \right\rangle. \tag{21}$$

Equation 21 can be solved by setting its derivative with respect to $\mathbf{I}_{Bi}$ to 0:

$$2(\mathbf{I}_{Bi} - \mathbf{I}) + \rho^{k-1} \mathbf{D}^T (\mathbf{DS} - \mathbf{X}^{k-1}) + \mathbf{D}^T \mathbf{Y}^{k-1} = 0. \tag{22}$$

We then introduce 2D-FFT to speed up the solution of the above equation:

$$\mathbf{I}_{Bi}^k = \mathscr{F}^{-1} \Big(\frac{\mathscr{F}(\mathbf{I}) + \frac{\rho^{k-1}}{2} \Psi}{1 + \frac{\rho^{k-1}}{2} (\mathscr{F}^*(\mathbf{D}_x) \mathscr{F}(\mathbf{D}_x) + \mathscr{F}^*(\mathbf{D}_y) \mathscr{F}(\mathbf{D}_y))} \Big), \tag{23}$$

where $\mathscr{F}$ denotes 2D-FFT, $\mathscr{F}^{-1}$ denotes 2D-IFFT, $\mathscr{F}^*$ denotes the conjugate operator and $\Psi = \mathscr{F}^*(\mathbf{D}_x) \mathscr{F}(\mathbf{X}_x^{k-1} - \frac{\mathbf{Y}_x^{k-1}}{\rho^{k-1}}) + \mathscr{F}^*(\mathbf{D}_y) \mathscr{F}(\mathbf{X}_y^{k-1} - \frac{\mathbf{Y}_y^{k-1}}{\rho^{k-1}})$.

(2) $\mathbf{X}$ Sub-Problem

$$\mathbf{X}^k = \underset{\mathbf{X}}{\text{argmin}} \lambda \left\| \mathbf{W}^{k-1} \cdot \mathbf{X} \right\|_1 + \frac{\rho^{k-1}}{2} \left\| \nabla \mathbf{I}_{Bi}^k - \mathbf{X} \right\|_2^2 + \left\langle \mathbf{Y}^{k-1}, \nabla \mathbf{I}_{Bi}^k - \mathbf{X} \right\rangle. \tag{24}$$

The closed form solution of Eq. 24 can be obtained by performing the following shrinkage operation:

$$\mathbf{X}^k = \mathscr{T}_{\frac{\lambda \mathbf{W}^{k-1}}{\rho^{k-1}}}(\nabla \mathbf{I}_{Bi}^k + \frac{\mathbf{Y}^{k-1}}{\rho^{k-1}}), \tag{25}$$

where $\mathscr{T}_{\alpha>0}(x)$ represents the shrinkage operator and $\mathscr{T}_\alpha(x) = sgn(x)\max(|x| - \alpha, 0)$.

(3) $\mathbf{Y}$, $\mathbf{W}$ *and* ρ

$$\mathbf{Y}^k = \mathbf{Y}^{k-1} + \rho^{k-1}(\nabla \mathbf{I}_{Bi}^k - \mathbf{X}^k), \tag{26}$$

$$\mathbf{W}^k = \frac{1}{(\nabla \mathbf{L}^k)^\gamma}, \mathbf{L}^k = log(\mathbf{I}_{Bi}^k), \tag{27}$$

$$\rho^k = \eta \rho^{k-1}, \eta > 1. \tag{28}$$

Since FFT considerably accelerates the first sub-problem, the whole filtering process is much faster.

Similarly, we can use FFT to accelerate the optimization of Eq. 9. First, we transform Eq. 9 into an equivalent form:

$$\beta^* = \min_\beta \|\beta - \ln I_H / \ln t\|_2^2 + \lambda \|\nabla \beta\|_2^2. \tag{29}$$

As the above problem only involves quadratic terms, we can directly have an analytical solution:

$$\beta - \frac{\ln \mathbf{I_H}}{\ln \mathbf{t}} + \lambda \mathbf{D}^\mathsf{T} \mathbf{D} \beta = 0. \tag{30}$$

By introducing 2D-FFT, the optimal β can be efficiently obtained as:

$$\beta^* = \mathscr{F}^{-1}(\frac{\mathscr{F}(\frac{\ln \mathbf{I_H}}{\ln \mathbf{t}})}{1 + (\mathscr{F}^*(\mathbf{D}_x)\mathscr{F}(\mathbf{D}_x) + \mathscr{F}^*(\mathbf{D}_y)\mathscr{F}(\mathbf{D}_y))}). \tag{31}$$

4.2 Interactive Segmentation

While image segmentation algorithms based on deep learning have achieved very promising results [10], it is still not easy to implement them on mobile devices

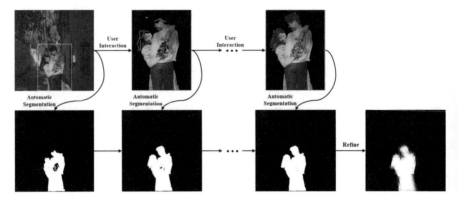

Fig. 8 Interactive image segmentation

due to limited computing resources. Moreover, since the interaction between a user and his or her phone is almost dominated by finger touching and swiping, GrabCut technology is very suitable for the proposed application.

As shown in Fig. 8, the adopted interactive image segmentation process can be performed through the following steps. First, a user drags a rectangular box on the screen in which the "object" is selected. The segmentation is then implemented in the backend. Considering segmentation errors can occur after the first round of interaction, the user is allowed to use the brush tool for further interactions. The user can brush the screen to further indicate which areas should be anchored as the object of interest or the background. The segmentation result is then updated based on the additional information from the new interactions until the user is satisfied with the segmentation result. Finally, the binary mask is refined based on the guided filter for seamless fusion.

4.3 Experimental Results

In this section, we demonstrate results of the naturalness-preserving low-light enhancement and mixed pencil drawing generation techniques. We tested the apps on a mid-level Android phone in which all algorithms were implemented on the phone CPU with unoptimized code. In general, the most computationally expensive procedure is pencil drawing generation. For example, an image of 1080*1080 resolution takes around 4 s.

Some results are shown in Figs. 9 and 10. We can see that the generated visual effects well satisfy the proposed objective. More results can be seen in Figs. 11 and 12.

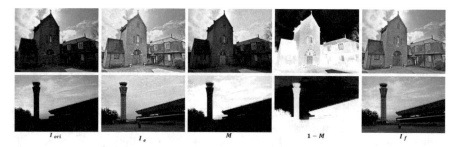

Fig. 9 Low-light image enhancement based on the fusion model

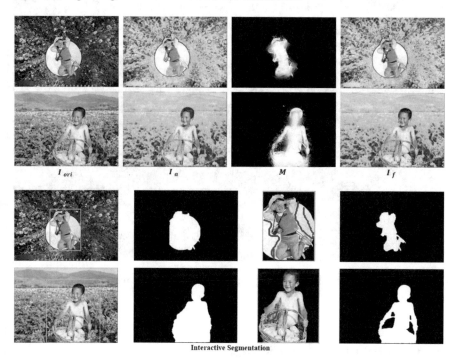

Fig. 10 Pencil drawing image generation based on the fusion model

It is worth noting that the proposed general model is quite versatile, and therefore more diversified results can be obtained. For example, as shown in Fig. 13, we can replace pencil-drawn backgrounds with cartoon-like rendering effects.

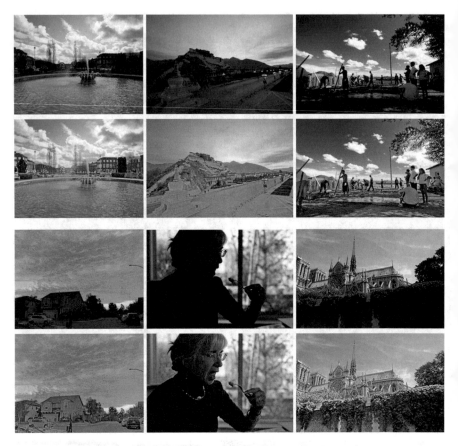

Fig. 11 More examples of low-light image enhancement based on the fusion model

5 Conclusion and Discussion

In this chapter, we proposed a general framework for fusion-based image enhancement. Based on this framework, we constructed different image enhancement models to generate photorealistic and non-photorealistic visual effects. First, by constructing a lightness-aware fusion map, we achieved naturalness-preserving low-light enhancement. Second, by introducing semantic segmentation, the segmentation mask can be used to guide the fusion of the photorealistic target and the non-photorealistic background, producing the mixed reality-virtuality effect. For an efficient mobile application, we used FFT to accelerate the filtering process, and used the interactive segmentation to facilitate user control. Prototype Android APPs can be downloaded from the Internet.

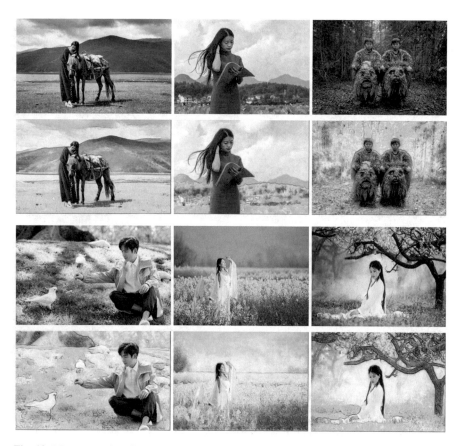

Fig. 12 More examples of pencil drawing image generation based on the fusion model

There are some points worth further exploration. During image segmentation, some complicated segmentation errors may require multiple interventions by the user, which will impact the overall user experience. We plan to investigate image segmentation algorithms to achieve more accurate segmentation with less user involvement. Currently, the software runs on a CPU in a single thread. With the advancements of mobile devices, useful techniques such as GPU-based parallel computing or multi-threaded implementations can be considered.

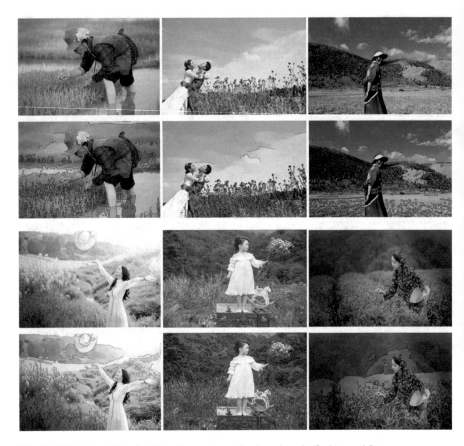

Fig. 13 More examples of cartoon image generation based on the fusion model

Acknowledgments This research is partially supported by National Nature Science Foundation of China under Grant Number 61772171, 61632007.

References

1. Kou, F., Wei, Z., Chen, W., Wu, X., Wen, C., Li, Z.: Intelligent detail enhancement for exposure fusion. IEEE Trans. Multimedia **20**(2), 484–495 (2018)
2. Ma, K., Li, H., Yong, H., Wang, Z., Meng, D., Zhang, L.: Robust multi-exposure image fusion: a structural patch decomposition approach. IEEE Trans. Image Process. **26**(5), 2519–2532 (2017)
3. Fu, X., Zeng, D., Huang, Y., Liao, Y., Ding, X., Paisley, J.: A fusion-based enhancing method for weakly illuminated images. Signal Process. **129**, 82–96 (2016)

4. Feng, Z., Zhou, Z., Hong, R., Hao, S., Ge, Y., Wang, M.: Single low-light image enhancement by fusing multiple sources. In: 2018 IEEE Fourth International Conference on Multimedia Big Data (BigMM), pp. 1–4. IEEE, Piscataway (2018)
5. Hao, S., Guo, Y., Wei, Z.: Lightness-aware contrast enhancement for images with different illumination conditions. Multimed. Tools. Appl. **78**, 3817–3830 (2019)
6. Lu, C., Xu, L., Jia, J.: Combining sketch and tone for pencil drawing production, In: Proceedings of the Workshop on Non-Photorealistic Animation and Rendering (2012)
7. Hao, S., Guo, Y., Hong, R., Wang, M.: Scale-aware spatially guided mapping. IEEE Multimedia **23**(3), 34–42 (2016)
8. Qiu, J., Liu, B., He, J., Liu, C., Li, Y.: Parallel fast pencil drawing generation algorithm based on GPU. IEEE Access **7**, 83543–83555 (2019)
9. Li, Y., Fang, C., Hertzmann, A., Shechtman, E., Yang, M.: Im2Pencil: controllable pencil illustration from photographs, In: Proceedings of the Conference on Computer Vision and Pattern Recognition. IEEE, Piscataway (2019)
10. Hao, S., Zhou, Y., Guo, Y.: A brief survey on semantic segmentation with deep learning. Neurocomputing **406**, 302–321 (2020)
11. Mortensen, E.N., Barrett, W.A.: Intelligent scissors for image composition. In: 22nd Annual Conference on Computer Graphics and Interactive Techniques, Association for Computing Machinery, pp. 191–198 (1995)
12. Boykov, Y.Y., Jolly, M.P.: Interactive graph cuts for optimal boundary & region segmentation of objects in N-D images. In: Eighth IEEE International Conference on Computer Vision, pp. 105–112. IEEE, Piscataway (2001)
13. Rother, C., Kolmogorov, V., Blake, A.: "GrabCut": Interactive foreground extraction using iterated graph cuts. In: ACM SIGGRAPH 2004, Association for Computing Machinery, pp. 309–314 (2004)
14. Zhang, S., Liew, J., Wei, Y., Wei, S., Zhao, Y.: Interactive object segmentation with inside-outside guidance. In: Proceedings of the Conference on Computer Vision and Pattern Recognition, pp. 12234–12244. IEEE, Piscataway (2020)
15. Lee, C., Lee, C., Kim, C.: Contrast enhancement based on layered difference representation of 2D histograms. IEEE Trans. Image Process. **22**(12), 5372–5384 (2013)
16. Hao, S., Han, X., Guo, Y., Xu, X., Wang, M.: Low-light image enhancement with semi-389 decoupled decomposition. IEEE Trans. Multimed. **22**(12), 3025–3038 (2020)
17. Wang, R., Zhang, Q., Fu, C., Shen, X., Zheng, W., Jia, J.,: Underexposed photo enhancement using deep illumination estimation, In: Proceedings of the Conference on Computer Vision and Pattern Recognition. IEEE, Piscataway (2019)
18. He, K., Sun, J., Tang, X.: Guided image filtering. IEEE Trans. Pattern Anal. Mach. Intell. **35**(6), 1397–1409 (2013)
19. Guo, X., Li, Y., Ling, H.: LIME: Low-light image enhancement via illumination map estimation. IEEE Trans. Image Process. **26**(2), 982–993 (2017)
20. Farbman, Z., Fattal, R., Lischinski, D., Szeliski, R.: Edge-preserving decompositions for multi-scale tone and detail manipulation. In: ACM SIGGRAPH 2008, pp. 1–10. Association for Computing Machinery (2008)

Open-Domain Textual Question Answering Systems

Zhen Huang, Xinxin Su, Shiyi Xu, and Minghao Hu

Abstract Open-domain textual question answering (QA) systems have been a hot topic in Natural Language Processing (NLP) for quite some time. These systems are designed to find answers from a large amount of textual sources, such as Wikipedia or search engines. Due to the rapid development of deep learning, the performance of QA systems have been significantly improved, especially on machine reading comprehension. In this chapter, we provide an overview of open-domain QA systems, then introduce models on paragraph ranking, candidate answer extraction, and answer selection.

Keywords Question answering · Reading comprehension · Semantic retrieval · Answer selection · Deep learning

1 Introduction

Open-domain textual question answering (QA) is a classical and hot task in the area of Natural Language Processing (NLP), which can be tracked to the origin of artificial intelligence, namely the famous Turing test [1]. This area of research has evolved continually in the last 60 years, and many new techniques have been introduced [2].

Open-domain QA can be classified into categories based on different dimensions, such as structured, semi-structured, and unstructured depending on the data source. Here we focus on unstructured text. Generally, a technical architecture for QA consists of the paragraph ranking module, candidate answer extraction module, and final answer selection module [3]. Regarding a specific question, the paragraph rank-

Z. Huang (✉) · X. Su · S. Xu
Science and Technology on Parallel and Distributed Laboratory, National University of Defense Technology, Changsha, China
e-mail: huangzhen@nudt.edu.cn; xinxinsu@nudt.edu.cn; xushiyi18@nudt.edu.cn

M. Hu
PLA Academy of Military Science, Beijing, China

© The Author(s), under exclusive license to Springer Nature Switzerland AG 2021
T. McDaniel, X. Liu (eds.), *Multimedia for Accessible Human Computer Interfaces*,
https://doi.org/10.1007/978-3-030-70716-3_4

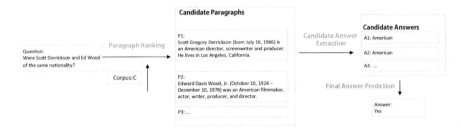

Fig. 1 The technical architecture of open-domain QA systems. For example, the question is "Were Scott Derrickson and Ed Wood of the same nationality?". The paragraph ranking module retrieves several related documents and then selects several candidate paragraphs. Next, the reading comprehension module extracts multiple candidate answers. The final answer prediction module gives the most promising prediction, "Yes", as the final answer

ing module first retrieves several the most relevant paragraphs. From these candidate paragraphs, the answer extraction module locates a few candidate answers. Finally, these answers are fed into the final answer selection module to predict the most credible answer.

2 Overview of Open-Domain Question Answering Systems

For an open domain QA system, the corpus C is predefined, and consists of a set of paragraphs, denoted as $P = \{p_1, p_2, \ldots, p_i, \ldots, p_n\}$. For each question, denoted as $Q = \{q_1, q_2, \ldots, q_j \ldots, q_m\}$, relevant paragraphs may be returned through the paragraph ranking module.

Selected paragraphs are fed into the candidate answer extraction module employing a Reading Comprehension (RC) model to extract answers, from which candidate answers, denoted as $A = a_1, \ldots, a_i$, are obtained. Each answer is denoted as a start position a_i^s and an end position a_i^e. The true label answer of each question starts from y_i^s and ends at y_i^e.

The final answer selection module will aggregate candidate answers, and the answer with the maximum probability will be chosen. The structure is shown in Fig.1, and one question is processed as an example.

3 Paragraph Ranking

Retrieving several of the most relevant paragraphs of a given question is the first step of open-domain QA systems. This task can be divided into two subtasks: retrieving and ranking. Some QA datasets have every answer to each question located in one paragraph, while in some, answers are located in several paragraphs. The latter is a more popular topic, and relatively, more complex.

Traditional retrieval methods, such as TF-IDF and BM25 [4–6], can rank documents according to the statistical features of words between question and documents, while the semantic features of sentences are ignored. These methods are simple and have low computational complexity. In contrast, deep learning models [7, 8] can capture more complex semantic features. But such models utilized to compute similarity between two texts are usually processing short sequences that are similar in length. These models are therefore unsuitable for the matching task between questions and paragraphs in open-domain QA systems.

Traditional methods tend to feed more paragraphs to the RC model, ensuring the correct answer is not missed. One problem is the sharp reduction in answer prediction accuracy because often most of the paragraphs considered to be correct don't contain answers. These paragraphs may even mislead the model.

3.1 Multi-Level Fused Sequence Matching Model

Yang Liu et al. [9] proposed a multi-level fused sequence matching (MFS) model, which leveraged a deep neural network to filter noise paragraphs for open-domain QA. The model performed better than previous text matching models as it has a more complex structure and can fully capture semantic features of paragraphs.

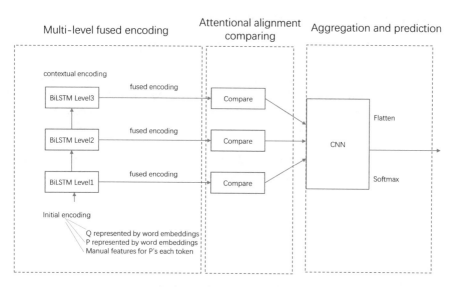

Fig. 2 An overview of the MFS model. Initial encoding, contextual encoding and comparison features are combined. CNN receives the aggregated features, and final prediction (classification) is made

Figure 2 shows an overview of MFS, which consists of three layers: (1) multi-level fused encoding layer to fuse the contextual features at different levels, including word-embedding features, manual features and contextual features, (2) alignment and comparison layer leveraging the attention mechanism to align question and paragraph so as to obtain the comparison features between them, and (3) aggregation and prediction layer, which leverages a CNN to integrate the features at all levels and makes the final classification.

3.1.1 Multi-Level Fused Encoding

The 300-dimensional Glove [10] word-embeddings are utilized as the representation of word-level tokens, denotes $emb(p_i)$ and $emb(q_i)$ for the paragraphs and questions respectively. The initial encoding $H_0(Q)$ for Q is $emb(q_i)$ and $H_0(P)$ for P is $emb(p_i)$. Manual features include $f(p_i)$, which are concatenated to $emb(p_i)$, and include part-of-speech (POS), name entity recognition (NER) tags, term frequency (TF), and a flag indicating whether the token appeared in the sequence Q.

To obtain the higher-level semantic information of each token in the sequence, the encoder employs multi-layer Bidirectional Long Short-Term Memory (BiLSTM) [11] to process the initial word-embeddings of each token, which can be formulated as Eq. 1.

$$H_{k+1}(P) = \text{BiLSTM}_P(H_k(P)) \tag{1}$$

$H_{k+1}(Q)$ is obtained in a similar way, which can be formulated as Eq. 2:

$$H_{k+1}(Q) = \text{BiLSTM}_Q(H_k(Q)) \tag{2}$$

It should be noted that the manual features are added only to P; the initial vector of P and Q is different in dimension, so the BiLSTM codings for Q and P are different. $H_k(.)$ is the k-th level semantic encoding for each token and is the input of $H_{k+1}(.)$, and compared to $H_k(.)$, $H_{k+1}(.)$ represents more global semantic information.

To make full use of the semantic features at all levels, the encoder fuses different levels of contextual semantic encoding and corresponding initial word-embeddings as Eq. 3.

$$\tilde{H}_k(P) = \begin{bmatrix} H_k(P) \\ emb(P) \end{bmatrix}, \quad \tilde{H}_k(Q) = \begin{bmatrix} H_k(Q) \\ emb(Q) \end{bmatrix}, \quad k = 1, 2, \dots \tag{3}$$

3.1.2 Attention Model with Alignment and Comparison

Since the sequence length of questions are usually shorter than paragraphs, the model should align the sequences of questions and paragraphs before comparison

[12, 13]. Before alignment, similarity between $p_i \in P$ and $q_j \in Q$ can be measured as:

$$P_k = \text{ReLU}(W\tilde{H}_k(P) + b), \quad Q_k = \text{ReLU}(W\tilde{H}_k(Q) + b)$$

$$E_k := [e_{ij}^{(k)}] = P_k^T Q_k \qquad (4)$$

where W and b are learnable parameters, E is a $m \times n$ sized similarity matrix to measure the similarity between Q and P.

Then at the k-th level, the attentional representation P_k' which is aligned with P and generated by the semantic information of Q can be calculated as:

$$A_k : [\alpha_{ij}^{(k)}], \quad \alpha_{ij}^{(k)} = \frac{\exp(e_{ij}^{(k)})}{\sum_j \exp(e_{ij}^{(k)})}$$

$$P'_k = A_k Q_k^T \qquad (5)$$

After alignment, the comparison features of the two sequences on the k-th level are compared using Eq. 6. The symbol $\odot$ denotes element-wise multiplication.

$$sub_k = (P_k - P'_k) \odot (P_k - P'_k), \quad mul_k = P_k \odot P'_k \qquad (6)$$

3.1.3 Aggregation and Prediction

After capturing the abundant information in the previous layers, the final step is to aggregate these features, and make a final prediction with the fused features.

At each level, there are four features: P_k, P'_k, sub_k and mul_k. These four features have the same size, so they can be stacked as a 4-channel 2D feature map, with each channel corresponding to a feature. In Eq. 7, stacking all the K levels will obtain a $4K$-channel feature map FM_k. $Concat(\cdot, \cdot)$ applies the concatenation operation on the channel.

$$FM_k = Concat(P_k, P'_k, sub_k, mul_k)$$

$$FeatureMap = Concat(FM_1, FM_2, \ldots, FM_K) \qquad (7)$$

All features are aggregated by a multi-layer 2D-CNN. The small size of the model parameters reduces the size of the feature map and accelerates the training process.

$$v = \max_{row} CNN(FeatureMap) \qquad (8)$$

where $CNN(\cdot)$ is a multi-layer 2D-CNN. After multiple passes of CNN processing, the $FeatureMap$ continually shrinks, and finally converts into an x-channel map, where x is the number of convolutional kernels in the final CNN layer. Within each channel, using max pooling along the rows which corresponds to the length of the sequence, the map is compressed into a vector. In Eq. 8, v is a 1-dimensional vector with x channels, which is utilized to make a prediction.

$$v' = Flatten(v)$$
$$p = \text{softmax}(W_p v' + b_p)$$
(9)

The model then evaluates the relation between Q and P through a full connection layer and softmax function. $Flatten(\cdot)$ transforms the matrix into a vector through concatenating each row, where (W_p, b_p) are learnable parameters.

3.2 Evaluation

The Multi-level Fused Sequence Matching Model is evaluated on two different datasets: SNLI [14], a public dataset for textual entailment; and PF, a semantic matching dataset constructed with question-answer pairs of SQuAD [15] and contexts of Wikipedia through distant supervision. The MFM model is trained on the PF dataset as a filter of the DrQA pipeline. Using accuracy as the evaluation metric for the semantic matching task, the model performs best on PF and very competitive on SNLI compared to DrQA-Reader [16] and CA-model [17]. For open-domain QA tasks, when the model uses recall as the evaluation metric on the filtered candidate paragraphs, the results of open-domain QA compared to DrQA are improved. This indicates that open-domain QA can be improved by removing several noise candidates.

4 Candidate Answer Extraction

The candidate answer extraction module extracts the candidate answers from the candidate paragraphs filtered through the first module. The candidate answer extraction module consists of three parts: (1) a feature encoding layer to encode the text with word-embeddings and pretrained models, (2) an interaction attention layer to aggregate the semantics of questions and paragraphs using an attention mechanism, and (3) a candidate answer prediction layer using feature aggregation methods.

In reality, most of the retrieved passages in the first step do not contain true answers, and they are also long and complex for the RC models to extraction. In the process of locating answers, the importance of every paragraph varies, but previous RC models access all paragraphs and treat every passage equally, even paragraphs that provide negative information.

4.1 Dynamic Semantic Discard Reader

Wang Xu et al. [18] proposed a Dynamic Semantic Discard Reader (DSDR), a novel reading model which improves the candidate answer extraction process by discarding noise information dynamically.

Figure 3 shows an overview of the DSDR model. The model can be divided into five layers: (1) an information encoding layer to encode the context of passages and questions through a BiLSTM, (2) an attention matching layer to align the sequence of passages and questions to further extract semantic information, (3) a dynamic discard layer to fuse the information of the aligned text pairs and discard irrelevant information through a feed-forward network, (4) a result aggregation layer to match the semantics of P and Q and obtain effective features through a neural network, and (5) a final prediction layer to calculate the probability distributions of the answer to the provided question through a Softmax function.

4.1.1 Feature Encoding

Based on the Glove word-embeddings, the encoder processes the embedded question Q and passage P, and leverages a BiLSTM to yield the context features using Eq. 10. The context representations are denoted as $P^c = \{p_1^c, p_2^c \dots p_m^c\} \in R^{d \times m}$ and $Q^c = \{q_1^c, q_2^c \dots q_n^c\} \in R^{d \times n}$. Vectors q_j^c and p_i^c denote the hidden states of the BiLSTM and d is the hidden dimension.

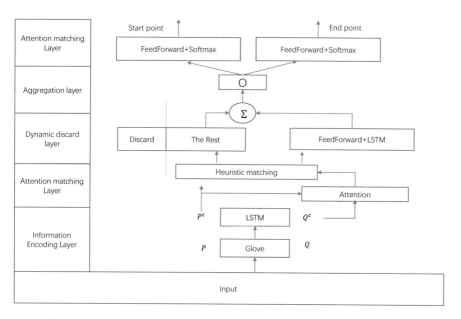

Fig. 3 The overview of the DSDR model, which consists of five layers

$$p_i^c = \text{BiLSTM}(p_i), \quad q_j^c = \text{BiLSTM}(q_j) \tag{10}$$

4.1.2 Attention Matching

The *question-aware attention* technique is utilized here to align the word fragment in passages and questions. The attention weights and the new representation of Q as the same dimension as P are obtain using Eq. 11.

$$\alpha = \text{Softmax}((P^c)^{\text{T}}(W^\alpha Q^c + b^\alpha \otimes e_n))$$
$$Q^\alpha = Q^c \alpha^T \tag{11}$$

where $b^\alpha \otimes e_n$ is a $d \times n$ matrix which indicates that the column vector b^α repeats n times. Each element of the attention weight matrix $\alpha \in R^{m \times n}$ represents the relevancy between all the tokens in Q and P.

Next, the model puts Q^α and P^c through matching representation processing. A heuristic algorithm is utilized to compute the semantic matching $I \in R^{4d \times n}$ between Q and P as Eq. 12, which shows the difference and relativism between questions and passages.

$$I = [P^c, Q^\alpha, P^c \odot Q^\alpha, P^c - Q^\alpha] \tag{12}$$

4.1.3 Dynamic Discard

The Dynamic Discard layer is the core of the DSDR model. The model discards noise information and retains only partial information, which has a positive effect on the final prediction stage.

First, the aligned matching matrix I is fed into a single-layer feed-forward neural network to obtain a joint information representation of the passages and questions.

$$F = \text{relu}(W^f I) \tag{13}$$

where $W^f \in R^{2d \times 4d}$ are trainable parameters, and $F \in R^{2d \times n}$ denotes the feature matrix, which can be treated as a fine-grained semantic matching process. Through the activation function, the joint feature I will be further fused.

The model then calculates the probability distribution of I to evaluate different information matching degrees between passages and questions.

$$(\lambda_1, \lambda_2, \ldots \lambda_{k+z}) = \text{softmax}(W^g I) \tag{14}$$

where $W^g \in R^{(k+z) \times n}$ are weight parameters. The output represents the information ranked by relevance, from most to least; only the first k-parts are chosen as effective information while the last z-parts are discarded as negative information.

4.1.4 Information Aggregation

In this layer, the semantic information of contexts will be further aggregated, incorporated by another BiLSTM.

$$H^F = \text{BiLSTM}(F) \tag{15}$$

where $H^F \in R^{d \times n}$ denotes aggregating the context information by each time step. Then, the partial key context information is chosen as k-parts.

$$O = \sum_{i=1}^{k} (\lambda_i \otimes e_d) \odot H^F \tag{16}$$

where $O \in R^{d \times n}$, considered to be the effective matching representation between passages and questions, will be utilized for prediction.

4.1.5 Prediction

Finally, the prediction layer utilizing feed-forward network predicts the start and end position of an answer span in the passage. The probability distribution of start points is calculated as Eq. 17.

$$
\begin{aligned}
A^s &= \tanh(W^s O + b^s \otimes e_n) \\
\gamma^s &= \text{Softmax}(W^{s1} A^s)
\end{aligned} \tag{17}
$$

where $W^s \in R^{d \times d}$, $W^{s1} \in R^d$ and $b^s \in R^d$ are learnable parameters. The result $\gamma^s \in R^n$ indicates the probability distribution of the start positions in the passage with length n words. The probability distribution $\gamma^e \in R^n$ of the end points is obtained in a similar way while $W^e \in R^{d \times d}$, $W^{e1} \in R^d$ and $b^e \in R^d$ are different parameters. Finally, the loss is calculated using a Maximum Likelihood (ML) [19] estimate.

$$\mathcal{L}(A_{true}|P, Q) = -\frac{1}{x} \sum_{i}^{x} (\log(\gamma^s_{y_i^s}) + \log(\gamma^e_{y_i^e})) \tag{18}$$

where A_{true} is the ground-truth answer of the question, x is the number of sampled passages, y_i^s and y_i^e denote the start and end indices of the answer in the x-th passage respectively, and $\gamma_{y_i^s}^s$ and $\gamma_{y_i^e}^e$ are corresponding probabilities.

In the test process, the maximum values of γ^s and γ^e are chosen, and the indices of the start position must be less than the end position.

4.2 Reinforced Mnemonic Reader

Neural attention is a frequently-used method to capture complex interactions between questions and relevant passages. As more attention layers are used, more features are captured, and so multi-layer attention architectures have been proposed [20, 21]. However, in these multi-layer architectures, the attention calculation of the current layer does not refer to the attention information of the previous layers, which leads to two distinct but highly related problems: *attention redundancy*, where multi-layer attention is distributed on the same text, and *attention deficiency*, where multi-layer attention fails to concentrate on important parts of the text, resulting in a lack of attention. For training methods, recent research [21] has proposed to use reinforcement learning algorithms to maximize the expectation of reward, which can be calculated as the degree of word overlap between the predicted answer and the ground-truth. However, this method may lead to *convergence suppression* when the baseline is better than the reward; the output will be negative after normalization, which will inhibit the convergence of the model.

To solve the above problems, Hu et al. [22] presented the Reinforced Mnemonic Reader (R.M-Reader) for Reading Comprehension. The model proposed a reattention mechanism to temporarily store the attention of the previous layer for use in the current layer to fine-tune the calculation of the attention distribution. Moreover, they proposed dynamic-critical reinforcement learning, which dynamically decides the reward and the baseline. The end-to-end architecture is shown in Fig. 4, which is composed of three main components: (1) *an encoder* to build the hidden representations of the questions and paragraphs, (2) *an iterative aligner* which adopts a multi-layered attention architecture based on the reattention mechanism to perform multiple rounds of alignment between questions and paragraphs, and (3) *an answer pointer* to predict the start and end positions of the answer sequentially.

4.2.1 RC with Reattention

The aligner aligns each context word with the entire question, and enhances the context representation with the attentive question information. Let $Q = \{q_i\}_{i=1}^n$ and $P = \{p_j\}_{j=1}^m$ be sets of hidden vectors, which denote questions and paragraphs, respectively. A similarity matrix $E \in R^{n \times m}$ for question-aware attention can be computed as:

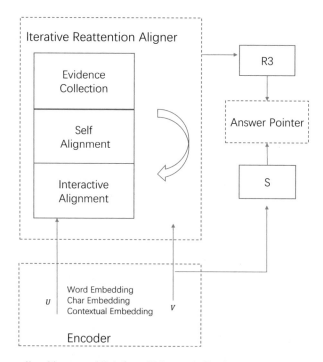

Fig. 4 The overall architecture of Reinforced Mnemonic Reader

$$E_{ij} = f(q_i, p_j) \tag{19}$$

where E_{ij} represents the semantic similarity between the i-th word of the question and the j-th word of the paragraph, and f is a similarity function. The Softmax function is then used to normalize the matrix by column to obtain a distribution of attention for each paragraph word for the entire problem. Based on this attention distribution, semantic fusion can be further carried out to obtain the question-aware paragraph representation $\boldsymbol{H} = \{h_j\}_{j=1}^{m}$.

Another similarity matrix of self-alignment aligns the context itself [23], which can capture long-term dependencies among context words, obtained in a similar way [24].

$$B_{ij} = \mathbf{1}_{i \neq j} f(h_i, h_j) \tag{20}$$

where $\mathbf{1}_{\{.\}}$ is an indicator function to ensure that the paragraph word does not calculate similarity with itself. The attentive information can then be integrated to form a self-aware paragraph representation $\boldsymbol{Z} = \{z_j\}_{j=1}^{m}$ to predict the answer.

The above process is a single-layer attention architecture. However, due to the small number of attention layers and shallow network depth, a model that is based on this mechanism is limited in capturing complex semantic interactions between questions and paragraphs. Therefore, a multi-layer attention architecture was proposed to enhance the network's presentation ability, which stacks several identical aligning layers. Specifically, let $Q^t = \{q_i^t\}_{i=1}^n$ and $P^t = \{p_j^t\}_{j=1}^m$ denote the hidden states of questions and paragraphs of the t-th layer. The corresponding question-aware context representation is denoted $H^t = \{h_j^t\}_{j=1}^m$. The two similarity matrices can be computed as below.

$$E_{ij}^t = f(q_i^t, p_j^t), \quad B_{ij}^t = 1_{i \neq j} f(h_i^t, h_j^t) \tag{21}$$

However, one problem with the multi-layer attention architecture is that each attention layer does not directly perceive the previous semantic similarity information. Historical attention information can only flow to subsequent layers by updating the hidden states. Two problems may be resulted: (1) *attention redundancy*, which refers to the situation where multiple attentions are distributed on the same text. Let softmax(x) denotes the Softmax function over vector x. Then the problem of attention redundancy can be formalized as $D(\text{softmax}(E_{:j}^t) \| \text{softmax}(E_{:j}^k)) < \sigma (t \neq k)$, where σ is a small bound and D is a function to measure the distribution distance. (2) *attention deficiency*, where multiple attention distributions fail to pay attention to the important parts of the input. This problem can be formalized as $D(\text{softmax}(E_{:j}^{t\,*}) \| \text{softmax}(E_{:j}^t)) > \delta$, where δ is another bound and softmax($E_{:j}^{t\,*}$) is the hypothetical ground-truth attention distribution.

To address these attention problems, the system temporally memorizes past attentions and explicitly utilizes them to refine the current attentions. The intuition behind this is that if the attention distribution of two words to the same text segment is highly similar, then the similarity between the two words should be also high. Therefore, the computation of reattention is defined as follows. Let E^{t-1} and B^{t-1} represent the temporarily stored similarity matrix of the previous layer. The similarity matrix of the current layer $E^t (t > 1)$ can then be calculated as

$$\begin{aligned} \tilde{E}_{ij}^t &= \text{softmax}(E_{i:}^{t-1}) \cdot \text{softmax}(B_{j:}^{t-1}) \\ E_{ij}^t &= (f(q_i^t, p_j^t) + \gamma \tilde{E}_{ij}^t) \end{aligned} \tag{22}$$

where γ is a learnable parameter, softmax($E_{i:}^{t-1}$) is the interactive attention distribution of the i-th question word aligned to the paragraph, and softmax($B_{:j}^{t-1}$) is the self attention distribution for the j-th paragraph word. In extreme cases when there is no overlap between the two distributions, the dot product E_{ij}^t will be 0. Otherwise, if the two distributions are identical and concentrated on one word, it will have the maximum value of 1. Therefore, the similarity between the question word i and paragraph word j can be explicitly measured by their historical attention distribution. In addition, due to the result of the dot product being relatively small compared to the similarity calculated based on the hidden states, γ is initialized with a hyper-parameter and kept trainable. The refined current layer similarity matrix can be obtained by adding the dot product result to the original similarity after γ magnification. Similarly, the refined matrix B^t can be calculated as Eq. 23, which will then be utilized in the calculation of the original multi-layer attention architecture.

$$
\begin{aligned}
\tilde{B}_{ij}^t &= \text{softmax}(B_{i:}^{t-1}) \cdot \text{softmax}(B_{j:}^{t-1}) \\
B_{ij}^t &= \mathbf{1}_{i \neq j}(f(h_i^t, h_j^t) + \gamma \tilde{B}_{ij}^t)
\end{aligned}
\tag{23}
$$

4.2.2 Dynamic-Critical Reinforcement Learning

To obtain the neural network model distribution $p(A|C, Q; \theta)$ $(p_{\theta(A)})$ for the extractive reading task, the standard Maximum Likelihood Estimation (MLE) training method is used to maximize the log probabilities of the ground-truth answer spans similar to Eq. 18.

However, this training method can only be optimized when it exactly matches the ground-truth answer span, and those text segments that are highly overlapped with the ground-truth answer do not have any supervision signals. To solve this problem, a training method based on reinforcement learning is introduced into the extractive reading task, where the task reward is measured as the word overlap degree between the randomly sampled answer and the ground-truth answer. To further reduce the variance of the reward, a baseline b is leveraged to normalize the reward, which is calculated as the word overlap between the greedy sampled answers and the ground-truth answers. Such a method is called Self-Critical Sequence Training (SCST). Specifically, let $R(A^s, A^*)$ $(R(A^s))$ denote the word overlap score between a sampled answer A^s and the ground-truth A^*. The training goal is then to maximize the expected reward after normalization:

$$
\mathcal{L}_{SCST}(\theta) = -E_{A^s \sim p_\theta(A)}[R(A^s) - R(\hat{A})]
\tag{24}
$$

where A^s is the randomly sampled answer, and $\hat{A}$ is the greedily sampled answer, which can be obtained by:

$$
\hat{A} = \arg \max_A p(A|C, Q; \theta)
\tag{25}
$$

The above formulation needs to traverse the entire set of candidate answers from the model distribution $p(A|C, Q; \theta)$, which is not feasible in actual calculations. Therefore, an approximate gradient $\nabla_\theta \mathcal{L}_{SCST}(\theta)$ can be estimated according to the REINFORCE algorithm as

$$
\begin{aligned}
\nabla_\theta \mathcal{L}_{SCST}(\theta) &= -E_{A^s \sim p_\theta(A)}[(R(A^s) - b)\nabla_\theta \log p_\theta(A^s)] \\
&\approx -(R(A^s) - R(\hat{A}))\nabla_\theta \log p_\theta(A^s)
\end{aligned}
\tag{26}
$$

where A^s and $\hat{A}$ are obtained by utilizing a single Monte-Carlo sampling through model distribution.

However, when the return value is worse than the baseline value, the normalized reward will be a negative number, which will cause the approximate gradient to be positive. As a result, the gradient will cause the model to descend in the opposite direction. The prediction of the ground-truth answer is hindered if the randomly sampled answer and the ground-truth answer partly overlap. This situation is referred to as the *convergence suppression* problem.

To solve this problem, the Dynamic Critic Reinforcement Learning (DCRL) training method is proposed. The core idea is to always ensure that the normalized reward is positive, which is achieved by dynamically determining the reward and baseline based on the values of random sampling and greedy sampling. Specifically, random sampling and greedy sampling are regarded as two different strategies in reinforcement learning: random sampling is used to encourage exploration, while greedy sampling focuses on exploitation. The word overlap between the two sampled answers and the ground-truth answer is then calculated according to the F1 function, where the sample with the higher score is always set as the reward, and the other as the baseline. In this way, the approximate gradient is calculated as follows:

$$
\begin{aligned}
\nabla_\theta \mathcal{L}_{DCRL}(\theta) = & - \boldsymbol{E}_{A^s \sim p_\theta(A)}[(R(A^s) - b)\nabla_\theta \log p_\theta(A^s)] \\
\approx & - \mathbf{1}_{\left\{R(A^s) \geq R(\hat{A})\right\}} (R(A^s) - R(\hat{A}))\nabla_\theta \log p_\theta(A^s) \\
& - \mathbf{1}_{\left\{R(\hat{A}) > R(A^s)\right\}} (R(\hat{A}) - R(A^s))\nabla_\theta \log p_\theta(\hat{A})
\end{aligned}
\tag{27}
$$

The normalized reward in the above formula is constantly positive so that superior answers are always encouraged. In addition, when the score of random sampling is higher than the greedy sampling, DCRL is equivalent to SCST.

Homoscedastic uncertainty is then utilized as task-dependent weights to combine MLE and DCRL objectives to stabilize reinforcement learning training.

$$
\mathcal{L} = \frac{1}{2\sigma_a^2}\mathcal{L}_{ML} + \frac{1}{2\sigma_b^2}\mathcal{L}_{DCRL} + \log \sigma_a^2 + \log \sigma_b^2
\tag{28}
$$

where σ_a and σ_b are learnable parameters.

4.2.3   End-to-End Architecture

As described above, the Reinforced Mnemonic Reader includes three main components:

1. Encoder

The encoder builds embedding representations for questions and paragraphs. It utilizes a 100-dimensional Glove embedding and a 1024-dimensional ELMo embedding to initialize word embeddings. A BiLSTM is leveraged to encode character sequences to yield character-level embeddings, which is obtained by concatenating the last hidden state of both directions. Next, exact matching binary features, POS features, and NER features for questions and paragraphs are added. By concatenating the above word embeddings, character embeddings, and features, the embeddings of questions and paragraphs can be represented as $X^Q = \{x_i^q\}_{i=1}^n$ and $X^P = \{x_j^c\}_{j=1}^m$. Moreover, to aggregate contextual semantic information in each word, a weight-shared BiLSTM is utilized:

$$Q = BiLSTM(X^Q), \quad P = BiLSTM(X^P) \tag{29}$$

where $Q = [q_1, q_2, \ldots, q_n] \in R^{2d \times n}$ and $P = [p_1, p_2, \ldots, p_n] \in R^{2d \times m}$ are the representations of question and paragraph respectively, and d is the dimension of the hidden state.

2. Iterative Aligner

The iterative aligner processes multi-round alignments between questions and paragraphs with a multi-layer attention architecture based on the reattention mechanism. The iterative aligner consists of three aligning blocks and each aligning block includes three modules.

(1) *a bi-directional alignment layer* that captures the interactive information between paragraphs and questions to form question-aware paragraph representations, (2) *a self alignment* that captures the iterative information within a paragraph to form self-aware paragraph representations, (3) *an evidence collection layer* that further fuses the contextual semantic information within paragraphs.

To effectively aggregate the weighted sum representation of the question into the paragraph representation, a heuristic aggregation function, fusion(x, y), is proposed as follows:

$$\tilde{x} = \text{relu}(W_r[x; y; x \circ y; x - y])$$
$$g = Sigmoid(W_g[x; y; x \circ y; x - y])$$
$$o = g \circ \tilde{x} + (1 - g) \circ x \tag{30}$$

Here, $[\cdot; \cdot]$ denotes the concatenation operation, $\circ$ denotes element-wise multiplication. W_r and W_g are the weight matrices, and the offset is omitted. The output vector is the linear interpolation of the input x and the intermediate vector $\tilde{x}$. g is a gate to control the proportion of $\tilde{x}$ in the output vector x.

For a single alignment block, the similarity matrix E is first calculated as Eq. 21 and an attended question vector is obtained by $\tilde{q}_j = Q \cdot \text{softmax}(E_{:j})$. Then, the question-aware context vectors $H = [h_1, \ldots, h_m]$ can be obtained as $h_j = \text{fusion}(p_j, \tilde{q}_j)$. Similarly, B is computed as Eq. 21. The weighted sum representation of the j-th word with respect to the entire paragraph is then computed as $\tilde{h}_j = H \cdot \text{softmax}(B_{:j})$. Similar to the fusion function $z_j = \text{fusion}(h_j, \tilde{h}_j)$, self-aware paragraph vectors $Z = [z_1, \ldots, z_m]$ are obtained. Finally, a BiLSTM is adopted to collect the evidence, with inputting Z, the output is the fully-aware paragraph vectors $R = [r_1, \ldots, r_m]$.

To solve the problem of attention redundancy and attention deficiency under the multi-layer attention architecture, two more alignment blocks are stacked with the reattention mechanism as follows.

$$
\begin{aligned}
R^1, Z^1, E^1, B^1 &= \text{align}^1(P, Q) \\
R^2, Z^2, E^2, B^2 &= \text{align}^2(R^1, Q, E^1, B^1) \\
R^3, Z^3, E^3, B^3 &= \text{align}^3(R^2, Q, E^2, B^2, Z^1, Z^2)
\end{aligned}
\tag{31}
$$

where $align^t$ denotes the t-th block. In the t-th block (t > 1), the inputs include the hidden states of question Q, the paragraph representation of the previous round R^{t-1}, and the similarity matrix E^{t-1} and B^{t-1} which were computed by the previous round. The attention distribution under the reattention mechanism E^t and B^t are computed as Eqs. 22 and 23 respectively. In additional, a residual connection in the last BiLSTM forms the final paragraph representations $R^3 = [r_1^3, \ldots, r_m^3]$: $r_j^3 = \text{BiLSTM}([z_j^1; z_j^2; z_j^3])$.

3. Answer Pointer

The answer pointer predicts the answer span sequentially. The system applies a variant of pointer networks as the answer pointer to predict the answer positions. First, the model summarizes the hidden state Q of the question into a fixed-size vector s as: $s = \sum_{i=1}^{n} \alpha_i q_i$, where $\alpha_i \propto \exp(\omega^T q_i)$. Then, taking the question summary vector s and the paragraph representation R^3 as input, the probability of the starting position $p_1(i)$ of the answer is heuristically calculated as

$$
p_1(i) \propto \exp(\omega_1^T \tanh(W_1[r_i^3; s; r_i^3 \circ s; r_i^3 - s]))
\tag{32}
$$

Next, a paragraph summary vector $l = R^3 \cdot p_1$ is computed based on the predicted distribution of the starting position of the answer, and a new question summary vector $\tilde{s}$ is updated by the fusion function mentioned above as $\tilde{s} = \text{fusion}(s, l)$. Finally, based on the latest question summary vector, the probability of the ending position of the answer $p_2(j|i)$ is computed

$$p_2(j|i) \propto \exp(\omega_2^T \tanh(W_2[r_j^3; \tilde{s}; r_j^3 \circ \tilde{s}; r_j^3 - \tilde{s}]))$$ (33)

4.3 Read and Verify System

For the final feature aggregation to predict candidate answers, SQuAD 1.0 ensures a correct answer in passages for each question. Eventually, some cases with no answer appeared in SQuAD as well as Open-domain QA. To deal with this issue, one additional "no-answer" probability of questions needs prediction by learning a large amount of linguistic phenomena between two texts. A share-normalization operation has been applied between the "no-answer" score and answer span scores. The approach predicts a probability that one question is unanswerable and outputs a candidate answer. One problem is that the answerability is not validated the second time. Obviously, verifying the reliability of predicted answers makes the result more credible.

The answer extraction module produces two scores, α and β, over the passage words that indicate the answer boundaries using a pointer network. To detect whether a question is unanswerable, a special no-answer score z can be predicted jointly.

$$\mathcal{L}_{joint} = -\log\left(\frac{(1-\delta)e^z + \delta e^{\alpha_a \beta_b}}{e^z + \sum_{i=1}^{l_p} \sum_{j=1}^{l_p} e^{\alpha_i \beta_j}}\right)$$ (34)

where a and b are the start and end positions of ground-truth, and θ is 1 if the question is answerable, and otherwise, 0. At test time, if the normalized no-answer score of a question exceeds some threshold, it will be detected as unanswerable.

Hu et al. proposed a novel Read and Verify system, which includes a no-answer reader and an answer verifier, as shown in Fig. 5. The neural no-answer reader extracts candidate answers and produces no-answer probabilities. The answer verifier infers the answer the second time by detecting if it is entailed by input snippets.

4.3.1 Reader with Auxiliary Losses

Previous no-answer readers can jointly perform answer extraction and no-answer detection. But there are two problems. For answer extraction, unanswerable questions have no candidate answers. For no-answer detection, utilizing the shared normalization between span scores and the no-answer score results in a conflict. Since the sum of these normalized scores is always 1, an over-confident span probability causes a less confident no-answer probability, and vice versa. To deal with these issues, two auxiliary losses are proposed. They will optimize each task independently.

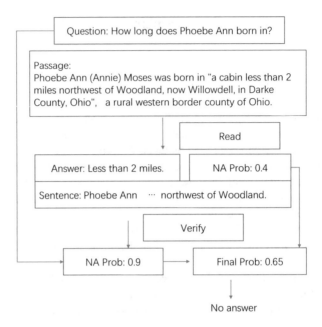

Fig. 5 An overview of the approach. A candidate answer is extracted and a no-answer probability (NA Prob) is produced as well. The answer verifier is then utilized to check whether the extracted answer is legitimate. Finally, previous results are aggregated and the final prediction is outputted

1. Independent Span Loss

Independent Span Loss is for answer extraction. The model extracts candidate answers for all questions. Therefore, besides answerable questions, there are also unanswerable cases that are positive examples, and the plausible answer is considered as the gold answer. U and V are the interdependent representations for passages and questions. To not interfere with no-answer detection, the system proposes to utilize a multi-head pointer network. Another pair of span scores is produced, denoted as $\tilde{\alpha}$ and $\tilde{\beta}$.

$$\tilde{o}_j = \tilde{\omega}_v^T v_j,$$

$$\tilde{t} = \sum_{j=1}^{l_q} \frac{e^{\tilde{o}_j}}{\sum_{k=1}^{l_q} e^{\tilde{o}_k}} v_j \qquad (35)$$

$$\tilde{\alpha}, \tilde{\beta} = \text{pointernetwork}(U, \tilde{t})$$

where multiple heads share the same network architecture but with different parameters. The augmented ground-truth answer boundaries are denoted $\tilde{a}$ and $\tilde{b}$, and an independent span loss is defined as:

$$\mathcal{L}_{indep-I} = -\log\left(\frac{e^{\tilde{\alpha}_{\tilde{a}}}e^{\tilde{\beta}_{\tilde{b}}}}{\sum_{i=1}^{l_p}\sum_{j=1}^{l_p}e^{\tilde{\alpha}_i}e^{\tilde{\beta}_j}}\right) \tag{36}$$

By simple mean pooling over the two pairs of softmax-normalized span scores, the final span probability is obtained.

2. Independent No-Answer Loss

The no-answer score z is normalized with the span scores. The no-answer detection will be weakened here, and so the system considers exclusively encouraging the prediction on no-answer detection. An independent no-answer loss is defined as:

$$\mathcal{L}_{indep-II} = -(1-\delta)\log\sigma(z) - \delta\log(1-\sigma(z)) \tag{37}$$

where σ is the sigmoid activation function. The model produces a more confident prediction on no-answer score z without considering the shared-normalization operation by utilizing this loss. Finally, the above losses are combined as Eq. 38.

$$\mathcal{L} = \mathcal{L}_{joint} + \gamma\mathcal{L}_{indep-I} + \lambda\mathcal{L}_{indep-II} \tag{38}$$

where two hyper-parameters, γ and λ, control the weight of two auxiliary losses.

4.3.2 Answer Verifier

The answer verifier infers the extracted answer by comparing the answer sentence with the question. The answer verifier recognizes the local textual entailment to support the answer. Defining the answer sentence as the context sentence that includes plausible or gold answers, three architectures are explored, shown in Fig. 6: (1) *a sequential model*, which accepts input as a long sequence, (2) *an interactive model*, which interdependently encodes two sentences, and (3) *a hybrid model*, which takes the two aforementioned approaches into account.

1. Model-I: Sequential Architecture

The answer sentence S, the question Q, and the extracted answer A are converted into an input sequence ordered as $X = [S, Q, \$, A]$. Then, the Generative Pre-trained Transformer (OpenAI GPT) performs the answer verification. Multiple transformer blocks are utilized to encode the sequence embeddings as h_i. The last token's activation $h_n^{l_m}$ is accepted by a linear projection layer followed by a softmax function to output the no-answer probability y.

Fig. 6 The Input structures for running three different models

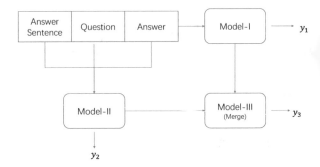

$$p(y|X) = \text{softmax}(h_n^{l_m} W_y) \tag{39}$$

A standard cross-entropy objective will minimize the negative log-likelihood.

$$L(\theta) = -\sum_{(X,y)} \log p(y|X) \tag{40}$$

2. Model-II: Interactive Architecture

For verifying the answer, capturing the interactions between two sentences can help recognize their local entailment relationships. First, the model utilizes Glove word-embeddings and runs a BiLSTM to encode the characters. The character-level embeddings are obtained by concatenating the two last hidden states. In addition, a binary feature is added to indicate if the answer includes the word. All embeddings along with aforementioned feature are concatenated and encoded by a weight-shared BiLSTM, yielding two series of contextual representations s_i and q_i. Two inference-aware sentence representations are produced as follows.

$$a_{ij} = s_i^T q_j$$
$$b_i = \sum_{j=1}^{l_q} \frac{e^{a_{ij}}}{\sum_{k=1}^{l_q} e^{a_{ik}}} q_j \tag{41}$$
$$c_i = \sum_{i=1}^{l_s} \frac{e^{a_{ij}}}{\sum_{k=1}^{l_s} e^{a_{kj}}} s_i$$

where b_i refers to the attended vector from question Q for the i-th word in answer sentence S, and vice versa for c_j. To separately compare the aligned pairs for finding local inference information, a weight-shared function F is utilized to model these aligned pairs as $\tilde{s}_i = F(s_i, b_i)$ and $\tilde{q}_i = F(q_i, c_i)$. F can have various forms, such as the BiLSTM and multilayer perceptron. Here, the model employs a heuristic function $o = F(x, y)$, similar to Eq. 30, but replacing $relu$ with $gelu$.

Next, the intra-sentence modeling layer is applied by capturing self correlations inside each sentence. The input are inference-aware vectors $\tilde{s}_i$ and $\tilde{q}_j$, which are first passed through another BiLSTM layer for encoding. The same attention mechanism that is utilized above is then used again between each sentence and itself. To ensure that a word is not aligned with itself, set $a_{ij} = -inf$ if $i = j$. Another function F produces self-aware vectors $\hat{s}_i$ and $\hat{q}_j$ respectively. A concatenated residual connection models the sentences with a BiLSTM to obtained $\bar{s}_i = \text{BiLSTM}([\tilde{s}_i; \hat{s}_i])$ and $\bar{q}_i = \text{BiLSTM}([\tilde{q}_j; \hat{q}_j])$. A mean-max pooling operation summarizes the final representation of two sentences, namely $\bar{s}_i$ and $\bar{q}_i$. All summarized vectors will be concatenated. There is a feed-forward classifier that consists of a projection sublayer with $gelu$ activation and a softmax output sublayer. It processes the concatenated vector and yields the no-answer probability. It optimizes the negative Maximum-likelihood objective function for training.

3. Model-III: Hybrid Architecture

The features extracted by Model-I and Model-II can be combined to obtain a better representation. The above two models are combined to form Model-III. The output vectors of two models are merged into a single joint representation. A unified feed-forward classifier outputs the no-answer probability. Such a design tests whether the performance can benefit from the combination of two architectures. In practice, the system employs a simple concatenation to merge the information from two sources.

4.4 Evaluations

DSDR is evaluated on two challenging datasets: Quasar-T [25], a popular QA problem dataset, and SearchQA [26], a large-scale dataset to test the full pipeline of a QA system. Using EM and F1 as evaluation metrics, on the Quasar-T dataset, DSDR performs better than several strong competing systems, such as GA [27], BiDAF [28] and R3 [29]. Also, on the SearchQA dataset, DSDR performs better than BiDAF, AQA [30] and R3, and even Human Performance.

R.M-Reader achieves competitive results on the dataset SQuAD 1.0 [15] in EM and F1 scores, outperforming several strong systems, such as SLQA [31] and SAN[32]. On two adversarial SQuAD datasets, on which models can be fooled by confusing sentences with wrong answers appended at the end of the context, R.M-Reader outperforms FusionNet [33], which obtained the best results by more than 6% in both EM and F1 score, indicating that R.M-Reader is more robust against adversarial attacks.

The Read and Verify system is evaluated on the dataset SQuAD 2.0 [34], a reading comprehension benchmark augmented with unanswerable questions. The system is comprised of the R.M-Reader, ELMo embeddings [35] and Verifier. The system performs better than SLQA in terms of the F1 score. The result indicates that two auxiliary losses have helped the model better identify the answer boundaries and coordinate the conflict between answer extraction and no-answer detection. Nevertheless, the system is good at recognizing negation and antonyms while performing less effectively on more difficult cases, such as impossible conditions and other neutral types.

5 Answer Selection Module

The final answer selection module predicts the final answer from multiple candidate answers utilizing feature aggregation. There are several methods, such as evidence aggregation, multi-steps aggregation, and fusion of knowledge bases and text, among others. Here, we introduce a multi-steps aggregation method, and illustrate an evidence aggregation method with logical computation.

For the entirety of open-domain QA systems, the three-steps pipeline of retriever, reader and reranker have improved overall performance, but it is greatly inefficient owing to re-encoded inputs for each module [36]. Moreover, the modules, trained separately, will pass errors step by step. The final module will suffer the greatest loss. The answer selection module can benefit from a unified system, because it, instead, leverages the information of upstream modules to help subsequent tasks.

5.1 RE^3QA: Retrieve, Read and Rerank

Hu et al. proposed RE^3QA [37], a unified QA system consisting of three components: (1) *an early-stopped retriever* for efficiently selecting a few relevant contexts, (2) *a distantly-supervised reader* for proposing multiple candidate answers, and (3) *an answer reranker* for rescoring candidates. The model is trained end-to-end and with pre-trained Transformer blocks, the inputs are encoded only once.

In the unified system, earlier blocks are trained to predict retrieving scores for all input snippets, while a few top-ranked segments of text will be transformed for later blocks. They are reranked utilizing their span representations extracted from the last block's hidden states. The architecture is shown in Fig. 7.

In the system, documents are first pruned to discard irrelevant information using TF-IDF and by choosing the top K paragraphs to form a new pruned document d with length L_d. Instead of reading the retrieved documents at paragraph-level or sentence-level, the system slides a window of length l with a stride r over d, and a set of text segments $C = \{c_1, \ldots, c_n\}$ are produced, where $n = \left\lceil \frac{L_d - l}{r} \right\rceil + 1$.

Next, segments are encoded along with the question utilizing a highly parallel encoding scheme: the pre-trained Transformer blocks. Concatenating the question,

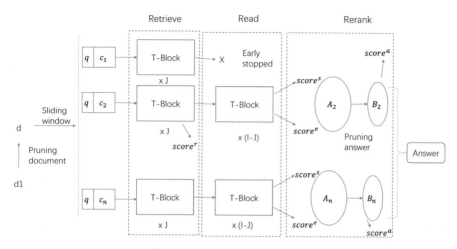

Fig. 7 The architecture of RE³QA. All input documents are pruned and split into multiple segments. A few top-ranked segments are reserved. For every selected segment, multiple candidate answers are proposed, and they will be pruned and reranked later. The system has three outputs per candidate answer: the retrieving, reading, and reranking scores

segment and several delimiters as $[[CLS]; q; [SEP]; c; [SEP]]$, the input $x = (x_1, \ldots, x_{L_x})$ to the network and the input embeddings $h^0 \in R^{L_x \times D_h}$ are obtained. D_h is the hidden size.

A series of I pre-trained Transformer blocks are employed. The input embeddings will be projected into a sequence of contextualized vectors as:

$$h^i = \text{Transformer Block } (h^{i-1}), \forall i \in [1, I] \tag{42}$$

While a parallel encoding scheme is very appealing, it is inefficient to fully encode all segments. The early-stopped retriever computes a $score^r \in R^2$ by summarizing h^J into a fixed-size vector with a weighted self-aligning layer followed by multi-layer perceptrons. Only top N ranked segments per instance are passed to the subsequent blocks. To ensure the model is focused on reading the most relevant context, N is relatively small.

Multiple candidate answers per segment are proposed. By projecting the final hidden states h^I element-wise, two sets of scores for the start and end positions of the answer, $score^s$ and $score^e$, are obtained. A reading score is computed as $s_i = score^s_{\alpha_i} + score^e_{\beta_i}$, where α_i and β_i denote the start and end indices of candidate answer a_i. The distantly-supervised reader finally yields a set of preliminary candidate answers $A = \{a_1, \ldots, a_M\}$ along with their scores $S = \{s_1, \ldots, s_M\}$ for the top M candidates.

5.1.1 Answer Reranker

The answer reranker resets the order of the candidate answers. First, a span-level non-maximum suppression algorithm will prune redundant candidate spans, and then the reranking scores are predicted for the remaining candidates utilizing their span representations.

1. Span-Level Non-maximum Suppression

In the process of predicting answers, predicting a unique span for an answer string is not required. It is possible that multiple candidates refer to identical texts. Other than the initial correct span, other spans on the same text will be false positives. The system presents a Span-level NMS (Algorithm 1) to delete the overlapped candidate answers set B.

Algorithm 1 Span-level NMS

Input: $A = \{a_i\}_{i=1}^{M}$; $S = \{s_i\}_{i=1}^{M}$; M^*
  A is the set of preliminary candidate answers
  S is the corresponding confidence scores
  M^* denotes the maximal size threshold
1: Initialize B = {}
2: while A $\neq$ {} and size(B) $\leq$ M^* do
3:    i = arg max S
4:    B = B $\bigcup$ {a_i}; A = A -{a_i}; S = S - {s_i}
5:    for a_j in A do
6:       if overlap(a_i, a_j) then
7:          A = A -{a_j}; S = S - {s_j}
8: return B

---

2. Candidate Answer Reranking

For a candidate answer a_i in B, based on its span representation, the model computes a reranking score. The representation is a weighted self-aligned vector, and is bounded by the span of the answer.

$$\eta = \text{softmax}(w_\eta h^l_{\alpha_i:\beta_i})$$

$$\text{score}^a_i = w_a \tanh\left(W_a \sum_{j=\alpha_i}^{\beta_i} \eta_{j-\alpha_i+1} h'_j\right) \tag{43}$$

where $score_i^a \in R^1$, and $h_{\alpha_i:\beta_i}^l$ is a shorthand for stacking a list of vectors h_j^l with $\alpha_i \leq j \leq \beta_i$.

To train the reranker, two kinds of labels for each candidate a_i are constructed. Hard label $y_i^{hard} \in R_{M^*}$ is the maximal exaction match score between a_i and the ground-truth answers. Soft label $y_i^{soft} \in R_{M^*}$ is computed with the maximal F1 score between a_i and gold answers so that the partially correct prediction can still have a supervised signal. If all elements of y^{hard} are 0, which means there is no correct prediction in B, the method replaces the least confident candidate with a gold answer. Finally, the reranking component is trained by minimizing the following objective.

$$\mathcal{L}_{CAR} = -\sum_{i=1}^{M^*} y_i^{hard} \log(\text{softmax}(score^a)_i)$$
$$+ \sum_{i=1}^{M^*} \left\| y_i^{soft} - score_i^a \right\|^2 \tag{44}$$

5.1.2 End-to-End Training

Rather than train each component separately, the whole system is trained as a unified network so that downstream components can benefit from the high-quality upstream outputs.

Specifically, a multi-task learning approach is taken, sharing the parameters of earlier blocks. The joint objective function is defined as:

$$\mathcal{J} = \lambda\mathcal{L}_{retriever} + \mathcal{L}_{reader} + \gamma\mathcal{L}_{reranker} \tag{45}$$

where λ and γ are weight hyper-parameters.

5.2 Multi-Type Multi-Span Network for DROP

In some simplified settings, several systems have achieved human parity in the field of reading comprehension. But when applied to more realistic scenarios, like various types of answers or requiring discrete reasoning abilities, the performance degrades significantly.

DROP [38], a new reading comprehension dataset, requires Discrete Reasoning Over the content of Paragraphs to obtain the final answer. Hu et al. therefore proposed the Multi-Type Multi-Span Network (MTMSN) [39], a neural reading comprehension model to support various answer types and text spans consisting of a multi-type answer predictor and a multi-span extraction method.

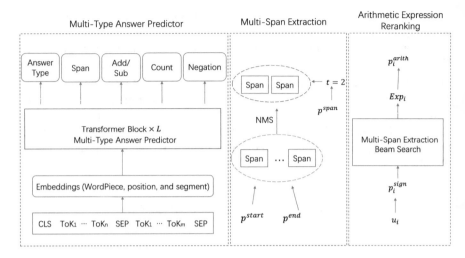

Fig. 8 The architecture of MTMSN. The predictor supports four kinds of answer types. One or several spans are proposed by a multi-span extraction method dynamically. The arithmetic expression reranking mechanism ranks expression candidates that are decoded by beam search for further validating the prediction

An illustration of the MTMSN architecture is shown in Fig. 8. The system employs BERT as its encoder and maps word-embeddings into contextualized representations utilizing pre-trained Transformer blocks. The multi-type answer predictor then produces four answer types based on the representations. To support multi-span extraction, the model explicitly predicts the number of answer spans. Next, non-overlapped spans are outputted until the specific amount is reached, and for the type of arithmetic expression, the reranking process is added to further confirm the prediction.

5.2.1 Multi-Type Answer Predictor

Rather than restricting one answer to be a span of text, discrete-reasoning reading comprehension task involves several answer types. The system proposes a multi-type answer predictor to selectively produce different kinds of answers such as span, count number, arithmetic expression and a new type, logical negation. Moreover, unlike prior work that separately predicts passage spans and question spans, the approach directly extracts spans from the whole input sequence.

1. Answer Type Prediction

The embeddings are calculated using Eq. 42 and the last four blocks ($H_{I-3}, \ldots, H_I$) are used as the input to the answer predictor, denoted as M_0, M_1, M_2, M_3 respectively. To predict the answer type, M_2 is split into a question representation Q_2 and a passage representation P_2 according to the index of intermediate [SEP] token. Then, two vectors are computed to summarize the question and passage information respectively as $h^{Q_2} = \text{softmax}(W^Q Q_2)Q_2$ and $h^{P_2} = \text{softmax}(W^P P_2)P_2$.

Next, the probability distribution to represent the different answer types is calculated as:

$$p^{type} = \text{softmax}(\text{FFN}[h^{Q_2}; h^{P_2}; h^{CLS}]) \tag{46}$$

Here, h^{CLS} is the first vector in the final contextualized representation M_3, and FFN denotes a feed-forward network consisting of two linear projections with a *GeLU* activation followed by a layer normalization in between.

2. Span

If the answer type is judged to be span, a gating mechanism and the standard decoding strategy are combined to predict starting and ending positions across the entire sequence.

Specifically, three vectors, $g^{Q_0}, g^{Q_1}, g^{Q_2}$, are computed to summarize the question information among different levels of question representations.

$$\beta^Q = \text{softmax}(\text{FFN}(Q_2)), \; g^{Q_2} = \beta^Q Q_2 \tag{47}$$

where g^{Q_0}, g^{Q_1} are computed over Q_0, Q_1 respectively in a similar way. The probabilities of starting and ending indices of the answer span are then computed from the input sequence as:

$$
\begin{aligned}
\bar{M}^{start} &= [M_2; M_0; g^{Q_2} \otimes M_2; g^{Q_0} \otimes M_0] \\
\bar{M}^{end} &= [M_2; M_1; g^{Q_2} \otimes M_2; g^{Q_1} \otimes M_1] \\
p^{start} &= \text{softmax}(W^S \bar{M}^{start}) \\
p^{end} &= \text{softmax}(W^E \bar{M}^{end})
\end{aligned}
\tag{48}
$$

where $\otimes$ denotes the outer product between the vector g and each token representation in M.

3. Arithmetic Expression

To model the process of performing addition or subtraction among multiple numbers mentioned in the passage, there is a three-way categorical variable (plus, minus, or zero) for each number to indicate its sign. As a result, an arithmetic expression that has a number as the final answer can be obtained and easily evaluated.

Specifically, for each number mentioned in the passage, its corresponding representation is gathered from the concatenation of M_2 and M_3, eventually yielding $U = (u_1; \ldots; u_N) \in R^{N \times 2*D}$ where N numbers exist. Then, the probabilities of sign (plus, minus, or zero) assigned to the i-th number are computed as:

$$p_i^{sign} = \text{softmax}(\text{FFN}[u_i; h^{Q_2}; h^{P_2}; h^{CLS}]) \qquad (49)$$

4. Count

Counting entities is modeled as a multi-class classification problem. To achieve this, the module first produces a vector h^U that summarizes the important information among all mentioned numbers, and then computes a counting probability distribution as:

$$\alpha^U = \text{softmax}(W^U U), \quad h^U = \alpha^U U$$
$$p^{count} = \text{softmax}(\text{FFN}[h^U; h^{Q_2}; h^{P_2}; h^{CLS}]) \qquad (50)$$

5. Negation

One obvious but important linguistic phenomenon that prior work fails to capture is *negation*. There are many cases in DROP that require performing logical negation on numbers. To model this phenomenon, the system assigns a new two-way categorical variable for each number to indicate whether a negation operation should be performed. The probability of logical negation on the i-th number is then computed as:

$$p_i^{negation} = \text{softmax}(\text{FFN}([u_i; h^{Q_2}; h^{P_2}; h^{CLS}]) \qquad (51)$$

5.2.2 Multi-Span Extraction

Although existing reading comprehension tasks focus exclusively on finding one span of text as the final answer, DROP loosens the restriction so that the answer to the question may be several text spans. Therefore, specific adaptation should be made to extend previous single-span extraction to the multi-span scenario.

The system proposes directly predicting the number of spans first and modeling it as a classification problem. This is achieved by computing a probability distribution on span amount as

$$p^{span} = \text{softmax}(\text{FFN}[h^{Q_2}; h^{P_2}; h^{CLS}]) \qquad (52)$$

To extract non-overlapped spans to the specific amount, the non-maximum suppression (NMS) algorithm is adopted like Algorithm 1.

5.2.3 Arithmetic Expression Reranking

As discussed in Sect. 5.2.1, the system models the phenomenon of discrete reasoning on numbers by learning to predict a plus, minus, or zero sign for each number in the passage. The signed numbers then compose an arithmetic expression. The final answer can be deduced by performing simple arithmetic computation.

However, since the sign of each number is only determined by the number representation and some coarse-grained global representations, the context information of the expression itself has not been considered. The model may therefore predict some wrong expressions (e.g., the signs that have maximum probabilities are either minus or zero, resulting in a large negative value). In order to further validate the prediction, the system adds one more step for arithmetic expression to rerank several highly confident expression candidates utilizing the representation summarized from the expression's context.

Specifically, Beam Search is utilized to produce top-ranked arithmetic expressions, which are sent back to the network for reranking. For each number in the expression, its corresponding vector is gathered from the representation U, and for the signs, an embedding matrix $E \in \mathrm{R}^{3 \times 2 * D}$ is initialized, and the sign-embeddings for each signed number are found.

Given the i-th expression that contains M signed numbers at most, number vectors $V_i \in \mathrm{R}^{M \times 2 * D}$ as well as sign-embeddings $C_i \in \mathrm{R}^{M \times 2 * D}$ can be obtained. Then, the expression representation along with the reranking probability can be calculated as:

$$
\alpha_i^V = \mathrm{softmax}(W^V(V_i + C_i)), \quad h_i^V = \alpha_i^V(V_i + C_i)
$$
$$
p_i^{arith} = \mathrm{softmax}(\mathrm{FFN}([h_i^V; h^{Q_2}; h^{P_2}; h^{CLS}]))
$$

$$(53)$$

5.3 Evaluations

On TriviaQA-wikipedia and TriviaQA-unfiltered datasets [40], RE^{3}QA both outperforms previous best approaches like CAPE [41] and HAS-QA [42] in terms of the F1 score. Further experiments on the SQuAD-document and SQuAD-open datasets, both modified versions of SQuAD, also show gains over previous results with respect to the F1 score.

Experiments show that the MTMSN model creates competitive results on the DROP dev and test set [43], even compared to $NABERT_{LARGE}$ [43], which employs $BERT_{LARGE}$ as an encoder. Those gains mainly come from numbers, the most frequent type. The type requires various types of symbolic, discrete reasoning operations and the multi-span category. This shows the validity of multi-span extraction method.

6 Conclusion

In summary, we have presented an overview of the Open-domain textual question answering systems, and introduced the technical architecture including paragraph ranking module, candidate answer extraction module and final answer selection module. Deep Learning technology is crucial for the performance of Open-domain textual QA. Although these systems are developing fast, many challenges remain, such as balancing accuracy, efficiency and scalability of ranking; complex machine reading comprehension models lacking interpretation, resulting in difficulty with evaluating performance; significant energy consumption with increasing model size; and more complex sub-tasks like reasoning across multiple snippets. Moreover, the distantly-supervised objectives in the training process also matter. Recent trends for open-domain textual QA also concentrate on several points, such as combining complex reasoning modules to deal with challenging sub-tasks, complexity improvement for searching small networks to improve the efficiency, and integration of multiple technologies from different fields to improve performance.

References

1. Turing, A.M.: Computing Machinery and Intelligence. Computation & Intelligence. American Association for Artificial Intelligence, Menlo Park (1995)
2. Yao, X.: Feature-driven question answering with natural language alignment (2014)
3. Huang, Z., Xu, S., Hu, M., Wang, X., Wang, C.: Recent trends in deep learning based open-domain textual question answering systems. IEEE Access PP(99), 1-1 (2020)
4. Robertson, S., Zaragoza, H.: The probabilistic relevance framework: BM25 and beyond. Found. Trends Inf. Retrieval 3(4), 333–389 (2009)
5. Zaragoza, H., Craswell, N., Taylor, M.J., et al.: Microsoft Cambridge at TREC 13: web and hard tracks. In: Trec (2004)
6. Ponte, J.M., Croft, W.B.: A language modeling approach to information retrieval. In: Research and Development in Information Retrieval, pp. 275–281 (1998)
7. Kato, S., Togashi, R., Maeda, H., Fujita, S., Sakai, T.: LSTM vs. BM25 for open-domain QA: A hands-on comparison of effectiveness and efficiency. In: Proceedings of the 40th International ACM SIGIR Conference on Research and Development in Information Retrieval, ser. SIGIR '17, New York, NY, pp. 1309–1312 (2017)
8. Seo, M., Kwiatkowski, T., Parikh, A., Farhadi, A., Hajishirzi, H.: Phrase-indexed question answering: A new challenge for scalable document comprehension. In: Proceedings of the Conference on Empirical Methods in Natural Language Processing (EMNLP), pp. 559–564 (2018)
9. Liu, Y., Huang, Z., Hu, M., Du, S., Peng, Y., Li, D., et al.: MFM: a multi-level fused sequence matching model for candidates filtering in multi-paragraphs question-answering. In: Pacific Rim Conference on Multimedia. Springer, Cham (2018)

10. Pennington, J., Socher, R., Manning, C.: Glove: global vectors for word representation. In: Conference on Empirical Methods in Natural Language Processing, pp. 1532–1543 (2014)
11. Hochreiter, S., Schmidhuber, J.: Long short-term memory. In: Supervised Sequence Labelling with Recurrent Neural Networks, pp. 1735–1780. Springer Berlin Heidelberg, Berlin (1997)
12. Tan, M., Xiang, B., Zhou, B.: LSTM-based deep learning models for non-factoid answer selection. Comput. Sci. (2015)
13. Yu, L., Hermann, K.M., Blunsom, P., et al.: Deep learning for answer sentence selection. Comput. Sci. (2014)
14. Bowman, S.R., Angeli, G., Potts, C., Manning, C.D.: A large annotated corpus for learning natural language inference. In: Proceedings of the 2015 Conference on Empirical Methods in Natural Language Processing (EMNLP) (2015)
15. Pranav, R., Jian, Z., Konstantin, L., Percy, L.: Squad: 100,000+ questions for machine comprehension of text (2016). Preprint. arXiv:1606.05250
16. Chen, D., Fisch, A., Weston, J., Bordes, A.: Reading wikipedia to answer open-domain questions. In: Proceedings of the Annual Meeting of the Association for Computational Linguistics (ACL), vol. 1, Vancouver, BC, pp. 1870–1879 (2017)
17. Wang, S., Jiang, J.: A compare-aggregate model for matching text sequences. In: Conference on ICLR (2017)
18. Wang, X., Huang, Z., Zhang, Y., Tan, L., Liu, Y.: DSDR: dynamic semantic discard reader for open-domain question answering, pp. 1–7 (2018)
19. Shuohang, W., Jing, J.: Machine comprehension using match-lstm and answer pointer. In: Proceedings of ICLR (2017)
20. Hsin-Yuan, H., Chenguang, Z., Yelong, S., Weizhu, C.: Fusionnet: Fusing via fullyaware attention with application to machine comprehension (2017). Preprint. arXiv:1711.07341
21. Caiming, X., Victor, Z., Richard, S.: Dcn+: Mixed objective and deep residual coattention for question answering (2017). Preprint. arXiv:1711.00106
22. Hu, M., Peng, Y., Huang, Z., Qiu, X., Wei, F., Zhou, M.: Reinforced mnemonic reader for machine reading comprehension (2017)
23. Wenhui, W., Nan, Y., Furu, W., Baobao, C., Ming, Z.: Gated self-matching networks for reading comprehension and question answering. In: Proceedings of ACL (2017)
24. Dirk, W., Georg, W., Laura, S.: Making neural qa as simple as possible but not simpler. In: Proceedings of CoNLL, pp. 271–280 (2017)
25. Bhuwan, D., Kathryn, M., William, W.C.: Quasar: Datasets for question answering by search and reading (2017). Preprint. arXiv:1707.03904
26. Matthew, D., Levent, S., Mike, H., Ugur, G., Volkan, C., Kyunghyun, C.: Searchqa: a new q&ataset augmented with context from a search engine (2017). Preprint. arXiv:1704.05179
27. Bhuwan, D., Hanxiao, L., Zhilin, Y., William, W.C., Ruslan, S.: Gated-attention readers for text comprehension (2016). Preprint. arXiv:1606.01549
28. Seo, M., Kembhavi, A., Farhadi, A., et al.: Bidirectional attention flow for machine comprehension (2016)
29. Shuohang, W., Mo, Y., Xiaoxiao, G., Zhiguo, W., Tim, K., Wei, Z., Shiyu, C., Gerald, T., Bowen, Z., Jing, J.: R3: Reinforced reader-ranker for open-domain question answering (2017). Preprint. arXiv:1709.00023
30. Christian, B., Iannis, B., Massimiliano, C., Andrea, G., Neil, H., Wojciech, G., Wei, W.: Ask the right questions: active question reformulation with reinforcement learning (2017). Preprint. arXiv:1705.07830
31. Wang, W., Yan, M., Wu, C.: Multi-granularity hierarchical attention fusion networks for reading comprehension and question answering. In: Proceedings of ACL (2018)
32. Liu, X., Shen, Y., Duh, K., Gao, J.: Stochastic answer networks for machine reading comprehension. In: Proceedings of ACL (2018)
33. Hsin-Yuan, H., Chenguang, Z., Yelong, S., Weizhu, C.: Fusionnet: fusing via fullyaware attention with application to machine comprehension (2017). Preprint. arXiv:1711.07341
34. Rajpurkar, P., Jia, R., Liang, P.: Know what you don't know: unanswerable questions for squad. In: Proceedings of ACL (2018)

35. Peters, M.E., Neumann, M., Iyyer, M., Gardner, M., Clark, C., Lee, K., Zettlemoyer, L.: Deep contextualized word prepresentations. In: Proceedings of NAACL (2018)
36. Zhen, W., Jiachen, L., Xinyan, X., Yajuan, L., Tian, W.: Joint training of candidate extraction and answer selection for reading comprehension. In: Proceedings of ACL (2018)
37. Hu, M., Peng, Y., Huang, Z., Li, D.: Retrieve, read, rerank: towards end-to-end multi-document reading comprehension (2019)
38. Dua, D., Wang, Y., Dasigi, P., Stanovsky, G., Singh, S., Gardner, M.: Drop: A reading comprehension benchmark requiring discrete reasoning over paragraphs. In: Proceedings of NAACL (2019)
39. Hu, M., Peng, Y., Huang, Z., Li, D.: A multi-type multi-span network for reading comprehension that requires discrete reasoning (2019)
40. Joshi, M., Choi, E., Weld, D.S., Zettlemoyer, L.: Triviaqa: A large scale distantly supervised challenge dataset for reading comprehension. In: Proceedings of ACL (2017)
41. Ming, Y., Jiangnan, X., Chen, W., Bin, B., Zhongzhou, Z., Ji, Z., Luo, S., Rui, W., Wei, W., Haiqing, C.: A deep cascade model for multi-document reading comprehension. In: Proceedings of AAAI (2019)
42. Pang, L., Lan, Y., Guo, J., Xu, J., Su, L., Cheng, X.: Has-qa: Hierarchical answer spans model for open-domain question answering. In: Proceedings of AAAI (2019)
43. Dua, D., Wang, Y., Dasigi, P., Stanovsky, G., Singh, S., Gardner, M.: Drop: A reading comprehension benchmark requiring discrete reasoning over paragraphs. In: Proceedings of NAACL (2019)
44. Geoffrey, H., Oriol, V., Jeff, D.: Distilling the knowledge in a neural network. In: Proceedings of NIPS Workshop (2014)

Part II
Auditory Technologies for Accessible Human Computer Interfaces

Speech Recognition for Individuals with Voice Disorders

Meredith Moore

Abstract Voice has become a common form of interacting with computing systems. Automatic speech recognition (ASR), voice interfaces, and interactive dialogue systems are already established as popular technologies. Speech-based interaction will continue to grow in the future and generally, voice-interaction is here to stay. The goal of this chapter is to provide an overview of the field of ASR for individuals with voice disorders including a briefing on foundational acoustic and phonetic concepts as well as some of the basics of voice disorders. After introducing these foundations, the field of ASR is reviewed focusing on the characterization of different ASR algorithms. The primary contribution of this chapter is the introduction of a new nomenclature to discuss systems that recognize speech from individuals with voice disorders. This new characterization of ASR systems focuses on how the system handles speech from individuals with voice disorders, introducing the terms *disorder-independent, disorder-dependent,* and *disorder-adaptive* speech recognition systems. This chapter takes this new characterization one step farther by establishing a leveling system that describes the difficulty of the speech recognition problem based on the amount of both implicit (noise derived from the voice itself) and explicit (noise added from the environment or recording equipment) noise in the speech sample. Through these new characterizations and nomenclature, this chapter works to more accurately categorize the work in the field. After defining a clearer system of classification of strategies for accomplishing difficult speech recognition, approaches to model speech at the different levels are described. Pulling from the most successful methods of dealing with explicit noise in speech recognition systems, we evaluate the field of disordered speech recognition, identify key strategies for recognizing disordered speech, and posit which methodologies from the field of explicit-noise-robust ASR systems might be successful in the domain of disordered speech recognition. The chapter ends in a discussion around how speech disorders present an accessibility challenge to voice interfaces and argues that this accessibility barrier will only continue to grow with

M. Moore (✉)
Drake University, Des Monies, IA, USA
e-mail: meredith.moore@drake.edu

© The Author(s), under exclusive license to Springer Nature Switzerland AG 2021
T. McDaniel, X. Liu (eds.), *Multimedia for Accessible Human Computer Interfaces*,
https://doi.org/10.1007/978-3-030-70716-3_5

the proliferation of voice-based technologies if we don't take action now to make these technologies inclusive.

Keywords Voice disorder · Speech recognition · Levels · Nomenclature

1 Motivation and Introduction

The primary goal of automatic speech recognition (ASR) is to interface effectively with computers through speech. To optimize the usability of such interfaces, ASR systems must include as many different groups of users as possible. The number of speech interfaces and services enabled through voice-interaction continues to grow. However, these systems are optimized for users with 'normal' speech patterns and often act as a barrier to access for individuals with voice disorders, speech disorders, or atypical speech patterns. In this chapter, key concepts in the field of ASR for individuals with voice disorders are defined as well as a new nomenclature to discuss algorithms that attempt to recognize speech from individuals with voice disorders. Pulling from the literature that attempts to build more robust ASR systems, this chapter describes techniques that have been previously used to more accurately recognize speech from noisy and low-resourced datasets. This chapter will also discuss techniques that have been particularly successful in recognizing speech from individual's with voice disorders.

1.1 Voice Interaction Is Here to Stay

The field of ASR has shown a dramatic improvement in the past several years. This significant change is possible because of the many large speech datasets that contain labeled speech as well as the powerful advances in deep learning techniques. This improvement has fueled a booming industry of consumer-facing devices that enable voice-based interaction. Advancements in ASR and natural language processing (NLP)—the field of understanding, deciphering, and interpreting human language at a syntactic and semantic level—have influenced the integration of voice interaction into the technology that is used every day by consumers such as mobile phones, smartwatches, or devices that are tied to our home environments like smart home sensors, and digital assistant equipped speakers. Interacting with phones, watches, and homes via voice has become more and more standard and the utility of these integrations continues to grow.

The volume of research disseminated involving voice-based interaction has increased significantly over the last 10 years. Take the foremost journal in Human-Computer Interaction—The Association for Computing Machinery's Computer-Human Interaction (CHI). This conference has been held annually since 1985. In Fig. 1, the number of papers with titles or abstracts including the keywords *voice*,

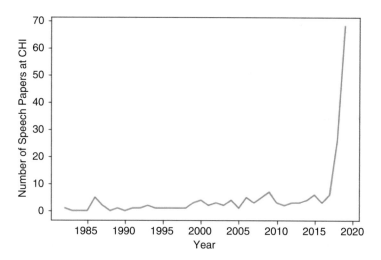

Fig. 1 Number of speech papers at ACM's CHI conference over time

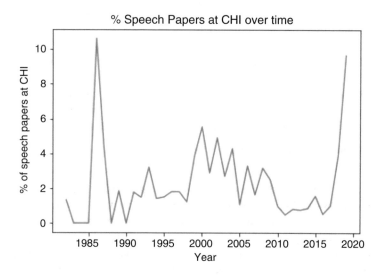

Fig. 2 Percent of speech papers at ACM's CHI conference over time

and *speech* is shown over time. The percent of the papers at CHI that contained *voice* and *speech* over time is shown in Fig. 2. In Fig. 2, it is evident that there was a spike in the percent of papers relating to speech and voice-based technologies in 1986. This increased representation for voice-based technologies in 1986 is largely due to ASR systems being developed to the point where they were potentially usable as an input modality for computers. This advancement in the ability of computing systems to recognize speech drove an influx of research papers positing how to develop systems that are controlled by speech interaction.

Recently, consumers are buying technology that is voice-enabled at a sharply increasing rate. More than 270 smart speaker models have been made available to consumers since the first Amazon Echo product shipped in 2014. Speech and voice disorders present an accessibility challenge to voice interfaces now that will grow with their proliferation if steps aren't taken to resolve these barriers. This chapter focuses on establishing the background knowledge of ASR systems through the lens of building ASR systems that are accessible to individuals with voice and speech disorders.

1.2 Accessibility Considerations in Voice Interaction

Despite the growing field of voice-based interaction, some users are left out of the conversation. It is estimated that 17.9 million U.S. adults (7.6%) have reported having a problem with their voice in the past 12 months. Of those individuals, some 9.4 million (4.0%) reported having a problem with their voice that lasted for a week or more [3]. However, voice and speech disorders don't only affect adults, it is estimated that 5% of children between the ages of 3 and 17 have a speech disorder lasting a week or longer. Children—estimated 8–9%—often experience speech sound disorders particularly articulation disorders or phonological disorders [41].

Systems reliant on speech as input are inaccessible to individuals with speech and voice disorders [38]. Why aren't these systems accessible to individuals with voice disorders? There are two primary reasons for this inaccessibility:

1. Insufficient data representing individuals with voice disorders
2. Lack of effective modeling techniques

In general, the more data used to train a deep learning model, the better the model will perform. Applying this generalization to the task of recognizing speech from individuals with speech and voice disorders, it makes sense that because there is very little publicly available data that represents speech from these speakers, the models that are trained on normative speech datasets do not perform well on disordered speech [38]. The speech from individuals with speech and voice disorders is significantly different enough from 'normative' speech that the models that are built to recognize 'normative' speech do not accept the level of variability shown in disordered speech.

2 Definitions and Concepts

In the pursuit of clarity, let's start by defining some of the prominent terminologies that will be used throughout this chapter. These are commonly defined terms in the field. Later on in this chapter, new terms that build on some of these concepts will be introduced to more precisely talk about the field of ASR for people with voice disorders.

- **Automatic Speech Recognition**: also known as speech recognition, or ASR, is the task of recording a speech signal and transforming the speech waveform into the text that was spoken aloud.
- **Voice Disorder**: a disorder that happens when characteristics of an individual's voice—the tone, pitch, volume, or overall quality—are inappropriate for how they see themselves. This definition of self may include the speaker's gender, culture, age, or even their geography [2, 28].
- **Speech Disorder**: The process of articulating words and sounds is known as speech. Speakers with speech disorders may not be able to make sounds precisely leading to unclear words and decreased intelligibility, have a different voice quality—sounding a bit raspy or hoarse—or have breaks or pauses in their speaking patterns leading to a not entirely fluent sound (called stuttering).
- **Dysarthria**: a class of neuromotor speech disorders which happen when the muscles responsible for speech are weakened due to brain damage. Dysarthria presents with a variety of possible symptoms. Dysarthric speech can sound slow, slurred, fast, soft, breathy, or raspy. This speech disorder can be a result of several different primary disorders including but not limited to Amyotrophic Lateral Sclerosis (ALS), stroke, brain injury, tumors, Huntington's, Cerebral Palsy, Multiple Sclerosis, or muscular dystrophy.
- **Robust ASR**: The propensity to accurately recognize highly variable speech is referred to as the **robustness** of an ASR system. Robust ASR systems can recognize speech that has a large amount of variability in it, whether that variability comes from background noise levels, different recording devices, or differences in the speech itself.

3 A Brief Introduction to Phonetics and Acoustics

The field of ASR is built on top of decades of research in acoustics, linguistics, and phonetics. To build systems that recognize and even understand speech and language, we need to understand the basics of how speech is produced and understood. The following sections outline healthy speech production as well as some common places where breakdowns in this process happen leading to voice or speech disorders. How this speech is perceived as well as common pre-processing steps taken before inputting to an ASR system are also described.

3.1   Speech Production

Speech production includes all of the steps by which thoughts are translated into speech—starting with generating thoughts, forming words within the rules of syntax and grammar, and then forming the specific muscle movements necessary to articulate the words using the vocal cords, lungs, nose, mouth, and tongue [5, 57]. Speaking is an incredible ensemble of very precise motor tasks resulting in a series of sounds that can travel relatively large distances. In physics, a sound is a vibration that propagates as an acoustic wave (an oscillation in pressure) through a transmission medium (gas, liquid, or solid). As humans, we experience sounds through the reception of these waves and their interpretation within the brain.

Models of speech production can help lead to a better understanding of how to computationally model speech [26]. One of the prevalent speech production models, the **source-filter model**, posits that speech is a combination of a sound source (the vocal cords), and an acoustic filter (the vocal tract). The sound source is represented by the pulsing signal—referred to as the excitation signal—created by the oscillation of the vocal cords, while the acoustic filter refers to how changes in the shape and placement of the vocal tract organs change the output of the sound. For example, if you start by saying /o/ as in 'stew', but open your lips, the sound will change. This is because you changed the acoustic filter. When the speaker moves their speech articulators (lips, tongue, mouth, etc), the shape of the vocal tract changes, causing different resonances to be formed—in the field of phonetics and acoustics, this is also referred to as the *frequency response*. The frequency responses of these resonances are known as *formants*. Formants are very important in the human ability to recognize speech [22]. The source-filter model is an approximation of how human speech works, and this model has been foundational in the speech recognition and synthesis fields [35].

3.1.1   Production of Disordered Speech

When an individual has a speech disorder, it means that some part of the speech production pathway is not working correctly. Speech disorders lead to a degradation of the speech quality, making the speech less intelligible to both humans and ASR systems. Disordered speech can be produced through problems with the functioning of the muscles that control the vocal cords, the tongue, the lips, or the lungs of the speaker. Producing speech requires an impressive ensemble of exact movements, and even small distortions in the neuromuscular control of the muscles along the speech production pathway can result in a significant degradation in the intelligibility of the speech [46].

Dysarthria is a common class of speech disorder associated with neuromotor conditions like Parkinson's disease and cerebral palsy as well as brain damage due to stroke or head injuries. Individuals with dysarthric speech exhibit a massive variability in the ability to articulate speech clearly. Common features of dysarthric speech include deviations in the time domain—leading to speech that sounds either slow, distorted, or sometimes rushed—as well as general difficulty in parsing out phonemes due to poor precision of the speech articulators. Differences in speech quality from the ability to control the volume of the voice to a nasal or breathy quality are also commonly seen in dysarthric speakers.

Voice disorders lead to **dysphonic speech** which can often be characterized similarly to dysarthric speech. Dysphonic speech, however, is often rooted more in the vocal cords than the speech articulators leading to slightly more intelligible speech than dysarthria, generally. The variability mainly stems from deviations in the tension in the vocal cords. If the vocal cords are loose—often due to spasms in the muscles that control the tension of the vocal cords, the speaker has speech that has a breathy quality and very low volume. If the vocal cords are tight—also often due to spasms in the muscles that control the tension of the vocal cords—the speaker's voice sounds tight, creaky, and often the speech is sped up to fit sentences into one breath. It is common for individuals with speech and voice disorders to change their prosody—the cadence, volume, or emphasis of how they speak—to be better understood by listeners [31].

3.2 Speech Perception

Speech perception is the process by which speech and language are heard, processed, and understood. Speech is perceived via both auditory and visual modalities [32]. Verbal communication and interaction are some of the defining characteristics of the human race [17]. The act of speaking involves producing a stream of meaningful sounds. Understanding these sounds starts by being able to discern *phonemes*. A **phoneme** is the smallest perceptible unit of speech from which through pattern recognition, one word can be distinguished from another. From phonemes, we can build the basis of recognizing and distinguishing words and therefore language.

From a young age, humans start learning to perceive speech. Speech perception is a relative concept—the language that is spoken to you as a child affects the development of the ability to detect certain phonemes. As we learn the language that surrounds us, we lose the ability to detect phonemes that are not part of that language [6]. Perceiving and understanding speech becomes more difficult if a speaker has an accent or atypical speech patterns. However, humans are quick learners and adapt readily to better understand atypical speech patterns [10]. This means that speech perception is not only relative but also a dynamic concept.

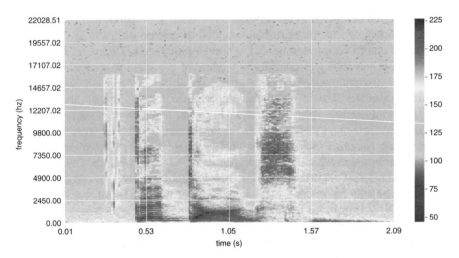

Fig. 3 An example of a spectrogram of a speech sample saying 'good dog'

3.3 Speech Parameterization Methods

The goal of ASR systems is to find the most likely word sequence. To this end, many ASR algorithms require that speech be parameterized—condensed down to relevant speech features. As the sampling rate of speech is so high—commonly 44,100 samples per second—it is common practice to reduce the size of the input by combining the input in different ways that are relevant to the frequency and spectral parts of the speech. There are many techniques to accomplish this goal, and below some of the more common techniques are discussed.

One rudimentary technique of parameterizing speech is to use **windowing**—a technique where a speech signal is sectioned off into short, overlapping segments (generally on the order of 10 ms) and summarized. At this level, the signal in the speech remains relatively stationary, and the resulting features can represent the phonetic and acoustic content of the speech.

Another common technique for parameterizing speech is to use **Mel-Frequency Cepstrum Coefficients (MFCCs)**. MFCCs are based on the short-term Fourier transform (SFT) of the speech waveform and attempt to replicate some of the psycho-acoustic properties of the human auditory system. Other speech parameterization methods include speech articulation features [15] and pitch information [16].

Formant analysis is another common technique for pre-processing speech [61]. Estimating the **formants** involved in a specific utterance can lead to a better understanding of what and how a speech sample was said. Formants are the distinct frequency components of speech, and as such are measured in Hz. Formants can be visualized using spectrograms and can be estimated by finding the local maxima of the spectrum. Formants provide information about the articulation of the speech, and when combined with lip and mouth position, words can be interpreted. In individuals with voice disorders, it is relatively common to see shifts in the formants of their speech in comparison to control speech.

A slightly more modern technique for parameterizing speech, spurred by the development of convolutional neural networks for computer vision, is to use a common visual representation of speech—the **spectrogram**. Spectrograms are a visual way of representing the information in speech and are analogous to sheet music, where the frequency of the voice is shown over time. Spectrograms encode information such as the loudness (intensity) of different frequencies over time. Figure 3 shows a spectrogram of the author saying 'good dog'. The x-axis represents the different frequencies, while the y-axis represents time. The intensity of the frequency at a given time is shown by the color of the signal, where reds indicate high intensity, and blues indicate lower intensity.

More recently, rather than parameterizing speech before inputting it to an ASR system, researchers have attempted speech recognition by inputting the raw speech signals. The idea here is that, much like has happened in the field of computer vision, by applying deep learning techniques, maybe the explicit knowledge that the field has been trying to infuse the data with attempts to parameterize speech can be implicitly discovered by the latent variables in deep learning. Training machine learning models on raw speech data presents some problems, notably the size of the signal. While speech is a one-dimensional signal, the sampling rate is commonly 44,100 samples per second. To process this many inputs at a real-time speed is quite difficult without speech parameterization methods.

3.4 Markers of Disordered Speech

In Fig. 4, two different spectrograms are shown, both holding the prolonged vowel $/i/$. The spectrogram on the top is of a speech sample from a control speaker (no voice disorder), while the spectrogram on the bottom is from a speaker with a voice disorder. Visually, it is relatively easy to see how this specific voice disorder causes the vowels to sound less 'stable' than the control speaker's vowel. Using information like this to be able to identify and compensate for a voice disorder in a speech recognition task is an important part of building disorder-robust ASR systems.

While there are many diverse measurements relating to the extent to which a voice is disordered, the main concept that these ratings usually try to model is **intelligibility**—the ability of a spoken utterance to be perceived, understood and internalized by the communication partner. While on the surface, intelligibility seems like a pretty straight forward concept, it has proven to be quite tricky to model effectively. This is partly due to the subtle complexity of the concept of intelligibility. Intelligibility is both dynamic—the more we hear someone's voice the more we get used to how they communicate, we change our prosody based on environmental factors—and relative—someone with an accent similar to the speech that you were raised around will be easier for you to understand than a

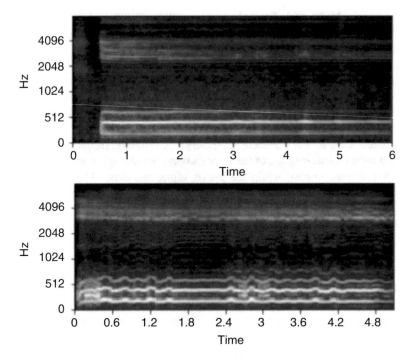

Fig. 4 A comparison of two sustained phonations of the vowel /i/. The spectrogram on top is from an individual without a voice disorder while the spectrogram below is from an individual with a voice disorder, more specifically, spasmodic dysphonia

foreign accent. Most voice disorders are characterized by a decrease in intelligibility. Generally, the lack of intelligibility has a significant impact on an individual's life, causing difficulty with completing activities of daily living.

To recognize disordered speech, it will be helpful to be able to identify disordered speech. There has been quite a bit of research on this topic in the speech-processing and clinical fields. From this literature, there exist a few standard features that have consistently been shown to be correlated with voice disorders. These features include jitter, shimmer, harmonic noise ratio and the cepstral peak prominence [52, 56, 62]. These features are values that can be calculated with relative ease and have led to accurate classification of disordered speech [13]. Formants provide information about the articulation of the speech and have been used to classify voice disorders [40]. Having a set of features that can identify disordered speech may help identify disordered speech and apply different methods of speech recognition for these voices.

To build systems that can recognize disordered speech, it will be important to be able to recognize and potentially quantify or cluster disordered speech. The markers discussed above such as changes in the jitter, shimmer, harmonic noise ratio, and cepstral peak prominence, as well as a general decrease in intelligibility, can be used to identify disordered speech.

4 Automatic Speech Recognition Overview

To understand the different ASR systems, and gain an overall understanding of how ASR systems work with the eventual goal of understanding how and why these systems can be made more accessible to individuals with voice disorders, it is first prudent to understand some of the characterizations of different ASR systems. In the following sections, some of the more important parameters of ASR systems are discussed.

4.1 Characterization of ASR Systems

4.1.1 Speaker Dependence

An important parameter in building an ASR system to recognize disordered speech is what level of dependence the system will have on the speaker:

An ASR system is **speaker dependent** when it is trained using samples from a single user. Speaker dependent systems are more successful in recognizing speech from individuals with speech and voice disorders, however, they require a significant amount of data from the speaker who will be using the system, and do not generalize well to other speakers.

An ASR system is **speaker independent** when it will recognize speech from any speaker. The result is a system that is more flexible to a broad range of speakers, however, speaker-independent systems require a vast amount of speech data from many diverse speakers. In general, speaker-independent models are not very successful at recognizing disordered speech. One explanation of the poor performance of speaker-independent systems on disordered speech is that disordered speech is not part of the training data that the system is trained on.

The middle ground between speaker-dependent and speaker-independent systems is what is referred to as 'speaker adaptive' ASR systems. A **speaker-adaptive** ASR system is first trained on data similar to that of speaker-independent systems— a vast amount of data that is representative of many diverse voices—and then later the last layers of the neural network are re-trained on a specific speaker's voice. In this capacity, some of the advantages of speaker-independent models are preserved, and while some data is necessary from the end-user of the system, the amount of data necessary to fine-tune a speaker-adaptive model is significantly less than the amount of data needed to train a speaker-dependent system.

4.1.2 Continuity

Originally, ASR systems were built such that they recognized **discrete** words—that is, isolated words spoken one at a time. This kind of interaction is great for simple tasks like controlling a simple interface or providing simple commands, however, it is unnatural for humans to put significant space between words, and thus, not a good user experience.

Continuous speech recognition refers to the idea of recognizing natural speech—speech that does not necessarily have space in between each word. Continuous speech recognition allows the user to speak in a more normal cadence than discrete speech recognition. The ideal ASR system recognizes continuous speech, however, there still is some utility in discrete speech recognition systems, especially if the speech is particularly difficult to understand.

4.1.3 Vocabulary Size

Another important parameter for building ASR systems for individuals with voice disorders is the size of the vocabulary that the system will recognize. While originally, speech recognition systems were built to recognize small vocabulary sets, usually including the alphabet, digits, and some simple commands, Large Vocabulary Continuous Speech Recognition (LVCSR) is the goal of most ASR systems [51].

LVCSR has yet to be achieved for individuals with voice disorders. The most successful ASR systems for individuals with voice disorders use significantly smaller vocabularies. These vocabularies are generally limited to digits, commonly used words, and simple directions, and in most cases are designed as discrete systems.

4.2 Nomenclature of Disordered Speech Recognition

Along with these classifications of the different levels of difficulty of the ASR task based on the amount of implicit and explicit noise, this chapter also introduces a new vocabulary to discuss models that recognize speech from individuals with disordered speech.

Within the general field of ASR, there are several different ways to classify speech recognition models, primarily dealing with the characterizations explained above. Building upon the previously defined terminology of *speaker dependent, speaker-independent, and speaker adaptive* models laid out in Sect. 4.1, new variants of these concepts are proposed relating not only to the speaker but to speech disorders as a whole, to facilitate more inclusive voice-based systems. The new vocabulary is as follows:

- **Disorder-Robust ASR**: This refers to the field of ASR that deals with building models that are robust to the implicit noise found in speech from speakers with voice and speech disorders.
- **Disorder-Dependent ASR**: This refers to ASR systems that are trained only on data from a specific type of disordered speech. For example, if a system was built to understand speech from individuals with Spasmodic Dysphonia, the resulting model would be a disorder-dependent approach to disorder-robust ASR.
- **Disorder-Independent ASR**: A disorder-independent ASR system refers to a system for which the recognition accuracy of speech from individuals with voice disorders is greater than or equal to that of individuals without voice disorders.
- **Disorder-Adaptive ASR**: Disorder-adaptive ASR refers to ASR systems that are initially trained on the LVCSR data—large vocabulary, continuous speech from many speakers—and then are later adapted to represent a particular disorder.

With this new characterization of disorder-robust ASR systems, it is relatively easy to see how this scaffold could help lay the foundation for the development of new, better disorder-robust ASR systems.

4.3 The Ideal System

From the nomenclature and characterizations above, the goal of building ASR systems for users with voice disorders is defined as achieving a **disorder-independent, large vocabulary, continuous** system such that the recognition accuracy of speech from individuals with voice disorders is greater than or equal to that of individuals without voice disorders. This system would be not only disorder-independent but would also work on continuous speech and for a very large vocabulary. Toward this goal, a classification of the difficulty of tasks in the field of ASR is introduced below.

4.4 Levels of Difficulty in ASR Tasks

When input speech is clear and the data is clean—generally obtained from speakers who are near the microphone—ASR systems have been able to achieve human-level performance. However, this formulation has a lot of variables and if there is background noise, an increased distance from the microphone—leading to decreased signal to noise ratio—or less clarity in the original signal, the performance of ASR systems quickly declines.

In this chapter, noise generated from anything external to the speaker's voice—the distance from the microphone, presence of background noise, etc.—will be referred to as **explicit noise** while any noise coming directly from the speaker's voice—differences in the timing, quality, or ability of the speaker to articulate speech clearly—will be referred to as **implicit noise**.

Previously, any ASR task that dealt with data that had significant noise—either natural to the environment where the data was collected or artificially added—was referred to as **robust automatic speech recognition**. However, this definition does not differentiate between different sources of noise. Most of the literature surrounding *robust ASRs* deals with ways to make ASR systems robust to *explicit noise*. Literature in this field will take the clean speech, corrupt it by adding noise at different signal-to-noise-ratios, and then build systems that will accurately recognize the data with artificial explicit-noise.

Not all speech recognition tasks are created equal—the level of noise in the signal impacts the difficulty of achieving accurate speech recognition. To make this distinction clear, a new nomenclature of referring to ASR tasks based on four levels is presented. As demonstrated in Table 1, the main difference between these levels is the amount of explicit or implicit noise (Fig. 5).

Table 1 Definition of different levels of ASR problems based on the amount of implicit and explicit noise

	Type of noise		
Level	Explicit	Implicit	Problem description
1	Low	Low	Clean/clear data
2	High	Low	Noisy/clear data
3	Low	High	Clean/unclear data
4	High	High	Noisy/unclear data

Fig. 5 A guide to the proposed levels of difficulty in ASR tasks. Levels 1–4 are characterized by different levels of explicit and implicit noise. Level 1 is the least difficult task, progressing to the most difficult task of level 4

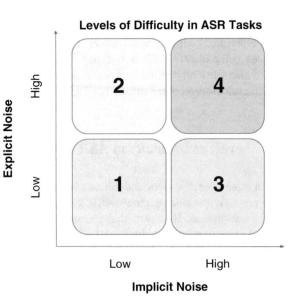

4.4.1   Level 1 ASR

Level 1 ASR deals with data that has small amounts of explicit and implicit noise meaning the data is both relatively free of background noise and spoken with a clear, intelligible voice. Level 1 ASR problems have largely been solved as demonstrated by the vast field of different smart speakers and digital assistants.

4.4.2   Level 2 ASR

Level 2 ASR tasks consist of data that has a large amount of explicit noise, but a small amount of implicit noise. This means that there may be background noise (either artificially added or naturally present upon the data collection process), but little implicit noise—the speaker's voice is generally clear and intelligible. Level 2 ASR tasks include most robust ASR tasks.

4.4.3   Level 3 ASR

Level 3 ASR tasks are the opposite of level 2 tasks—they have little explicit noise, but significant implicit noise. Level 3 tasks include most disordered speech recognition tasks, where the speaker's voice implicitly has a significant amount of noise that generally leads to a decreased intelligibility.

4.4.4   Level 4 ASR

Level 4 ASR tasks are the most difficult of the possible ASR tasks, where there is both significant explicit and implicit noise. This includes situations where the speaker's voice is not particularly clear or intelligible and there also exists some background noise, either artificial or natural.

5   A Level by Level Guide of ASR Modeling Approaches

5.1   Level 1 ASR: Clear and Clean Speech Recognition

5.1.1   Multimodels

The traditional model of ASR systems relies on multiple models to complete the task of ASR. These models take speech as an input, pre-process the speech—possibly extracting relevant features from the speech—and then pass either the features or the raw speech into the recognition algorithm. The recognition algorithm generally utilizes a language model and an acoustic model. **Acoustic models** are learned from a set of audio recordings and their corresponding transcripts. Acoustic models take speech broken into short, overlapping time frames as an input, and for each frame outputs a prediction of which phoneme was spoken. By concatenating the most likely phonemes from one frame to the next, the output of the acoustic model is a list of the most likely phonemes.

Using a lexicon and a language model, that list of phonemes is converted into the most likely sequence of words. A **lexicon** acts as a dictionary and provides context for which phonemes make up a given word, while **language models** contain the probability distribution over sequences of words—providing context to distinguish between words and phrases that sound similar. In general, the language model is responsible for representing the syntactic and semantic content of the speech while the combination of the lexicon and the acoustic model is responsible for handling the relationship between the input speech signal and which phonemes were said.

The primary objective of speech recognition is to build a statistical model to predict the text sequences W (say 'take the dog for a walk') from a sequence of feature vectors X. This problem is often formulated as a Maximum a Posterior Estimate as shown in Eq. 1.

$$W^* = \arg\max_W P(W|X) \tag{1}$$

From this formulation, Bayes' Theorem is applied, which leads to Eq. 2.

$$W^* = \arg\max_W \frac{P(X|W)P(W)}{P(X)} . \tag{2}$$

From Eq. 2, $P(X)$ can be removed because $P(X)$ does not vary with respect to W. What is left is the formulation shown in Eq. 3

$$W^* = \arg\max_W P(X|W)P(W) \tag{3}$$

Equation 3 takes into account the probability of the features given the sequence of words $P(X|W)$—also referred to as the **acoustic model**—and the probability of the sequence of words $P(W)$—often referred to as the **language model**. Acoustic models model the relationship between the audio signal and the linguistic content of the speech—generally phonemes or words—while language models deal with the syntactic and semantic composition of the words. Acoustic models are generally trained with the input being the acoustic features and the output being either words or phonemes while language models are trained on large datasets of text and output the probability that a sequence of words would be used together. Together, acoustic and language models make up the class of ASR systems referred to as **multimodels** with acoustic models going from speech to phonemes, and language models predicting the words that the phonemes were saying.

Figure 6 shows how a multimodel system works, taking speech as an input, applying speech parameterization, pre-processing, and feature extraction method-

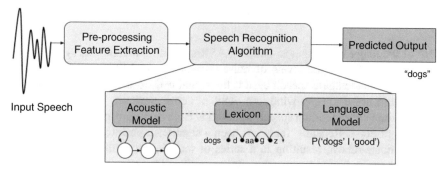

Fig. 6 An example of a multimodel, a combination of an acoustic model, language model, and lexicon for ASR

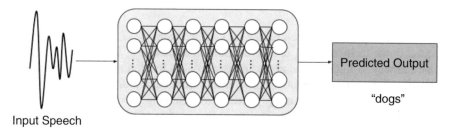

Fig. 7 A depiction of end-to-end (E2E) speech recognition. The idea is that there is little pre-processing of the data, and one model takes on the task of both acoustic modeling and language modeling to go straight from input speech to a predicted output sequence of words

ologies before passing the input into the general speech recognition algorithm. The general ASR algorithm includes the input being passed into the acoustic model to generate a prediction of which phonemes exist at each window of speech, which is then passed through a lexicon mapping which phoneme combinations are likely to be which words, and then that is passed into a language model which takes into account the semantics and syntax of the language to modify the predictions. From here, the predicted sequence of words is then output.

5.1.2 End-to-End Models

ASR models that don't rely on a combination of multiple models and make predictions based solely on the input speech data are referred to as **end-to-end ASR** (E2E) systems. Figure 7 shows an example of this kind of model. Generally, deep neural networks are used to make E2E systems. E2E models also require a lot of labeled speech data—a luxury that is not possible for disordered speech recognition.

5.2 Level 2 ASR: Noisy but Clear Speech Recognition

One of the major challenges in building ASR systems is making the system robust enough to deal with the levels of noise recorded in real-life speech recordings. Humans can understand speech even if the signal is distorted with a lot of noise— background noise, music, wind, etc. ASR systems, however, have a much more difficult time understanding speech signals that have been corrupted with even small amounts of noise. Recently, there has been a significant push to build ASR models that are noise-robust, resulting in a series of techniques resulting in more robust ASR systems. A few of these techniques are outlined below:

5.2.1 Data Augmentation

As the primary problems behind the lack of accessibility of ASR systems can be boiled down to insufficient data and insufficient modeling techniques, it follows that one way to improve the accessibility of ASRs for non-normative voices is to collect and disseminate annotated speech data from these individuals.

Another less time-consuming pathway to obtaining more speech data that is representative of non-normative voices is to use state-of-the-art machine learning models (such as generative adversarial networks, or variational autoencoders) to generate artificial disordered speech. This technique is referred to as **data augmentation** and has recently become a popular method for generating more data to help build robust solutions to problems where the data representing these problems is sparse. Generative Adversarial Networks have enabled the creation of realistic training data. By synthesizing speech, and then including that speech in the training data from which the ASR system is trained, lower word error rates can be achieved [20, 48]. This technique has been used for several different subsets of data, for example, in [53], the authors generated speech for children to help make their ASR system more robust to child speech.

5.2.2 Transfer Learning

In machine learning, **Transfer Learning** is a field that focuses on applying knowledge gained while solving one problem, to a different but related problem [59]. Transfer learning has been used in the domain of speech recognition to recognize speech that has different levels of noise. In [8], they train the model on data that is noisy and employ a few techniques to make sure that it will perform just as accurately on speech that is not noisy.

Another example of transfer learning in the speech recognition domain is training a model on adult speech, but then applying this knowledge to the problem of recognizing child speech. In [54], they do just that, evaluating different transfer learning methodologies for applying knowledge gained from adult speech recognition to child speech recognition. Some techniques that they evaluated include different speaker normalization and adaptation techniques.

Domain adaptation is a subfield of transfer learning and refers to the ability to apply an algorithm trained in a 'source domain' to a different but related 'target domain' [59]. In domain adaptation, the source and target domains have the same feature space (for this chapter, the feature space would be speech), but different distributions—say child and adult speech, whispered and loud speech, noisy and clear speech, or disordered and normative speech, while in transfer learning the domain feature spaces do not have to be the same.

Domain adaptation techniques include reweighting algorithms and searching for a common representation space. Domain adaptation has been used as a way to make ASR systems more robust to different domains of speech [11, 19].

5.2.3 Multimodal ASR

The McGurk effect shows that speech is perceived using not only auditory information but also visual information [32]. This makes sense as speech generation and perception are inherently bi-modal processes based on audio-visual representations. This means that there is information about what is said in the visual modality of speech.

The visual modality does not experience degradation due to background noise or different kinds of microphones as speech does—a characteristic that makes the addition of visual data to ASR systems attractive. The visual data generated from speech includes lip motion, head movement, facial expressions, and body gestures. The primary form of visual information incorporated into audio-visual automatic speech recognition systems (AVSR) is lip information. The importance and clarity of this visual component of speech increases for the speech from individuals with voice disorders [23].

Hidden Markov Models (HMMs) have been successful in implementing AVSR systems originally [12, 42], however, most AVSR models have transitioned into using deep-learning-based frameworks [21, 44, 45].

5.3 Level 3 ASR: Clean but Unclear Speech Recognition

Many of the methods that have been employed in Level 2 ASR are also useful in recognizing speech from speakers who may have unclear or disordered speech.

5.3.1 Data Augmentation

There have been a few attempts to artificially augment the amount of disordered speech data. While level 2 tasks have utilized Generative Adversarial Networks

(GANs) to augment the amount of speech data used, there exists too much variability and too little data to successfully implement GANs to augment disordered speech. Because of this, the primary methodology of artificially augmenting disordered speech datasets is to warp the time-domain of healthy speech to get it to sound more like disordered speech [58]. With the growing amount of disordered speech data available, hopefully, GANs will be able to be implemented to create artificial accurate representations of disordered speech to be used to train models to be more robust to disordered speech.

5.3.2 Multimodal Techniques

Utilizing multiple modalities to improve the performance of speech recognition systems has applications beyond level 2 ASR tasks. There have been a few papers that have explored using multimodal techniques to improve the performance of ASR systems on speakers with voice disorders [9, 29, 36].

5.3.3 Voice Conversion and Speaker Normalization

In [7], the task of voice conversion (VC) is used to convert dysarthric speech into speech that is more intelligible using convolutional neural networks. This is a relatively new approach to improving the intelligibility of disordered speech. The idea is that by applying this conversion to speech both humans and computers will be able to understand individuals with voice disorders more readily.

In [4], the researchers built a system to take in disordered speech and output speech that is more easily understood by both humans and computers. The way that they accomplished this was by collecting speech from individuals with speech/voice disorders and pairing each utterance with an artificially synthesized speech sample. They then trained a neural network to convert the input of disordered speech into the intelligible synthesized speech. The authors were able to achieve this speaker normalization with not only voice-disorder speech, but also differences in speech accent, prosody, and voices. Removing these kinds of variation in speech is known as *speaker normalization*. This process has been shown to improve the intelligibility of speech but also removes some of the emotion or other characteristics that make the speech personalized.

5.4   Level 4 ASR

There hasn't been much work completed on noisy disordered speech recognition, however, it is a problem which the solution will likely build off of innovations in Level 2 and level 3 ASR problems. While it isn't entirely practical to attempt solving Level 4 ASR problems while there is so much work to be done on Levels 1, 2, and 3, it's worth considering what the next step would be as these problems begin to have more satisfactory solutions. One potential way of testing the performance of current state-of-the-art ASR models of level 4 ASR tasks would be to simply corrupt some of the disordered speech samples described below with noise, and see how well these systems recognize the speech.

6 Disordered Speech Datasets

As identified above, one of the aspects of ASR of voice disorder speech that makes this task difficult is the limited amount of data available to use to train these systems. Below, we outline the prominent datasets that are available to use to train models to represent speech and voice disorders. A summary of these datasets can be found in Table 2.

6.1 Acoustic Datasets

6.1.1 Dysarthric Speech Dataset for Universal Access (UASPEECH)

The Universal Access Speech (UASPEECH) dataset from the University of Illinois [25] was published in 2008 and consists of speech samples from 15 individuals with dysarthrias, and 13 age and gender-matched control voices. The vocabulary used in UASPEECH consists of command words (up, left, down, right, etc.), common

Table 2 A table of relevant disordered speech datasets and their characteristics. **#D** refers to the number of speakers with disordered speech while **#C** refers to the number of control speakers

Dataset	#D	#C	Vocabulary	Data type	Speech type
[25] UASPEECH	15	13	765 isolated words (digits, letters, un/common words)	Audio	Dysarthria
[49] TORGO	8	7	Non words, short words, restricted and unrestricted sentences	Audio Articulatory	Dysarthria
[33] Nemours	11	0	74 nonsense sentences, two connected-speech paragraphs	Audio	Dysarthria
[43] HomeService	5		131 words, commands	Audio	Dysarthria
[39] UncommonVoice	48	9	Vowels, sentences, spontaneous speech	Audio	Dysphonia
[50] Parkinson's	20		Non words	Features	Parkinson's

words (the, and, I, you, etc.), the phonetic alphabet (alpha, bravo, charlie, etc.), digits 1–10, and 300 uncommon words. There are a total of 765 words for each speaker, three repetitions of each of the commands, letters, digits, and common words, and only one instance of the 300 uncommon words per speaker. The speech from UASPEECH was collected using a 'beep' sound to segment the instances of speech, and because of this, there is a lot of silence in the dataset.

6.1.2 The TORGO Database

The University of Toronto's TORGO database is a database that includes not only acoustic data, but also articulatory data [49]. This dataset consists of speech samples from eight individuals with dysarthria and seven control voices. The vocabulary of TORGO consists of non-words (vowel sounds, phoneme repetitions, etc.), short words (computer command words), words from the two common intelligibility assessments [14, 60], common words used in Britain, and words that have contrasting phonemes from [24]. The dataset also contains both read sentences, as well as spontaneous speech from image descriptions. One of the drawbacks of the TORGO database is that it includes the confounding variable of the recording equipment for the articulatory data. This equipment includes placing sensors on the tongue, lips, and mouth which very likely hindered speech to some degree. However, if knowing the specific details of how a dysarthric speaker articulates their speech is important, the TORGO database is the only database that provides this data publicly.

6.1.3 The Nemours Database of Dysarthric Speech

One of the original databases of dysarthric speech is the Nemours database. This database is a collection of 814 short sentences made up of words that don't make sense together, 74 sentences that make sense, and two paragraphs of connected speech. This database contains speech samples from 11 speakers with different degrees of dysarthria, all of whom are male [33]. The fact that this dataset only contains speech samples from males is potentially problematic, especially if this was one of the main datasets used to build an ASR system. It is important to have data representative of not only male dysarthric speakers but also female dysarthric speakers.

6.1.4 The HomeService Corpus

The HomeService Corpus was created by researchers at the University of Sheffield and provides the audio recorded during interactions between speakers with severe dysarthria and their environment [43]. HomeService consists of around 10 h of data from 5 individuals with severe dysarthria, including a vocabulary of 131 words, and a total of 9360 interactions.

The HomeService corpus was created to facilitate voice-based interaction with the environment for individuals with severe dysarthria. The recordings are of particular interest because they were recorded 'in-the-wild', and not in a sound studio. This means that the level of noise experienced in this dataset is equivalent to what a live dysarthric speech recognition system would experience. There are general benefits to training a recognition model on the data from the environment in which the model will be tested/used.

6.1.5   UncommonVoice

Inspired by Mozilla's Common Voice, in [39] UncommonVoice is a crowdsourced dataset of disordered speech. It includes speech from 57 individuals, 48 of whom have voice disorders. Speakers recorded nonwords, TIMIT sentences, and spontaneous speech (image descriptions). UncommonVoice consists of around 10 h of data and continues to grow. UncommonVoice also includes responses to a survey including information about how speakers with voice disorders have treated their voices, and how they would assess their voice on the day of recording.

UncommonVoice was built to have the functionality to act as a longitudinal dataset to learn more about how disordered speech changes over time, specifically with regards to voice treatments. The use of Botulinum toxin injections to treat the primary speech disorder found in this dataset—Spasmodic Dysphonia—is particularly important to this data, and the effects of this treatment can be evaluated using this dataset. The goal of UncommonVoice was to provide representation to the group of people with voice disorders to make more inclusive and accessible voice-based technologies.

One of the main downsides to UncommonVoice is that it was collected in a crowdsource manner, leading to data collected from many different microphones. This leads to a higher level of variability in the data. Also, speakers in Uncommon-Voice self-identified whether or not they had a voice disorder as well as what their diagnosis was, potentially leading to some inconsistencies in the data.

6.1.6   Parkinson's Disorder Speech Dataset

In this dataset of Parkinson's speech, speech data from 20 individuals with Parkinson's disease was collected. This dataset collected non-word utterances from the speakers. The data that was released as part of this freely and publicly available dataset are features that were extracted from the speech data [50]. The main drawback of this dataset is that you don't have the raw speech signals to work with, and instead have to work off of the features that they chose to extract. While this data is still important and useful, it is not as flexible as many researchers desire.

7   Utility and Applications of Disorder-Robust ASR

The goal of improving the recognition accuracy and decreasing the word error rate of ASR systems when the input is from disordered speech is not only to generally improve the accessibility of voice-based technology. There are other important applications of inclusive ASR technologies such as building robust clinical metrics to be able to facilitate speech and voice therapy and rehabilitation, building novel voice-assistive technologies, and generally improving everyday voice interactions for individuals with voice disorders.

7.1   Clinical Metrics

There exists a history of ASR systems being utilized to assess and evaluate speech and voice disorders. The word error rate (WER), or conversely, the word recognition rate is commonly used as proxy metrics for intelligibility. The word error rate (WER) is defined, as shown in Eq. 4, as the number of substitutions S, insertions I, and D divided by the total number of words in a phrase N. It is worth mentioning that WER is an unbounded metric in that an ASR system could insert more words in the prediction than there are in the transcript, causing the WER to be greater than one.

$$WER = \frac{S + I + D}{N} \qquad (4)$$

Word recognition rate (RR) is a metric that defines the accuracy of the ASR—the number of words recognized R divided by the number of total words N as depicted in Eq. 5.

$$RR = \frac{R}{N} * 100 \qquad (5)$$

The evaluation of intelligibility often requires gathering participants to listen to speech samples and orthographically transcribe—that is, write down/type out what they hear. It is easy to imagine that this form of evaluating intelligibility is time-consuming, expensive, as well as relatively subjective. In pursuit of a cheaper and faster way of evaluating the intelligibility of speech, researchers have employed the use of ASR systems. Research has found that ASR systems generally perform worse on recognizing speech from individuals with voice disorders than humans do [34], however, there is a pretty strong correlation between ASR recognition rate and human recognition rate—meaning that the speakers whom humans found most difficult to understand, the speech recognition system also found difficult to understand.

It has become relatively common practice for ASR systems to be utilized to evaluate the severity of speech disorders, as well as to measure the progress of speech and voice therapies [27, 30]. ASR systems have become integral parts of speech and voice disorder assessment tools [1], for both adults and children [55].

7.2   Voice Assistive Technologies

While ASRs have proven to be useful as a way for individuals with physical disabilities to interface with technology—smart homes, smartwatches, mobile devices, etc.—individuals with voice disorders are often not able to effectively interface with these systems via voice [18].

In a survey of 471 individuals with voice disorders, the primary impacts of having a voice disorder were evaluated resulting in three main areas of life that voice disorders disrupt: inhibition of social interactions, reduced emotional well being, and difficulties finding, keeping, and advancing in jobs [37]. In this same survey, five specific situations were described as particularly difficult for individuals with voice disorders:

1. Speaking on the phone
2. Speaking in environments with significant background noise (restaurants, parties, outdoors, etc.)
3. Ordering at a drive-thru
4. Meeting new people for the first time
5. Using auto-attendant phone-menu systems that require speech input.

These five situations provide areas of opportunity for the development of voice-assistive technologies. Very few voice-assistive technologies exist—the majority of what is available as voice-assistive technologies are voice amplifiers. While these amplifiers are helpful when individuals with voice disorders are unable to project their voice with enough volume to be understood—particularly in noisy environments—if there are other problems with the voice outside of the ability for the individual to project, then the amplifier ends up amplifying a still relatively unintelligible voice.

In [37], individuals with voice disorders made it clear that if it was an option, they would prefer to communicate using their voice, and that they generally wanted to be able to speak 'like normal'. These two findings suggest that systems that enhance the intelligibility of disordered speech could meet the needs of individuals with voice disorders quite nicely.

Recently, there has been a small focus on the development of these intelligibility-enhancing systems as demonstrated by Chen et al. [7] and Biadsy et al. [4]. Voice-normalization techniques are still relatively new, and there remains plenty of room for growth in this field.

7.3   Improvement of Everyday Voice Interactions

One of the main motivations for working on the problem of disorder-robust ASR is
to improve the everyday user experience of voice-based interactions for users with
and without disordered speech.

Universal Design is the concept that new technologies should be designed such
that everyone, regardless of ability should be able to use the system without adaptation or modification. Designing for everyone generally improves the accuracy/utility
of the system not just for those who were originally excluded, but also for other users
[47].

In this case, by designing voice-based technology so that it can be used by
everyone without adaptation, meeting the explicit needs of individuals with voice
disorders, the implicit needs of people without voice disorders—such as being able
to be understood when a temporary illness makes the speaker's voice scratchy/less
intelligible—are met.

Other applications of voice-based technology that would be very useful and
convenient for individuals with voice disorders are voice-based automotive
interactive/hands-free systems and improving the experience of using auto-
attendant (automatic phone menu) systems. Secondarily, improving the recognition
of disordered speech would also improve the accuracy of automatic captioning
systems, and generally the accessibility of digital assistants.

8   Conclusions

Voice-based interaction with technology has grown immensely over the past decade.
Voice-interaction is here to stay. As it stands, voice-based interaction is largely
inaccessible to individuals with atypical speech—whether it's from a speech or
voice disorder. Speech and voice disorders present an accessibility challenge to
voice interfaces now that will grow with their proliferation if steps are not taken
to resolve these barriers.

The root cause of the decreased performance of ASR systems on disordered
speech can be traced to two main problems, insufficient data, and insufficient
modeling techniques. These root problems can be exploited to start developing
solutions that will lead to more inclusive voice-based technologies.

This chapter provides a brief introduction to the applicable area of acoustics and
phonetics as they apply to disorder-robust ASR, as well as an overview of the field
of ASR.

To provide scaffolding for other disordered speech recognition research to stand
upon, this chapter presents a new nomenclature for the field of disorder-robust
ASR systems. Terms introduced include a new characterization of ASR systems concerning how the system deals with voice disorders—*disorder-dependent*,
disorder-independent, or *disorder adaptive*—as well as a new scaffold of different

kinds of tasks in ASR based on the type (implicit or explicit) and amount of noise in the data. This segmentation of the field allows relevant methods established in one level to be passed up and applied to other levels that present more noise.

Using this new leveling guide, this chapter explores common modeling techniques in each level ASR task, leading to an exploration of the field of noise-robust ASR systems as well as disorder-robust ASR systems, and a projection into the future of noisy-disordered speech recognition.

After establishing this new nomenclature and fitting some of the more relevant previous works into this system, this chapter then describes the humble library of disordered speech datasets, as well as the goals, advantages, and disadvantages of using each dataset.

Then, after a thorough discussion of the field of disorder-robust ASR systems, this chapter goes on to discuss the utility and applications of disorder-robust ASR in the fields of clinical metrics, voice assistive technologies as well as the general improvement of everyday voice-based technologies.

References

1. Alsulaiman, M.: Voice pathology assessment systems for dysphonic patients: detection, classification, and speech recognition. IETE J. Res. **60**(2), 156–167 (2014)
2. Aronson, A.E., Bless, D.M.: Clinical Voice Disorders. Thieme Publishers Series. Thieme (2009)
3. Bhattacharyya, N.: The prevalence of voice problems among adults in the united states. Laryngoscope **124**(10), 2359–2362 (2014)
4. Biadsy, F., Weiss, R.J., Moreno, P.J., Kanvesky, D., Jia, Y.: Parrotron: an end-to-end speech-to-speech conversion model and its applications to hearing-impaired speech and speech separation. In: Proc. Interspeech 2019, pp. 4115–4119 (2019)
5. Browman, C.P., Goldstein, L.: Articulatory phonology: an overview. Phonetica **49**(3–4), 155–180 (1992)
6. Burfin, S., Pascalis, O., Tada, E.R., Costa, A., Savariaux, C., Kandel, S.: Bilingualism affects audiovisual phoneme identification. Front. Psychol. **5**, 1179 (2014)
7. Chen, C.-Y., Zheng, W.-Z., Wang, S.-S., Tsao, Y., Li, P.-C., Lai, Y.-H.: Enhancing intelligibility of dysarthric speech using gated convolutional-based voice conversion system. In: Proc. Interspeech 2020, pp. 4686–4690 (2020)
8. Chin, T.-W., Zhang, C., Marculescu, D.: Improving the adversarial robustness of transfer learning via noisy feature distillation (2020). ArXiv, abs/2002.02998
9. Christensen, H., Cunningham, S.P., Fox, C., Green, P., Hain, T.: A comparative study of adaptive, automatic recognition of disordered speech. In: INTERSPEECH (2012)
10. Dahan, D., Drucker, S.J., Scarborough, R.A.: Talker adaptation in speech perception: adjusting the signal or the representations? Cognition **108**(3), 710–718 (2008)
11. Denisov, P., Thang Vu, N., Ferras, M.: Unsupervised domain adaptation by adversarial learning for robust speech recognition (2018). ArXiv, abs/1807.11284
12. Dupont, S., Luettin, J.: Audio-visual speech modeling for continuous speech recognition. IEEE Trans. Multimedia **2**(3), 141–151 (2000)
13. Eadie, T.L., Doyle, P.C.: Classification of dysphonic voice: acoustic and auditory-perceptual measures. J. Voice **19**(1), 1–14 (2005)
14. Enderby, P.M.: Frenchay Dysarthria Assessment. College-Hill Press, San Diego (1983). Includes index

15. Frankel, J., King, S.: Asr-articulatory speech recognition. In: Seventh European Conference on Speech Communication and Technology (2001)
16. Fujinaga, K., Nakai, M., Shimodaira, H., Sagayama, S.: Multiple-regression hidden markov model. In: 2001 IEEE International Conference on Acoustics, Speech, and Signal Processing. Proceedings (Cat. No. 01CH37221), vol. 1, pp. 513–516. IEEE, Piscataway (2001)
17. Greenberg, S., Ainsworth, W.A.: Speech processing in the auditory system: an overview. In: Speech Processing in the Auditory System, pp. 1–62. Springer (2004)
18. Hawley, M.S.: Speech recognition as an input to electronic assistive technology. Br. J. Occup. Ther. **65**(1), 15–20 (2002)
19. Hsu, W., Zhang, Y., Glass, J.: Unsupervised domain adaptation for robust speech recognition via variational autoencoder-based data augmentation. In: 2017 IEEE Automatic Speech Recognition and Understanding Workshop (ASRU), pp. 16–23 (2017)
20. Hu, H., Tan, T., Qian, T.: Generative adversarial networks based data augmentation for noise robust speech recognition. In: 2018 IEEE International Conference on Acoustics, Speech and Signal Processing (ICASSP), pp. 5044–5048 (2018)
21. Huang, J., Kingsbury, B.: Audio-visual deep learning for noise robust speech recognition. In: 2013 IEEE International Conference on Acoustics, Speech and Signal Processing, pp. 7596–7599. IEEE, Piscataway (2013)
22. Hunt, M.J.: Delayed decisions in speech recognition–the case of formants. Pattern Recogn. Lett. **6**(2), 121–137 (1987)
23. Keintz, C.K., Bunton, K., Hoit, J.D.: Influence of visual information on the intelligibility of dysarthric speech. Am. J. Speech Lang. Pathol. (2007)
24. Kent, R.D., Weismer, G., Kent, J.F., Rosenbek, J.C.: Toward phonetic intelligibility testing in dysarthria. J. Speech Hearing Disorders **54**(4), 482–499 (1989)
25. Kim, H., Hasegawa-Johnson, M., Perlman, A., Gunderson, J., Huang, T.S., Watkin, K., Frame, S.: Dysarthric speech database for universal access research. In: Interspeech, vol. 2008, pp. 1741–1744 (2008)
26. King, S., Frankel, J., Livescu, K., McDermott, E., Richmond, K., Wester, M.: Speech production knowledge in automatic speech recognition. J. Acoust. Soc. Am. **121**(2), 723–742 (2007)
27. Kitzing, P., Maier, A., Åhlander, V.L.: Automatic speech recognition (ASR) and its use as a tool for assessment or therapy of voice, speech, and language disorders. Logopedics Phoniatrics Vocology **34**(2), 91–96 (2009)
28. Lee, L., Stemple, J.C., Glaze, L., Kelchner, L.N.: Quick screen for voice and supplementary documents for identifying pediatric voice disorders. Lang. Speech Hearing Serv. Sch. **35**(4), 308–319 (2004)
29. Liu, S., Hu, S., Wang, Y., Yu, J., Su, R., Liu, X., Meng, H.: Exploiting visual features using bayesian gated neural networks for disordered speech recognition. In: INTERSPEECH, pp. 4120–4124 (2019)
30. Maier, A., Haderlein, T., Stelzle, F., Nöth, E., Nkenke, E., Rosanowski, F., Schützenberger, A., Schuster, M.: Automatic speech recognition systems for the evaluation of voice and speech disorders in head and neck cancer. EURASIP J. Audio Speech Music Process. **2010**(1), 926951 (2009)
31. Mayo, C., Aubanel, V., Cooke, M.: Effect of prosodic changes on speech intelligibility. Thirteenth Annual Conference of the international Speech Communication Association, (2012) http://www.isca-speech.org/archive/interspeech_2012/i12_1708.html
32. McGurk, H., MacDonaldJ.: Hearing lips and seeing voices. Nature **264**(5588), 746–748 (1976)
33. Menendez-Pidal, X., Polikoff, J.B., Peters, S.M., Leonzio, J.E., Bunnell, H.T.: The nemours database of dysarthric speech. In: Proceeding of Fourth International Conference on Spoken Language Processing. ICSLP '96, vol. 3, pp. 1962–1965 (1996)
34. Mengistu, K.T., Rudzicz, F.: Comparing humans and automatic speech recognition systems in recognizing dysarthric speech. In: Canadian Conference on Artificial Intelligence, pp. 291–300. Springer, Berlin (2011)
35. Milner, B., Shao, X.: Speech reconstruction from mel-frequency cepstral coefficients using a source-filter model. In: Seventh International Conference on Spoken Language Processing (2002)

36. Miyamoto, C., Komai, Y., Takiguchi, T., Ariki, Y., Li, I.: Multimodal speech recognition of a person with articulation disorders using AAM and MAF. In: 2010 IEEE International Workshop on Multimedia Signal Processing, pp. 517–520. IEEE, Piscataway (2010)
37. Moore, M.: "I'm Having Trouble Understanding You Right Now": A Multi-Dimensional Evaluation of the Intelligibility of Dysphonic Speech. PhD thesis, Arizona State University, 2020
38. Moore, M., Venkateswara, H., Panchanathan, S.: Whistle-blowing ASRs: evaluating the need for more inclusive automatic speech recognition systems. In: Proceedings of the Annual Conference of the International Speech Communication Association, INTERSPEECH, vol. 2018, pp. 466–470 (2018)
39. Moore, M., Papreja, P., Saxon, M., Berisha, V., Panchanathan, S.: UncommonVoice: a crowdsourced dataset of dysphonic speech. In: Proc. Interspeech 2020, pp. 2532–2536 (2020)
40. Muhammad, G., Alsulaiman, M., Mahmood, A., Ali, Z.: Automatic voice disorder classification using vowel formants. In: 2011 IEEE International Conference on Multimedia and Expo, pp. 1–6. IEEE, Piscataway (2011)
41. National Institute of Deafness and Other Communication Disorders (NIDCD). Statistics of voice speech and language disorders. National Institute on Deafness and Other Communication Disorders Fact Sheets (2016)
42. Nefian, A.V., Liang, L., Pi, X., Xiaoxiang, L., Mao, C., Murphy, K.: A coupled HMM for audio-visual speech recognition. In: 2002 IEEE International Conference on Acoustics, Speech, and Signal Processing, vol. 2, pp. II–2013. IEEE, Piscataway (2002)
43. Nicolao, M., Christensen, H., Cunningham, S., Green, P., Hain, T.: A framework for collecting realistic recordings of dysarthric speech - the homeService corpus. In: Proceedings of the Tenth International Conference on Language Resources and Evaluation (LREC'16), pages 1993–1997, Portorož, Slovenia, May 2016. European Language Resources Association (ELRA)
44. Ninomiya, H., Kitaoka, N., Tamura, S., Iribe, Y., Takeda, K.: Integration of deep bottleneck features for audio-visual speech recognition. In: Sixteenth annual conference of the international speech communication association (2015)
45. Noda, K., Yamaguchi, Y., Nakadai, K., Okuno, H.G., Ogata, T.: Audio-visual speech recognition using deep learning. Appl. Intell. 42(4), 722–737 (2015)
46. Ogar, T., Slama, H., Dronkers, N., Amici, S., Gorno-Tempini, M.L.: Apraxia of speech: an overview. Neurocase 11(6), 427–432 (2005)
47. Panchanathan, S., Chakraborty, S., McDaniel, T.: Social interaction assistant: A person-centered approach to enrich social interactions for individuals with visual impairments. IEEE J. Sel. Top. Signal Process. 10(5), 942–951 (2016)
48. Qian, Y., Hu, H., Tan, T.: Data augmentation using generative adversarial networks for robust speech recognition. Speech Commun. 114, 1–9 (2019)
49. Rudzicz, F., Namasivayam, A.K., Wolff, T.: The torgo database of acoustic and articulatory speech from speakers with dysarthria. Lang. Resour. Eval. 46(4), 523–541 (2012)
50. Sakar, B.E., Isenkul, M.E., Sakar, C.O., Sertbas, A., Gurgen, F., Delil, S., Apaydin, H., Kursun, O.: Collection and analysis of a parkinson speech dataset with multiple types of sound recordings. IEEE J. Biomed. Health Inf. 17(4), 828–834 (2013)
51. Saon, G., Chien, J.: Large-vocabulary continuous speech recognition systems: A look at some recent advances. IEEE Signal Process. Mag. 29(6), 18–33 (2012)
52. Shahnaz, C., Zhu, W., Ahmad, M.O.: A new technique for the estimation of jitter and shimmer of voiced speech signal. In: 2006 Canadian Conference on Electrical and Computer Engineering, pp. 2112–2115 (2006, May)
53. Sheng, P., Yang, Z., Qian, Y.: Gans for children: A generative data augmentation strategy for children speech recognition. In: 2019 IEEE Automatic Speech Recognition and Understanding Workshop (ASRU), pp. 129–135 (2019)
54. Shivakumar, P.G., Georgiou, P.: Transfer learning from adult to children for speech recognition: evaluation, analysis and recommendations. Comput. Speech Lang. 63, 101077 (2020)

55. Smith, D., Sneddon, A., Ward, L., Duenser, A., Freyne, J., Silvera-Tawil, D., Morgan, A.: Improving child speech disorder assessment by incorporating out-of-domain adult speech. In: Proc. Interspeech 2017, pp. 2690–2694 (2017)

56. Teixeira, J.P., Fernandes, P.O.: Acoustic analysis of vocal dysphonia. Procedia Comput. Sci. **64**, 466–473 (2015). Conference on ENTERprise Information Systems/International Conference on Project MANagement/Conference on Health and Social Care Information Systems and Technologies, CENTERIS/ProjMAN / HCist 2015 October 7–9, 2015

57. Tremblay, S., Shiller, D.M., Ostry, D.J.: Somatosensory basis of speech production. Nature **423**(6942), 866–869 (2003)

58. Vachhani, B., Bhat, C., Kopparapu, S.K.: Data augmentation using healthy speech for dysarthric speech recognition. In: Proc. Interspeech 2018, pp. 471–475 (2018)

59. Venkateswara, H., Panchanathan, S.: Introduction to Domain Adaptation, pp. 3–21. Springer International Publishing, Cham (2020)

60. Walshe, M., Miller, N., Leahy, M., Murray, A.: Intelligibility of dysarthric speech: perceptions of speakers and listeners. Int. J. Lang. Commun. Disord. **43**(6), 633–648 (2008)

61. Wilkinson, N.J., Russell, M.J.: Improved phone recognition on TIMIT using formant frequency data and confidence measures. In: Seventh International Conference on Spoken Language Processing (2002)

62. Yumoto, E., Gould, W.J., Baer, T.: Harmonicsâtoânoise ratio as an index of the degree of hoarseness. J. Acoust. Soc. Am. **71**(6), 1544–1550 (1982)

Socially Assistive Robots for Storytelling and Other Activities to Support Aging in Place

Jordan Miller and Troy McDaniel

Abstract This chapter addresses how socially assistive robots can assist older adults as they age in place. When examining challenges with aging in place, isolation is found across all locations a person chooses to grow old. Isolation arises due to a reduction in social network, reduction in the amount of time spent outside the home, or lack of social contact. We examine different technological solutions to assist older adults who decide to age inside their home and how they can be used to keep individuals safe. We then examine different systems to help older adults connect to their community and solutions to address isolation. Finally, we explore socially assistive robots and how they are being used to assist older adults. We feel socially assistive robotics will become increasingly popular as advancements in natural language processing are made which will allow robots to converse naturally with their users.

Keywords Aging in place · Gerontechnology · Socially assistive robots · Older adults

1 Introduction

People around the world are living longer as modern medicine progresses [3]. According to 2019 news reports, couples are waiting longer in life to have children or not having them at all [26]. By 2050, it is expected that there will be 9.3 billion people on Earth with 2 billion people aged 65 or older [63]. These trends together have created a population shift. This shift will create novel problems around the world due to insufficient numbers of medical professionals entering the field to care

J. Miller
Arizona State University, Tempe, AZ, USA
e-mail: jlmill41@asu.edu

T. McDaniel (✉)
Arizona State University, Mesa, AZ, USA
e-mail: troy.mcdaniel@asu.edu

© The Author(s), under exclusive license to Springer Nature Switzerland AG 2021
T. McDaniel, X. Liu (eds.), *Multimedia for Accessible Human Computer Interfaces*,
https://doi.org/10.1007/978-3-030-70716-3_6

145

for older adults [34]. It is predicted that by 2020 there will be a shortage of nearly two million healthcare workers [63]. Robots can be used to fill this gap and assist healthcare workers in their daily activities [45].

There is a growing interest in placing technology in homes to make them "smart" to automate or assist with many aspects of daily life, including assisting older adults with remaining inside their homes for as long as possible. Smart home infrastructure often includes a multitude of sensors found throughout the house, from on the stove to alert when left on too long, to on windows to alert when left opened. Examples of other devices include smart thermostats and the now ubiquitous robot vacuum. These technologies can significantly reduce the workload inside the home, decreasing the burden of household chores, which often become more difficult and dangerous with age. Safety features allow individuals aging inside their home and their loved ones to often feel more at ease due to alerts when an abnormal situation arises, e.g., a faucet in the bathroom was left on for an unusual amount of time, or the front door was opened during the early morning hours. By allowing older adults to remain safe and healthy in their own home, the burden on understaffed healthcare workers will be lifted and their time can be better served assisting older adults who need more assistance.

The CDC defines aging in place as a person spending the remainder of his or her days in the dwelling of his or her choosing [25]. When choosing where to age in place, a person can choose from a variety of locations. These include their own home, an assisted living facility, a nursing home or a loved one's home. However, many people desire to stay inside their own homes instead of moving due to the memories associated with their homes or the stigma associated with care facilities [65]. Clarity surveyed 804 seniors currently not living in care facilities and 89% said it is very important to them to remain inside their homes [11]. Clarity then asked about their greatest fears, and 13% said they feared transitioning into a nursing home and 3% fear dying [11]. The location a person chooses to age in is often the same location he or she will parish. Therefore, it is paramount to design technologies for assisting older adults in a way that ensures they can maintain comfort and safety in their homes for as long as possible.

Each of these locations offer a set of challenges to address along with common hurdles shared by all locations. When people choose to age inside their homes, they believe they are sufficiently healthy to stay or they have made changes in the home to address common safety concerns. The most common changes include making floors flush, adding grab bars to the shower and toilet, fixing loose carpet, and repairing broken stair rails [68]. These issues can be easily addressed; however, not all challenges include a simple solution. Many older adults choose to age in place in a home that is outdated and not ideal for aging. Common features representative of these houses include two-story homes, not having a bedroom and bathroom on the first floor, and narrow doorways [14]. Clarity reports 75% of the adults surveyed are "very or somewhat concerned" about their health if they choose to remain inside the home and 55% are "very or somewhat concerned" about other safety and security issues [11]. Technology can assist the elderly who are aging at home to feel safe and secure while empowering a healthier old age.

Finances are a challenge in all locations people choose to age. Seniors who struggle with finances are incapable of making significant changes to accommodate their homes for safety, or they require support from a long-term care facility but are unable to afford it [14]. Many seniors who are "very or somewhat concerned" about the safety features of their homes will be unable to afford repairs and will ultimately live in an unsafe environment.

Pearson et al. [53] predict that by 2029, there will be 14.4 million seniors classified in the middle income class. Middle income seniors do not qualify for Medicare assistance and do not have the financial means to afford long-term care. Pearson et al. report around 80% of middle income seniors will need assistance, but 54% of this group will be incapable of affording care or receiving support.

The middle class will be incapable of upgrading their homes, and therefore be unable to bring property values high enough to cover long-term care. Knowing most seniors struggle with affording the care they need, technologist should deliberately implement low-cost, accessible solutions. Developing low-cost smart home solutions will ensure seniors are safe wherever they choose to age and can continue to live independently.

The second challenge found in all locations is isolation. Isolation is caused from being separated from others [17]. Isolation can arise when a person retires, loses friends, or becomes unable to attend social functions due to limited mobility. Mobility issues can be permanent or temporary, such as arthritis or a condition that can be remedied through a surgical procedure. Regardless, a person's mobility will be impacted. In cases where surgery is an option, depending on the severity of the condition, a person may never regain his or her full mobility.

Isolation can cause severe effects on a person's health and has been compared to smoking [13]. Santini et al. [61] report that isolation can have adverse consequences on a person's health including depression, poor sleep, cognitive decline, and eventually lead to premature death. Social disconnectedness predicts perceived isolation which correlates to feeling depressed and having anxiety. Isolation can quicken the aging of the brain, which can lead to needing assistance around the home or, in extreme cases, require a person to move into a long-term care facility. However, an individual may be unable to afford a long-term care facility if he or she is in the middle class income bracket, leaving the person aging inside an unsafe environment and unable to receive care.

Pearson et al. report that by 2029, most seniors will have fewer family caregivers due to individuals having less children which will increase the burden on younger family members [53]. Today's caregivers face challenges with finances, physical health, and mental health [30]. When fewer family caregivers are available to care for loved ones, new difficulties will be encountered by families. Younger family members may be unable to care for their older relatives due to couples waiting longer to have children, which might correspond with the age their parent would need assistance. This will leave adult children unable to care for their parents due to having young children at home who require attention. Additionally, a couple may have inadequate space or finances to support moving their aged family member into their home, leaving older adults aging in unsafe environments where isolation will only become more prevalent.

Social robots have the potential to address feelings of isolation to support aging in place. Surveys have explored what older adults think about robots and their preferences and views of technology. An important finding is that older adults are willing to accept robots for assistance [5, 7, 20]. Forlizzi et al. [20] call attention to products not being aesthetically pleasing, but Moyle et al. [49] notice that aesthetics are hardly taken into consideration when designing robotic applications. Older adults prefer a physical robot over a digital assistant for socializing due to feeling more engaged with the robot. Often, robots are designed to communicate using non-verbal cues to let users know they are being listened to, as opposed to digital assistants, which usually display a light to convey attention [6]. Robots developed to assist older adults do not need to resemble humans; older adults tend to associate the purpose of robots to providing assistance rather than focus on robots being lifelike [7]. Another design consideration is limiting how much robots move when users interacts with them; too much movement can hinder the user experience [55]. As social robots become more accepted, it is essential to understand the design features seniors want, otherwise, these users could be deterred from accepting new technology as a social companion.

Social robots have the potential to assist not only seniors, but also formal and informal caregivers. When designing technology to aid caregiving, consideration should be given to features that would make the jobs of caregivers both easier and less stressful. Broadbent et al. [7] report that caregivers desire robots to measure emotional levels, such as sadness. Caregivers expressed that a social robot should look different compared to a robot used for physical assistance. For example, a social robot should have a face, but no arms due to its main purpose of companionship. On the other hand, a robot to assist with physical labor, such as lifting people, should have arms, but no face since its purpose is to decrease the physical stress on a caregiver.

Caregivers expressed wanting robots to assist with routine tasks. Common tasks that have been identified are: taking blood pressure, monitoring the patient, and/or assisting the staff while not taking their jobs [7]. Enabling robots to assist caregivers in their daily routines will decrease workload. Robots have the potential to alleviate the caregiver gap by making interactions between caregivers and individuals more impactful. The remaining sections of this chapter include the following.

Section 2: Technology to Assist with Aging in Place provides an overview of existing technology to assist older adults who chose to age inside their homes. The technologies being developed are aimed at smart homes, and include various sensors embedded within houses for monitoring purposes. This section covers smart home technologies, systems to encourage fitness, and other devices to increase safety. Next-generation smart home safety features will allow older generations to stay inside their home longer and provide comfort to the individual and their family members.

Section 3: Technology for Communication provides an overview of technological solutions, both commercially-available systems and research prototypes, to address isolation including video calling, robotic pets, and haptic devices to support interpersonal interaction from a distance. These technologies are designed to make seniors feel connected with the world outside their homes. These devices are particularly beneficial to older adults with mobility issues or who live far from family members.

Section 4: Robots for Communication provides an overview of social robotics to overcome isolation. Most state-of-the-art robots include conversational capabilities, but most users desire more complex dialog interactions. Previous solutions are examined along with the current state-of-the-art. Finally, a discussion is provided on where the field is heading and how these technologies can assist with aging in place and address the problem of isolation.

2 Technology to Assist with Aging in Place

Technology is being developed to keep seniors at home longer while helping them stay safe. These technologies rely on the Internet of Things (IoT) using sensors throughout the home to monitor a resident and detect anomalies in daily routines including dangerous situations such as the risk of fire from leaving the oven or stove on too long. Clarity found that 65% of seniors are open and willing to use new technology, and 54% of people surveyed would consider using ambient monitoring technology inside the home [11].

Technology developers should remember that seniors are *willing* to try these technologies; however, *this does not mean they will continue to use a device if they feel their privacy is being violated.* Ensuring technology has high standards for privacy and does not make individuals feel they are being "watched" will be essential to adoption and long-term use. Individuals should be able to turn off a system whenever they are uncomfortable; this will ensure users feel and remain in control of their homes and lives. Being unable to control a device may make people feel that they are being forced into a lifestyle they do not desire. This may be why almost half of the individuals surveyed are hesitant about monitoring technologies, even though such devices would keep them in their homes longer. Research to better understand why almost half of seniors are unwilling to place these technologies inside their homes needs to be conducted so that we may begin to address these concerns.

2.1 Smart Homes and Safety

Smart Homes can enable older adults who are aging inside their homes to feel safe and connected to the outside world. Technology can detect falls and alert authorities, or a designated caregiver, that someone inside the home needs assistance. These same features can be used to assist stroke survivors or even detect a stroke as soon as it happens, enabling doctors to provide immediate care. Additionally, these homes can monitor a person with early stages of dementia and track the progression of the disease to allow interventions when necessary. Such processes will help keep a person inside his or her home as long as possible, reducing (1) time spent inside a care facility; (2) time an informal caregiver must spend caring for a loved one; and (3) money spent for care. Moreover, these processes will allow individuals living with dementia to maintain independence, increasing their sense of dignity for as long as possible.

Smart Homes often have features which can assist individuals with mobility impairments. Examples include the Roomba vacuum, using Samsung's smart plug to make devices voice-activated, the Ring doorbell, and the Nest thermostat. All of these devices can be used to assist an individual around the home through an app accessed on the phone. Evidence has been found, however, that older adults prefer technology to perform multiple tasks [20].

Intille et al. [28] developed a low-cost system to allow people to control their environment and create customized solutions for their specific needs by placing sensors along a roll of tape. Machine learning models were trained to learn daily routines to be able to recognize abnormal behavior. Upon detection of abnormal behavior, the system alerts a designated individual via a message. This early work shows the potential of sensors deployed in the home setting to facilitate the learning of daily routines of seniors. For example, if a person turns the bedroom light on around 7 AM everyday, the algorithm would recognize the absence of such a routine event as an outlier, and subsequently alert the specified individual about the abnormal behavior.

Kaye et al. [35] developed an at-home assessment tool to assist older adults who desire to age inside their homes. They report being the first to deploy hundreds of sensors into homes to track: frequency of ambulation, walking speed, and time spent in each room. The study took place over 2 years with 265 participants. Participants were asked to complete a weekly report on how often they fell. Kaye et al. hypothesized that the average reported number of falls each year is low due to seniors forgetting about falls in-between doctors visits. The results found were consistent with this hypothesis, reporting an annual fall rate 43% higher than the national average of 30%. At-home assessment tools can be utilized by doctors and medical staff to keep track of patients they do not see regularly. Such systems can allow medical staff to access weekly reports to determine if an individual needs an appointment sooner than originally planned, or to cancel unneeded appointments. This technology has the potential to allow doctors to track the progression of a disease on a weekly basis to determine how fast the condition is advancing and what kinds of intervention should take place and how often.

Rantz et al. [58] developed an in-home system to facilitate communication between individuals aging in place and their medical staff to detect early signs of illness. Sensors were placed on the stove, bed, and chairs. Pulse-Doppler Radar was used to detect falls and assess the risk of falling in individuals which can be an indicator of early signs of illness. This technology was aimed at assisting the oldest of the elderly who insist on living alone and do not require around the clock care.

By detecting falls, the system has the potential to bring attention to possible early illnesses which could be fatal at an older age.

Demir et al. [16] deployed sensors around the homes of adults living with dementia to detect half-completed tasks and alert a designated person when detected. The objective of this research was to test a prototype to assist people living with dementia who were unable to age inside a care facility. Sensors were chosen to avoid invading personal privacy. Four different types of sensors were placed throughout the home in the kitchen, the bedroom, the bathroom, and on the toilet. The sensors detected when a device was turned on but not turned off. The prototype was successful in detecting half-completed tasks. This technology can permit an individual living with dementia to continue to age inside his or her home as long as possible. By alerting caregivers and doctors of half-completed tasks, the progression of conditions may be better tracked, and more informed decisions can be made regarding the type of intervention needed. By making a better decision, the family can save money by paying for temporary in-home care and make adjustments along the way to better serve their loved one. Figures 1 and 2 depict an older woman leaving the stove on for an extended time.

Enshaeifar et al. [19] placed sensors in the home of a person living with dementia to alert medical professionals when something is abnormal. Sensors were placed in hallways, the living room, the kitchen, and on the doors to the bedroom and bathroom. The sensors allowed doctors to assess the location of the person inside the home. Additional sensors were used to monitor blood pressure, heart rate, and temperature, and alert a doctor early in case of any complications. Detecting early issues can save a person's life in extreme situations or prevent a situation from escalating. Many people living with dementia struggle with sundowners symptoms, which can cause paranoia at night and even lead to wandering outside the home. If an increase in blood pressure and heart rate is detected at night, doctors can intervene and attempt to calm the individual or send someone for assistance. If a

Fig. 1 Older woman leaving the kitchen with the stove on

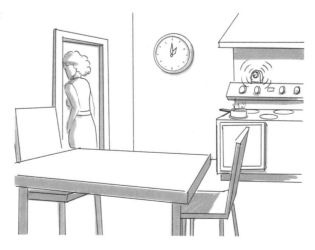

Fig. 2 Designated person
receiving text message

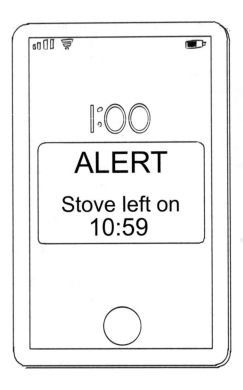

person wanders outside the home, the system can detect that he or she is not inside the home and send an alert.

Rostill et al. [60] augmented the homes of people living with dementia and their caregivers. The technology detected high blood pressure, low pulse rate, dehydration, becoming lost, amount of sleep, and amount of movement. A total of 408 people participated in the study. Half of the people received the system and the other half did not. Results from the study found all 204 people who received the technology welcomed it into their homes and reported that it was successful in assisting them. This finding allows technologist to understand what features should be included in a smart home environment for a person living with dementia and how to generalize such technological solutions to healthy older adults. Such systems should also be tested on other illnesses such as Parkinson's disease to explore efficacy, acceptance, and reactions. Rostill et al. have provided a strong foundation for future smart home technologies.

High heat can lead to health complications for older adults; yet few seniors trust the recommendations from the American National Weather Service to lower air conditioning when it is hot. Guo et al. [24] believe this mistrust is due to systems making recommendations the elderly do not see as applicable. Guo et al. are developing a sweating robot to indicate high levels of heat and encourage older adults to turn down the temperature. They believe this robot will introduce a level of trust seniors do not have in the National Weather Service. The robot communicates the temperature through sweating and releasing a scent to encourage seniors to decrease the temperature. These actions are universal to every language and culture making the robot easily adaptable to different regions worldwide.

Broadbent et al. [8] conducted a study using the RoboGen medicine management system to remind older adults to take their medication. RoboGen is designed to assist users with maintaining their own medication and health; however, the medication management system was found to be limited in terms of user friendliness. Broadbent et al.'s study aimed to evaluate the difference between RoboGen and a revised version called RoboGen2, designed to improve usability. Changes included a reduction in the number of clicks needed to complete tasks, changing labels with medical terminology, and a word completion feature that reduced the need for users to remember the full name of medications. Forty participants were recruited from a university campus. Participants were asked to enter prescriptions into both systems to compare which was easier to use. It was found that significantly more participants preferred the new system rather than the old one. Broadbent et al. reported that in RoboGen, numerous spellings of one medication were listed, sometimes with different dosage amounts. When older adults trust auto-generated recommendations, discrepancies could lead to taking more than the prescribed amount of medication, causing complications.

2.2 Technologies to Encourage Fitness

Exercise games, also known as exergames, are being explored to aid older adults in need of physical exercise or therapy, such as stroke survivors. Exergames allow users to perform task-specific exercises with personalized levels of difficulty. Exergames have been found to be beneficial to older adults, especially those who have limited mobility or cannot leave their home to go a local gym. Additionally, physical therapy at home can reduce costs and allow exercise to continue after or beyond outpatient rehabilitation.

Chen et al. [9] explored robots for assisting older adults with dancing to promote physical activity. Findings from a study revealed that participants enjoyed dancing with a robot and shared they would go out of their way to engage with robots in situations where they could learn new dance moves. Such an application has potential in care facilities to encourage fitness or physical therapy. Moreover, this application may encourage socialization between residents inside a home by improving dance skills and motivating dancing between residents.

Games are enabling older adults to exercise at home and within limited ranges of motion. Gerling et al. [21] developed a game which engages users in the process of growing plants. The game uses familiar movements such as raising arms straight above the body or out to the sides of the body. This example demonstrates how exergames can be used for physical therapy after required inpatient/outpatient sessions end. Exergames can often be customized in terms of controls and difficulty, and is a promising augmentation to gym visits. Common exercises range from strength training to improving balance and stability.

Fitness trackers can help older adults stay active longer as they age in place. Cooper et al. [12] report that most older adults are willing to use an activity tracker; however, the features of fitness devices are largely inaccessible to seniors. For older adults to successfully use these trackers, buttons and screens should be larger; wearables should be comfortable; and devices should provide continuous feedback. Fitness trackers can encourage users to be more active by allowing them to track progress. These devices work particularly well when progress can be monitored by clinicians and therapists to enable assessment of adherence to prescribed exercise.

Keizer et al. [36] used the NAO robot to train older adults through monitored exercise. The exercises were performed by mimicking a NAO robot. Future work is needed before this technology can be deployed on a larger scale, but overall user reaction to the robot was positive. Issues arose when interacting with the robot using speech. The main issues included: people often did not speak loud enough for NAO to hear them; some users could not hear NAO; and sometimes users interrupted NAO. Such a robotic application could be deployed into care facilities for use in group settings, which would allow the care staff to monitor all individuals at once and encourage socialization among residents. Mimicking NAO could encourage participation and even allow residents to enjoy attending physical therapy sessions.

Lotfi et al. [41] developed a robot capable of coaching individuals through exercises while providing feedback on performance. The robot was made from an iPad attached to the frame of a Double robot. A Microsoft Kinect was used to detect users. The robot was capable of determining whether a user is performing the prescribed workout correctly. Feedback was delivered through facial expressions and audio. If a workout is being performed incorrectly, visual feedback is displayed to provide guidance on how to adjust performance. Participants reported being satisfied with the product and expressed interest in using the device outside of the research study.

Piezzo et al. [54] used a Pepper robot, seen in Fig. 3, as a gait trainer for seniors. Their goal was to deploy Pepper into nursing homes to assist nurses with their daily routines and encourage interaction between patients. Pepper was capable of observing a person's gait to monitor balance, encouraging more ambulation, and providing guidance to a specific location. Encouragement was given via positive verbal praise. The screen on the torso of Pepper displayed the number of steps taken and the number of steps remaining to reach a goal. For this study, Pepper was operated via the Wizard of Oz approach to allow a deeper understanding of the acceptance of Pepper as a walking partner. All users preferred to walk behind Pepper, as opposed to follow at its side, feeling the robot served as a coach or guide. This application is useful for care facilities and hospitals. Often after surgery, nurses walk with patients to increase blood flow to reduce chances of clotting. Having Pepper supervise these walks, nursing staff can tend to other patients who may have more critical conditions.

Karunarathne et al. [33] used the Robovie-R3 robot, seen in Fig. 4, to evaluate older adults' acceptance of a robot-based walking partner. In this experiment,

Fig. 3 Pepper

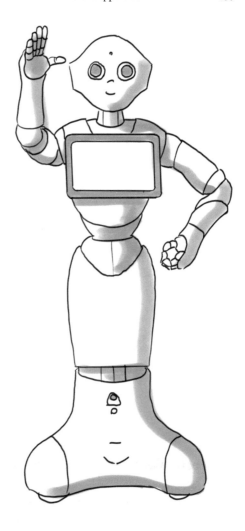

Karunarathne et al. recruited 20 participants to walk with Robovie-R3. All experiments happened outside on a university campus. Eighteen of the twenty participants sustained a side-by-side formation, but seven subjects eventually walked slightly in front of the robot. Two participants walked faster than Robovie-R3 leaving it behind. Five participants looked at the robot when walking with it and the remaining fifteen did not look at it. This study contradicts the previous study completed by Piezzo et al. where they found that the participants did not want to walk side-by-side with the robot. The differences in these findings could be related to the demographics of recruited participants. Karunarathne et al. did not specify whether older adults who require assistance were recruited; on the other hand, Piezzo et al. tested their robot inside a care facility. The variations in results highlight the importance of testing technology on a wide range of individuals to gain a general understanding of how to assist the older adult demographic.

Fig. 4 Robovie-R3

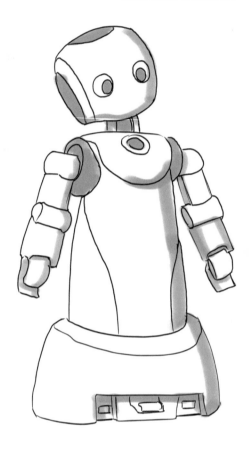

3   Technology for Communication

Today, there are countless technologies to facilitate communication between people
including smart phones, Web applications, social media, Amazon's Alex Show for
video interaction, among many others. More recent cutting-edge research prototypes
or commercial products include haptic devices to support interpersonal interaction
at a distance; robotic pets to decrease isolation; and telepresence robots often called
"Skype on Wheels". The previously mentioned devices have the potential to aid
older adults hoping to age in place; however, seniors are not usually tech savvy,
which can reduce their willingness to try and adopt new systems for communication.

Moyle et al. [49] studied the effectiveness of the Giraff telepresence robot inside
a care facility for enabling patients to connect with their loved ones via video-
calling. For example, a Giraff allows a senior to remote into the home of his or
her grandchildren for a birthday party, creating a sense of presence and togetherness
without being physically present. Such technologies can benefit seniors with limited
mobility or who are located in a different state than their family.

The Hug [18] uses haptics to communicate over long distances by simulating the feeling of a hug. The Hug device allows users to have a closed network of individuals they can send "hugs" to along with personalized messages. If the intended recipient does not answer the request, the sender can leave a voice recording. The Hug can be used by long distance families to communicate and provide feelings of connectedness.

Khosravi et al. [38] conducted a review on how older adults are confronting isolation through the use of technology. Khosravi et al. report that 50% of seniors who use the internet and email showed a decrease in feelings of isolation. They concluded that for seniors where no differences were noticed, a possible reason is the lack of extensive internet training. In seven studies reviewed by the survey, robots were used to decrease isolation, and six of these studies showed positive correlation. Other interventions mentioned include the use of video games, telepresence, and virtual reality. These devices demonstrate that technology has the potential to reduce perceived isolation among older adults who are socially isolated.

3.1 Robotic Pets

Robotic pets are being used to address feelings of isolation and increase communication among older adults living with dementia. Pet therapy is an effective method of calming patients; however, this type of intervention can be problematic due to the care and attention needs of real animals. These challenges can be addressed through robotic pets; e.g., Paro, depicted in Fig. 5.

Marti et al. [43] used Paro to help assist with behavioral issues in dementia patients. A therapist decided when to introduce Paro into therapy sessions for the study. Marti et al. reported that one patient's reaction seemed more pronounced compared to the other nine subjects when Paro was introduced. This particular participant had broken a hip and would frequently call out in pain; however, when Paro was introduced, the patient put all his effort into caring for Paro. This behavior allowed the therapist to guide conversations around Paro. This work demonstrates

Fig. 5 Paro

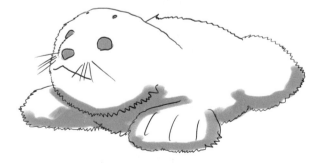

Fig. 6 Joy for All—robotic
pet

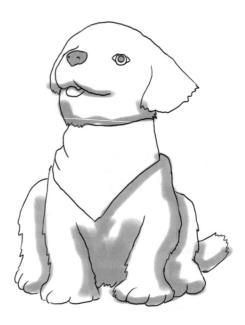

that robotic pets can be used to calm people who are living with dementia. In 2019,
the cost of Paro was $6000 [27].

Moyle et al. [48] conducted a study using Paro, and observed that participants
interacted with Paro much like one might interact with a real animal. Observations
included petting, caring for it, and talking lovingly to Paro. Moyle et al. expressed
the need for a conversational component in robots, noting that such features may be
inappropriate for robotic pets.

Leng et al. [40] conducted a systematic review of groups who had used Paro.
Six articles were reviewed that used Paro to examine behavioral and psychological
symptoms of dementia. Most participants in the studies preferred one-on-one
interaction with the robotic pet instead of group therapy sessions.

Joy for All makes inexpensive robotic pets [31] including a cat, puppy, and kitten,
all of which are commercially available. Figure 6 is an illustration of Joy for All's
robotic puppy. These pets interact with the user by barking or purring when spoken
to and petted. These low-cost solutions work well for older adults who cannot afford
a more expensive companion robot and/or for caregivers looking to increase social
interaction among seniors.

4 Socially Assistive Robots

Social robotics is an emerging field at the confluence of engineering and computer
science due to recent advancements in hardware, artificial intelligence, and robotics.
Most social robots use a simple interface to communicate with users and typically

respond to basic phrases. Social robots are also being used to facilitate specific activities, such as playing music, providing reminders, or challenging users with cognitive games. Limited applications use natural language processing to hold a simple conversation with a user.

Natural language processing (NLP) is a subfield of computer science dedicated to natural language interaction and communication between humans and computers [67]. NLP is still a difficult task for computers to perform: challenges include understanding irony, ambiguity, and vagueness; in other words, humans do not always directly express what they mean. Such issues make it difficult for a computer to have a veridical conversation with a human, but recent advancements are making strides toward this goal. Examples of NLP's progress include the iPhone digital assistant Siri, Amazon's Alexa, Microsoft's Cortana, and Google's digital assistant.

Each of the aforementioned applications listen to the user when instructed via a wake word, and perform a number of tasks such as set timers, send messages, or even tell jokes. In 2018, Google gave a presentation about their digital assistant being able to call and make appointments for their users. While this feature is currently available, not all calls can be completed without human intervention. However, there is consensus among researchers that a breakthrough in NLP is near, which will undoubtedly advance social robotics.

In this section, we discuss early work in the field of social robotics followed by the state-of-the-art from 2015 to 2020. We demonstrate the impact that NLP has had in social robotics.

4.1 Existing Technologies

In a pilot study, Tapus [64] developed an adaptive socially assistive robot called Bandit II. The motivation behind Bandit II is to improve users' cognitive attention through the following task: Bandit II plays a song, which the user must identify by pressing the corresponding button that indicates the song. Such interactions help improve the cognitive ability of seniors and can be used in care facilities to keep seniors' minds sharp.

Kanoh et al. [32] designed a robot to help relieve feelings of isolation and loneliness among older adults through conversation. The robot was tested in small groups with a facilitator and was shown to be capable of asking questions to stimulate conversation. However, many older adults had issues with hearing the robot, causing the facilitator to repeat questions, which led to less interaction between users and the robot. This finding demonstrates the importance of ensuring the voice of the robot is projected loudly and clearly. Many older adults loose hearing with age, therefore, the voice, volume, and capability to repeat phrases must be taken into consideration.

Martín et al. [44] used a NAO robot, shown in Fig. 7, to assist people living with dementia during therapy sessions. NAO engaged older adults through storytelling, music therapy, and by asking a series of prompted questions. Music therapy involved

Fig. 7 NAO

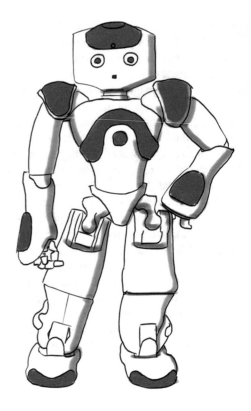

the robot singing and dancing to songs while encouraging patients to dance along. Martín et al. also used NAO to conduct physical therapy sessions consisting of patients mimicking the movements performed by the robot.

Research by Chu et al. [10] tested twin social robots called Jack and Sophie, see Fig. 8, inside four care facilities over a 5 year period from 2010 to 2014. Over this period, Chu et al. had 139 people living with dementia interact with these two robots. The robots were capable of setting reminders, singing songs, playing games, and telling stories. This longitudinal study showed that users enjoyed interacting with Sophie and Jack, and led to improvements in participants' conversational skills. This work demonstrates that social robots can be used to enhance the lives of older adults living with dementia and encourage socialization between residents in a care facility.

Abdollahi et al. [2] developed a companion robot, called Ryan, to interact with older adults living with dementia. Ryan can engage users through facial expressions, conversation, and by reminding users of their schedules. Ryan's torso is a display through which users can peruse a small photo album and play games, music, and videos. Conversations with Ryan include asking users simple questions or telling users a story about a photo selected from the album. Ryan demonstrates the potential

Fig. 8 Jack and Sophie

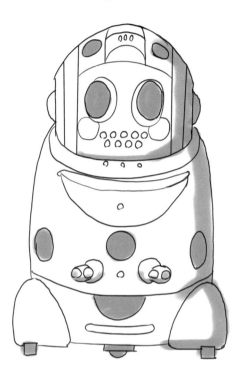

for social robots to be companions capable of carrying out more than one task that older adults prefer.

Portugal et al. [56] piloted a robot capable of navigating a care center for autonomous monitoring. The robot first detects faces, then navigates to users it recognizes. Once the robot approaches a known user, a conversation is initiated, and emotion are detected as the communication progresses. The robot is able to understand a small set of words, so most communication occurs via a touch screen on its torso. Users expressed a desire for the robot to express more speech and dialogue. Portugal et al. used a co-design process to ensure that users felt comfortable and interested in using the robot.

Paletta et al. [52] used Pepper to engage people living with dementia by encouraging exercise, social interaction, and cognitive training. A preliminary study was conducted where participants living with dementia, along with their caregivers, relatives, and trainers, were asked how they felt about using a social robot. All participants were unsure about the use of a social robot, but were interested in trying Pepper. Pepper was then used in a feasibility study where a person stands in front of Pepper and performs an activity. Results showed that people living with dementia are willing to accept social robots for multimodal training. Future work includes implementing a dialogue component for Pepper to motivate users in the next phase of development. This work demonstrates users are willing to accept social robots, especially when they provide different ways to engage the user.

Fig. 9 Eva

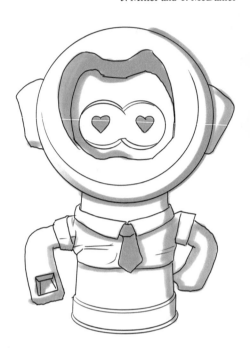

Khosla et al. [37] placed a robot, named Betty, inside the homes of individuals living with dementia. Betty is capable of telling a story, reading the news, providing daily reminders, dancing to songs, and engaging in cognitive games. Users interacted with the robot at least three times a day for 3 months. Four out of five participants reported feeling Betty was a friend. This finding demonstrates that most users will keep interest in companion robots over time, especially if they perform multiple tasks. Such robots can assist a person no matter where they age in place or be used in a hospital setting to keep patients company.

Magyar et al. [42] developed an autonomous dialog system for older adults living with dementia. The robot resembled a baby and was developed to be light to encourage users to hold onto the robot for extended periods of time. The robot assisted users in reducing symptoms of depression. This work builds upon the idea of using social robots to reduce feelings of isolation, and enables designers to focus on more complex conversational strategies.

Cruz-Sandoval et al. [15] developed a robot called Eva, illustrated in Fig. 9, to interact with those living with dementia. Eva is capable of handling simple conversations autonomously, but needs a human operator for more complex interactions. The human operator can change the expression on Eva's face, play songs, and provide customized messages. In a separate study, Cruz et al. reported that participants enjoyed interacting with Eva, and plan to work toward longer conversations with Eva.

Iwabuchi et al. [29] introduced Sota, a robot to reduce behavioral and psychological symptoms in people living with dementia. The robot was inspired by Paro;

Fig. 10 Jibo

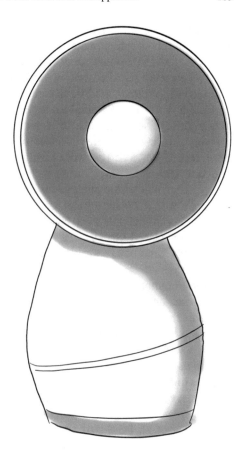

however, it includes a conversational feature. Sota is capable of greeting a user to initiate conversation, and prompts for a name to allow the user to be referred to explicitly during the communication. Sota can offer topics for conversation, including those designed to evoke emotion, and play Japanese word games. Sota demonstrates how customization in social robots makes human-robot interaction more enjoyable and personal when robots know information about the user.

Ostrowski et al. [51] used a robot called Jibo, shown in Fig. 10, in an assisted living facility for 3 weeks to facilitate human-to-human interaction. Jibo's features make the robot feel more like a companion compared to other robots. These features include simple question answering, playing music, dancing, sleeping at night, and taking naps. Jibo successfully increased feelings of connectedness among residents. More residents spent time in the common living areas engaging with the robot or having conversations with other residents related to the robot. An interesting observation is how residents interacted with the robot; many residents asked Jibo questions about how it was doing or other common conversation starters used in everyday social interactions. There were a few questions to Jibo about its functionality including requests for one-on-one sessions. This work demonstrates how social robots can promote curiosity and communication between humans.

Guiot et al. [23] tested a robot, named Buddy, inside the homes of seniors. People aged 66–91 were recruited; half of participants lived in care facilities while the other half did not. Informal and formal caregivers were also asked to participate, but in a co-design workshop. Participants tested the robot for 3 weeks inside their home. While Buddy can contribute to a person's enjoyment, all participants preferred the robot to have the safety feature of alerting their loved ones, or emergency personnel, if they fell. This work highlights the importance of ensuring older adults feel safe with technology inside their homes, and the opportunity for additional safety features to ensure older adults accept new technologies.

Simão et al. [62] used a small robot to communicate between two groups in a care facility. During the study, the robot was operated using a Wizard-of-Oz approach while users placed blocks on the robot to communicate different tasks. Some of the functions the blocks enabled included sending messages, recording messages, inviting others to lunch, and listening to music. The study results showed that users enjoyed communicating with each other between the groups: they recorded and shared messages about their loved ones; sang half of a song for the other group to complete; and quizzed each other on proverbs. Older adults were excited to use the robot, but desired more features such as arms for hugging and the ability to tell a staff worker they wished to go on a walk. The proposed technology was easy to use and allowed individuals inside care facilities to communicate with each other in different ways. The device also allowed residents to communicate at greater distances, which may have been more difficult previously given the limited mobility of many residents.

Baecker et al. [4] tested an algorithm on a NAO robot to provide emotional support for healthy older adults who experience loneliness. The robot responds to users by repeating what they say or using predefined responses to engage in reflective listening therapy. If the user skips a few days without interacting with the robot, the robot raises its arm to indicate a desire to talk. The robot starts a conversation by asking the user about his or her day. It was stressed to participants how the robot has limited capabilities to avoid the expectation discrepancy problem. This prototype provides a solid foundation for others to use when developing emotionally supportive robotic applications, and shows successful implementation of a conversation that can be used to engage users.

Ros et al. [59] used Pepper in day care facilities to encourage residents to play cognitive games. The games were personalized to each individual based on his or her preferences and goals. The sessions occurred in 15 min intervals or when the user requested to stop the session. The study focused on the design of the robot to understand how users would feel and respond. The biggest issue reported is that the robot spoke too fast. These systems have the potential to help older adults in care facilities maintain their cognitive function and reduce the onset of early aging from a lack of stimuli.

Mois et al. [46] tested a robot, called MARI, to improve the cognitive ability of participants living with dementia through piano lessons. MARI is small in size and

Fig. 11 MARI

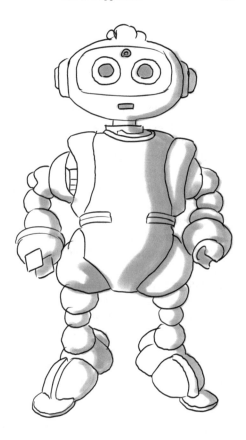

is operated via the Wizard-of-OZ approach. MARI was placed in front of a piano but would deliver the lessons via an online application. The study results indicated that MARI holds potential for cognitive training. Participants felt that MARI was highly qualified to teach piano lessons, especially as sessions increased in difficulty each week. This work is pushing the boundaries of socially assistive robotics and human-robot interaction (Fig. 11).

In [39], Lee et al. report on a social robot under development and its potential to assist socially isolated older adults during the COVID-19 pandemic. The robot, named Sunshine, is small and doll-like in appearance, aimed at mimicking a grandchild of 7 years of age using a chat-bot system. Sunshine is capable of reminding users about meals, medication, and appointments while also being able to play songs, tell stories, play Simon says, encourage reminiscence, and quote inspirational passages. Using Sunshine, a decrease in depression in older adults in South Korea was seen; however, further research is needed in different real-time situations.

Van Maris et al. [66] noticed that during a usability study using Pepper, many older adults had trouble understanding the robot. The study took place over 6 weeks inside a retirement village. The users did not have trouble with the robot when it was tested inside the lab. This study was completed using a Wizard-of-Oz approach with the aim of teaching users about the Seven Wonders of the World. Pepper explained one Wonder per session, and queried users about what they knew of the location and if they had visited prior. Pepper's responses were preset and prompted via a person to encourage conversations to continue. Fourteen participants were recruited at two different locations to interact with Pepper. At the first location, four participants were not provided subtitles of Pepper's dialogue, leading to all participants having difficulty understanding Pepper. At the second location, ten participants were provided subtitles of Pepper's dialogue, and almost all participants understood Pepper clearly; however, sometimes participants would respond to Pepper when they finished reading and not when Pepper was done speaking. This study highlights an important feature that should be given attention when designing social robotics. While subtitles are a simple solution to aid older adults in their understanding of robots' spoken output, it is not a long term solution and will not work for individuals with visual impairments.

Abbus et al. [1] developed an open-source crowd sourcing website that acted as the voice of Pepper in a virtual meeting with a user. The objective of the experiment was to understand how effective crowd sourcing is for using the robot in real-time when more complex conversation is needed instead of simpler dialogue. The aim was to address the current limitations of AI that make it challenging for machines to carry out veridical conversations with users. An actress was recruited to play the part of a distressed student and to converse with the robot via a web page. Having one, two, four, and eight workers in the queue to speak to the participant were tested to see which would be most successful. Increasing the number of workers in the queue did not improve dialogue.

Nault et al. [50] studied what sensory feedback older adults preferred and found more engaging when used for a memory game. They tested auditory, haptic, and multimodal feedback. The pilot study was ran using nine participants where they were asked to touch Pepper's left/right hand, left/right foot, or head based on Pepper's orders. In the haptic condition, when the location was touched, Pepper would vibrate. In the auditory condition, Pepper would beep when the location was touched. In the mutilmodal (haptic and auditory) condition, Pepper would perform both feedback responses. While the auditory feedback condition produced superior performance, some participants complained of feeling rushed.

Ghafurian et al. [22] conducted online surveys during the COVID-19 pandemic and found a shift in acceptance of social robots. Important tasks people wanted social robots to perform included playing games, exercising, participating in conversations, playing music, and receiving reminders. Participants wanted their social robot to recognize them, show emotions, and have a specific feature that users prefer such as being optimistic. Loneliness was reported to be a factor that would increase the probability that someone would buy a social robot.

4.2   How Robots Can Address Isolation

Mordoch et al. [47] conducted an in-depth review of contributions to social robotics, finding evidence that robots are effective at providing companionship. It is easy to imagine the benefits of advancements in AI and NLP that will enable more complex conversation and interaction. Adding such a feature to social robots will address feelings of isolation felt by older adults since there is evidence that older adults who interact with a social robot for an extended period of time view the robot as a friend [37]. Such innovations will help older adults age in place and promote social interactions to avoid the detrimental effects of social isolation, loneliness, and depression.

Pu et al. conducted a review on the effectiveness of social robots, finding that this technology reduces feelings of isolation, decreases stress, and increases engagement [57]. Social robots can be a peer, companion, or assistant [45]. Having a social robot serve as a companion, robotics has the potential to address isolation in older adults; but it is important that older adults are aware that these applications should not replace human contact [45]. However, for older adults without a social network, deceased loved ones, or certain cognitive disorders, social robots have the potential to prevent health-related impacts caused by depression. Social robots can also serve as companions in hospital rooms for patients who must stay for an extended period of time. Many patients are unable to have visitors due to distance or visiting hours; this does not, however, mean that the patient is ready to be alone for the night. Social robots can keep these patients company at any hour in unfamiliar environments.

Social robots can be deployed for larger settings such as care facilities. Studies have demonstrated that placing a robot inside a room encourages conversation with the robot and among residents; and assistive robots used during group therapy sessions have been found to stimulate conversation. Additionally, socially assistive robots can address the healthcare worker shortage as well as assist healthcare workers in their work. Applications for such robots include measuring depression levels, taking vitals, ensuring each resident has performed his or her daily physical fitness, or even assisting patients in walks. As the cost of robots continues to decrease or low-cost solutions are implemented, each resident of a care facility will be able to have his or her own social robot. Inside the home, these low-cost robotic solutions will be ideal for an informal caregiver who requires assistance.

Social robots could have assisted in the 2020 COVID-19 pandemic when residents across care facilities were required to self-isolate in their own rooms and outside visitors were not allowed. During this time, older adults were isolated more than the rest of the general population and were discouraged from even interacting with family members. Older adults, who already suffer from isolation and depression, likely had increased symptoms. Social robots could have assisted and comforted many older adults to maintain mental health. Many caregivers were also negatively impacted during COVID-19 due to required social isolation, especially from loved ones. Caregivers were already struggling with social isolation before the pandemic, but the situation was exacerbated due to the extreme caution they had to take in caring for high risk individuals.

Robotic applications have the potential to address the challenges associated with isolation, such as depression and anxiety, by filling the void left by having a small social network. Individuals who have a small social network due to limited mobility or living far from friends and family, have the most potential to benefit from these technologies. As costs lower, and AI and NLP continue to advance, social robots will be capable of holding a conversation that mimics human interaction, i.e., is veridical, interactive, and emotionally intelligent. Such innovations will ensure social robots are widely accepted, and their benefits are recognizable. This trend is already happening; more and more social robots feature some level of conversation, and older adults desire complex communication skills in robots.

Physical robots are essential to solving the issue of isolation among older adults; a preference has been seen for physical robots compared to digital assistants [6]. When designing for older adults, developers must keep in mind that seniors have decreased sensation including reduced vision and hearing. To combat this and ensure users find social robots user-friendly, features a robot should have are clearly visible screens (if used), clear speech and audio, and the ability to change the gender of its voice [7]. Customization will be beneficial to these products. Such personalizations will allow the robot to be fine-tuned to the preferences of the user and his or her personality, which will aid the robot in holding a conversation.

Robots should remember facts about users as well as past conversations to help create a more human-like conversational experience. Such interactions will facilitate bond building between humans and social robots, thereby improving trust. Recalling information from previous conversations will help the user feel less frustrated with the robot if a conversation overlaps or if the user begins telling a side-story, which is a human characteristic that often happens during a conversation.

Safety features should be required as a part of the design of social robots to ensure older adults trust the technology enough to adopt and accept it. One simple feature that is needed is an "off-switch", which would allow the user to disable the robot at any time, reinforcing that the user is in control at all times. Users will likely converse more with robots when they know that they are in control and can power off the machine at any time, especially when conversations become uncomfortable or the device malfunctions.

As shown, many robotic solutions have been developed without healthy older adults in mind or only healthy older adults in mind. Researchers should work to include a larger representation of the senior population during evaluation to ensure that what they develop will be marketable on a larger scale. It is likely some features of a socially assistive robot that are important to a healthy older adult will not be as important to older adults who are not healthy and vice versa. Understanding these limitations and overlap will be essential to developing technologies to assist with aging in place.

Acknowledgments The authors thank the Zimin Institute at Arizona State University and the National Science Foundation (Grant No. 1828010) for their funding support.

References

1. Abbas, T., Khan, V.J., Gadiraju, U., Barakova, E., Markopoulos, P.: Crowd of oz: A crowd-powered teleoperation system for enhanced human-robot conversations. In: Companion of the 2020 ACM/IEEE International Conference on Human-Robot Interaction, pp. 81–83 (2020)
2. Abdollahi, H., Mollahosseini, A., Lane, J.T., Mahoor, M.H.: A pilot study on using an intelligent life-like robot as a companion for elderly individuals with dementia and depression. In: 2017 IEEE-RAS 17th International Conference on Humanoid Robotics (Humanoids), pp. 541–546. IEEE, Piscataway (2017)
3. Ageing and health: https://www.who.int/news-room/fact-sheets/detail/ageing-and-health (2018)
4. Baecker, A.N., Geiskkovitch, D.Y., González, A.L., Young, J.E.: Emotional support domestic robots for healthy older adults: Conversational prototypes to help with loneliness. In: Companion of the 2020 ACM/IEEE International Conference on Human-Robot Interaction, pp. 122–124 (2020)
5. Beer, J.M., Smarr, C.A., Chen, T.L., Prakash, A., Mitzner, T.L., Kemp, C.C., Rogers, W.A.: The domesticated robot: design guidelines for assisting older adults to age in place. In: Proceedings of the Seventh Annual ACM/IEEE International Conference on Human-Robot Interaction, pp. 335–342 (2012)
6. Breazeal, C.L., Ostrowski, A., Singh, N., Park, H.W.: Designing social robots for older adults. Bridge **49**(1), 22–31 (2019)
7. Broadbent, E., Tamagawa, R., Patience, A., Knock, B., Kerse, N., Day, K., MacDonald, B.A.: Attitudes towards health-care robots in a retirement village. Australas. J. Ageing **31**(2), 115–120 (2012)
8. Broadbent, E., Montgomery Walsh, R., Martini, N., Loveys, K., Sutherland, C.: Evaluating the usability of new software for medication management on a social robot. In: Companion of the 2020 ACM/IEEE International Conference on Human-Robot Interaction, pp. 151–153 (2020)
9. Chen, T.L., Bhattacharjee, T., Beer, J.M., Ting, L.H., Hackney, M.E., Rogers, W.A., Kemp, C.C.: Older adults' acceptance of a robot for partner dance-based exercise. PloS One **12**(10), e0182736 (2017)
10. Chu, M.T., Khosla, R., Khaksar, S.M.S., Nguyen, K.: Service innovation through social robot engagement to improve dementia care quality. Assistive Technol. **29**(1), 8–18 (2017)
11. Clarity: Aginig in place in America: https://www.slideshare.net/clarityproducts/clarity-2007-aginig-in-place-in-america-2836029 (2007)
12. Cooper, C., Gross, A., Brinkman, C., Pope, R., Allen, K., Hastings, S., Bogen, B.E., Goode, A.P.: The impact of wearable motion sensing technology on physical activity in older adults. Exp. Gerontol. **112**, 9–19 (2018)
13. Cornwell, E.Y., Waite, L.J.: Social disconnectedness, perceived isolation, and health among older adults. J. Health Soc. Behav. **50**(1), 31–48 (2009)
14. Crary, D., (2011, November 11). Aging in place: Most seniors want to stay put. Retrieved April 27, 2021, from https://www.nbcnews.com/healthmain/aging-place-most-seniors-want-stay-put-1c9452940
15. Cruz-Sandoval, D., Favela, J.: A conversational robot to conduct therapeutic interventions for dementia. IEEE Pervas. Comput. **18**(2), 10–19 (2019)
16. Demir, E., Köseoğlu, E., Sokullu, R., Şeker, B.: Smart home assistant for ambient assisted living of elderly people with dementia. Procedia Comput. Sci. **113**, 609–614 (2017)
17. Dictionary, M.W.: https://www.merriam-webster.com/dictionary/isolation
18. DiSalvo, C., Gemperle, F., Forlizzi, J., Montgomery, E.: The hug: an exploration of robotic form for intimate communication. In: The 12th IEEE International Workshop on Robot and Human Interactive Communication, 2003. Proceedings. ROMAN 2003, pp. 403–408. IEEE, Piscataway (2003)

19. Enshaeifar, S., Zoha, A., Markides, A., Skillman, S., Acton, S.T., Elsaleh, T., Hassanpour, M., Ahrabian, A., Kenny, M., Klein, S., et al.: Health management and pattern analysis of daily living activities of people with dementia using in-home sensors and machine learning techniques. PloS One **13**(5), e0195605 (2018)
20. Forlizzi, J.: Robotic products to assist the aging population. Interactions **12**(2), 16–18 (2005)
21. Gerling, K., Livingston, I., Nacke, L., Mandryk, R.: Full-body motion-based game interaction for older adults. In: Proceedings of the SIGCHI Conference on Human Factors in Computing Systems, pp. 1873–1882 (2012)
22. Ghafurian, M., Ellard, C., Dautenhahn, K.: Social companion robots to reduce isolation: a perception change due to covid-19. Preprint. arXiv:2008.05382 (2020)
23. Guiot, D., Kerekes, M., Sengès, E.: Living with buddy: can a social robot help elderly with loss of autonomy to age well? In: 28th IEEE RO-MAN Internet Of Intelligent Robotic Things For Healthy Living and Active Ageing, International Conference on Robot & Human Interactive Communication, pp. 23–26 (2019)
24. Guo, Y., Tanaka, F.: Robot that sweats to remind the elderly of high-temperature. In: Companion of the 2020 ACM/IEEE International Conference on Human-Robot Interaction, pp. 221–223 (2020)
25. Healthy places terminology (2009). https://www.cdc.gov/healthyplaces/terminology
26. Howard, J.: Us fertility rate falls to 'all-time low,' cdc says (2019). https://www.cnn.com/2019/07/24/health/fertility-rate-births-2018-cdc-study/index.html
27. Hung, L., Liu, C., Woldum, E. et al.: The benefits of and barriers to using a social robot PARO in care settings: A scoping review. BMC Geriatrics **19**(232) (2019) https://doi.org/10.1186/s12877-019-1244-6
28. Intille, S.S., Larson, K., Tapia, E.M.: Designing and evaluating technology for independent aging in the home. In: International Conference on Aging, Disability and Independence. Citeseer (2003)
29. Iwabuchi, Y., Sato, I., Fujino, Y., Yagi, N.: The communication supporting robot based on "humanitude" concept for dementia patients. In: 2019 IEEE 1st Global Conference on Life Sciences and Technologies (LifeTech), pp. 219–223. IEEE, Piscataway (2019)
30. Johnson, R.W., Wang, C.X.: The financial burden of paid home care on older adults: Oldest and sickest are least likely to have enough income. Health Affairs **38**(6), 994–1002 (2019)
31. Joy for All: https://joyforall.com/ (2018)
32. Kanoh, M., Oida, Y., Nomura, Y., Araki, A., Konagaya, Y., Ihara, K., Shimizu, T., Kimura, K.: Examination of practicability of communication robot-assisted activity program for elderly people. J. Rob. Mechatronics **23**(1), 3 (2011)
33. Karunarathne, D., Morales, Y., Nomura, T., Kanda, T., Ishiguro, H.: Will older adults accept a humanoid robot as a walking partner? Int. J. Soc. Rob. **11**(2), 343–358 (2019)
34. Kavilanz, P.: The us can't keep up with demand for health aides, nurses and doctors (2018). https://money.cnn.com/2018/05/04/news/economy/health-care-workers-shortage/index.html
35. Kaye, J.A., Maxwell, S.A., Mattek, N., Hayes, T.L., Dodge, H., Pavel, M., Jimison, H.B., Wild, K., Boise, L., Zitzelberger, T.A.: Intelligent systems for assessing aging changes: home-based, unobtrusive, and continuous assessment of aging. J. Gerontol. B Psychol. Sci. Soc. Sci. **66**(suppl_1), i180–i190 (2011)
36. Keizer, R.A.O., Van Velsen, L., Moncharmont, M., Riche, B., Ammour, N., Del Signore, S., Zia, G., Hermens, H., N'Dja, A.: Using socially assistive robots for monitoring and preventing frailty among older adults: a study on usability and user experience challenges. Health Technol. **9**(4), 595–605 (2019)
37. Khosla, R., Chu, M.T., Khaksar, S.M.S., Nguyen, K., Nishida, T.: Engagement and experience of older people with socially assistive robots in home care. Assistive Technology, pp. 1–15 (2019)
38. Khosravi, P., Rezvani, A., Wiewiora, A.: The impact of technology on older adults' social isolation. Comput. Human Behav. **63**, 594–603 (2016)
39. Lee, O.E., Davis, B.: Adapting 'Sunshine,' a socially assistive chat robot for older adults with cognitive impairment: a pilot study. J. Gerontol. Soc. Work **63**(6-7), 696–698 (2020)

40. Leng, M., Liu, P., Zhang, P., Hu, M., Zhou, H., Li, G., Yin, H., Chen, L.: Pet robot intervention for people with dementia: a systematic review and meta-analysis of randomized controlled trials. Psychiatry Res. **271**, 516–525 (2019)
41. Lotfi, A., Langensiepen, C., Yahaya, S.W.: Socially assistive robotics: Robot exercise trainer for older adults. Technologies **6**(1), 32 (2018)
42. Magyar, J., Kobayashi, M., Nishio, S., Sinčák, P., Ishiguro, H.: Autonomous robotic dialogue system with reinforcement learning for elderlies with dementia. In: 2019 IEEE International Conference on Systems, Man and Cybernetics (SMC), pp. 3416–3421. IEEE, Piscataway (2019)
43. Marti, P., Bacigalupo, M., Giusti, L., Mennecozzi, C., Shibata, T.: Socially assistive robotics in the treatment of behavioural and psychological symptoms of dementia. In: The First IEEE/RAS-EMBS International Conference on Biomedical Robotics and Biomechatronics. BioRob 2006, pp. 483–488. IEEE, Piscataway (2006)
44. Martín, F., Agüero, C., Cañas, J.M., Abella, G., Benítez, R., Rivero, S., Valenti, M., Martínez-Martín, P.: Robots in therapy for dementia patients. J. Phys. Agents **7**(1), 48–55 (2013)
45. Mois, G., Beer, J.M.: Robotics to support aging in place. In: Living with Robots, pp. 49–74. Elsevier (2020)
46. Mois, G., Collete, B.A., Renzi-Hammond, L.M., Boccanfuso, L., Ramachandran, A., Gibson, P., Emerson, K.G., Beer, J.M.: Understanding robots' potential to facilitate piano cognitive training in older adults with mild cognitive impairment. In: Companion of the 2020 ACM/IEEE International Conference on Human-Robot Interaction, pp. 363–365 (2020)
47. Mordoch, E., Osterreicher, A., Guse, L., Roger, K., Thompson, G.: Use of social commitment robots in the care of elderly people with dementia: A literature review. Maturitas **74**(1), 14–20 (2013)
48. Moyle, W., Cooke, M., Beattie, E., Jones, C., Klein, B., Cook, G., Gray, C., et al.: Exploring the effect of companion robots on emotional expression in older adults with dementia: a pilot randomized controlled trial. J. Gerontol. Nurs. **39**(5), 46–53 (2013)
49. Moyle, W., Jones, C., Cooke, M., O'Dwyer, S., Sung, B., Drummond, S.: Social robots helping people with dementia: Assessing efficacy of social robots in the nursing home environment. In: 2013 6th International Conference on Human System Interactions (HSI), pp. 608–613. IEEE, Piscataway (2013)
50. Nault, E., Baillie, L., Broz, F.: Auditory and haptic feedback in a socially assistive robot memory game. In: Companion of the 2020 ACM/IEEE International Conference on Human-Robot Interaction, pp. 369–371 (2020)
51. Ostrowski, A.K., DiPaola, D., Partridge, E., Park, H.W., Breazeal, C.: Older adults living with social robots: Promoting social connectedness in long-term communities. IEEE Robot. Autom. Mag. **26**(2), 59–70 (2019)
52. Paletta, L., Fellner, M., Schüssler, S., Zuschnegg, J., Steiner, J., Lerch, A., Lammer, L., Prodromou, D.: Amigo: Towards social robot based motivation for playful multimodal intervention in dementia. In: Proceedings of the 11th PErvasive Technologies Related to Assistive Environments Conference, pp. 421–427 (2018)
53. Pearson, C.F., Quinn, C.C., Loganathan, S., Datta, A.R., Mace, B.B., Grabowski, D.C.: The forgotten middle: Many middle-income seniors will have insufficient resources for housing and health care. Health Affairs, Vol. **38**(5), 10–1377 (2019)
54. Piezzo, C., Suzuki, K.: Feasibility study of a socially assistive humanoid robot for guiding elderly individuals during walking. Future Internet **9**(3), 30 (2017)
55. Pollmann, K., Ruff, C., Vetter, K., Zimmermann, G.: Robot vs. voice assistant: Is playing with pepper more fun than playing with alexa? In: Companion of the 2020 ACM/IEEE International Conference on Human-Robot Interaction, pp. 395–397 (2020)
56. Portugal, D., Alvito, P., Christodoulou, E., Samaras, G., Dias, J.: A study on the deployment of a service robot in an elderly care center. Int. J. Soc. Rob. **11**(2), 317–341 (2019)
57. Pu, L., Moyle, W., Jones, C., Todorovic, M.: The effectiveness of social robots for older adults: a systematic review and meta-analysis of randomized controlled studies. Gerontologist **59**(1), e37–e51 (2019)

58. Rantz, M.J., Skubic, M., Miller, S.J., Galambos, C., Alexander, G., Keller, J., Popescu, M.: Sensor technology to support aging in place. J. Am. Med. Dir. Assoc. **14**(6), 386–391 (2013)
59. Ros, R., Espona, M.: Exploration of a robot-based adaptive cognitive stimulation system for the elderly. In: Companion of the 2020 ACM/IEEE International Conference on Human-Robot Interaction, pp. 406–408 (2020)
60. Rostill, H., Nilforooshan, R., Barnaghi, P., Morgan, A.: Technology-integrated dementia care: trial results. Nurs. Residential Care **21**(9), 489–494 (2019)
61. Santini, Z.I., Jose, P.E., Cornwell, E.Y., Koyanagi, A., Nielsen, L., Hinrichsen, C., Meilstrup, C., Madsen, K.R., Koushede, V.: Social disconnectedness, perceived isolation, and symptoms of depression and anxiety among older Americans (nshap): a longitudinal mediation analysis. Lancet Public Health **5**(1), e62–e70 (2020)
62. Simão, H., Pires, A., Gonçalves, D., Guerreiro, T.: Carrier-pigeon robot: Promoting interactions among older adults in a care home. In: Companion of the 2020 ACM/IEEE International Conference on Human-Robot Interaction, pp. 450–452 (2020)
63. Skouby, K.E., Kivimäki, A., Haukiputo, L., Lynggaard, P., Windekilde, I.M.: Smart cities and the ageing population. In: The 32nd Meeting of WWRF (2014)
64. Tapus, A.: Improving the quality of life of people with dementia through the use of socially assistive robots. In: 2009 Advanced Technologies for Enhanced Quality of Life, pp. 81–86. IEEE, Piscataway (2009)
65. Thomas, W., Blanchard, J.: Moving beyond place: Aging in community. Generations **33**(2), 12–17 (2009)
66. van Maris, A., Dogramadzi, S., Zook, N., Studley, M., Winfield, A., Caleb-Solly, P.: Speech related accessibility issues in social robots. In: Companion of the 2020 ACM/IEEE International Conference on Human-Robot Interaction, pp. 505–507 (2020)
67. Barbara J.G.,: Natural language processing, Artificial intelligence, **19**(2), 131–136, ISSN 0004-3702, (1982) https://doi.org/10.1016/0004-3702(82)90032-7 (https://www.sciencedirect.com/science/article/pii/0004370282900327)
68. Wiles, J.L., Leibing, A., Guberman, N., Reeve, J., Allen, R.E.: The meaning of "aging in place" to older people. Gerontologist **52**(3), 357–366 (2012)

Part III
Haptic Technologies for Accessible Human Computer Interfaces

Accessible Smart Coaching Technologies Inspired by Elderly Requisites

Swagata Das, Yuichi Kurita, and Ramin Tadayon

Abstract Ageing in place (at home) is gaining popularity due to the increasing proportion of the elderly population and stay at home lifestyle. Technology can be of great help to support ageing in place. Primarily, we need systems for telerehabilitation, exercise or necessary physical training, support for weakly functioning body parts and self-assessment. This chapter introduces state-of-the-art devices for each of the mentioned categories that can support and enhance the quality of life (QoL) of older adults. Wearable technologies that are suitable for at-home usage are discussed next that use a low-pressure type McKibben actuator called the pneumatic gel muscle (PGM). PGMs are utilized to design a soft exoskeleton jacket for remote human interaction to achieve a wearable solution for telerehabilitation. The force induced by the system and the latencies involved are reported. PGMs are further used to design a wearable balance exercise device. The effectiveness of the device is evaluated using a single-leg stance test. Another system using PGMs to support swing motion is elaborated. This design is evaluated using various parameters of the lower limb. The stealth adaptive exergame design framework is explained along with an exergame enabling adjustable load. Finally, a brushed body area assessment system is discussed.

Keywords Wearable force-feedback · Balance exercise · Swing support · Exergames · Bathing skill

S. Das (✉) · Y. Kurita
Hiroshima University, Hiroshima, Japan
e-mail: swagatadas@hiroshima-u.ac.jp; ykurita@hiroshima-u.ac.jp

R. Tadayon
Arizona State University, Mesa, AZ, USA
e-mail: rtadayon@asu.edu

© The Author(s), under exclusive license to Springer Nature Switzerland AG 2021
T. McDaniel, X. Liu (eds.), *Multimedia for Accessible Human Computer Interfaces*,
https://doi.org/10.1007/978-3-030-70716-3_7

1   Introduction

The accomplished Irish playwright, George Bernard Shaw, once said, "We do not stop playing because we grow old. We grow old because we stop playing." Ageing is an inevitable process. Compared to 1990, the world's aged population (65+ years old) is projected to rise by 166.67% in 2050, which will account for 16% of the world's total population [1]. Science and technology have gifted an increased life expectancy, but it also calls for a good quality of life (QoL) during the latter years of our lives. Being active is an important aspect to sustain the essence of health and satisfaction in the process of ageing. With the recent onset of the COVID-19 pandemic, older adults are especially at high risk, due to which regular hospital visits are cut short, and the concept of *ageing in place* is being extensively promoted by policymakers [2]. The term *Ageing in place* has been used to define the concept of living in the community rather than in residential care, thus promoting some level of independence [3].

Technology can play a major role in implementing *ageing in place* [4, 5]. In particular, we need more cutting edge technologies that support telerehabilitation, home-based physical training, physical assistance to achieve uninterrupted living conditions, and self-assessment. In this chapter, we will introduce some recently developed technologies that belong to these categories of application and are also suitable for usage by older adults.

2   A Review of Accessible Technology in Healthcare

Technology has played an essential role in delivering accessible care to patients. Technological advances in modern medicine can be categorized into five main areas: electronic health records, personalized healthcare, telehealthcare, surgical technology and immersive learning through artificial intelligence (AI) and mixed reality (MR). This section discusses some of the recent advances in the areas of personalized healthcare and telehealthcare. With respect to technology in personalized healthcare, we will emphasize the fields of rehabilitation, sports and wearables. In terms of telehealthcare, our focus will be telerehabilitation and wearables. Since wearable technology is an overlapped area, it will be addressed as a single topic called wearable exoskeletons.

Personalized Rehabilitation The importance of personalized rehabilitation for gait impairments in Parkinson's disease (PD) was reported in [6]. This individualized approach may be based on a set of behavioural markers applicable to therapy for various motor and non-motor features in PD. A training support system for personalized upper limb motor rehabilitation was developed to enable therapists to implement training trajectories and training programs tailored to address the individual requirements of the patients [7]. Personalized rehabilitation techniques were tested for post reverse shoulder arthroplasty (RSA) rehabilitation and found productive in improving clinical outcomes and decreasing the rate of complications [8]. Machine learning has a significant role in personalizing the rehabilitation process. The potential of personalized rehabilitation assessment using a combination of expert's knowledge and machine learning models to improve conventional rehabilitation practices was explained in [9]. A personalized cognitive virtual reality (VR)-enabled rehabilitation tool called AGATHE was developed and tested by researchers to offer customized rehabilitation sessions, based on simulated activities of daily living (ADL) [10]. The motivation behind this work was to let the patients become a partner in developing the tool. Another personalized gamified exercise through a recommender system was developed to tackle the issue of gradually declining interest in therapeutic sessions [11]. VR was also used to design a Virtual CoMBaT (Center of mass-assisted balance tasks) system [12]. This system was designated for individualized and adaptive balance rehabilitation exercises depending on the user's performance. The importance of individually different rehabilitation approaches for children with disabilities, including autism spectrum disorder, was carefully and systematically discussed in [13]. Personalized rehabilitation was referred to as the ultimately needed goal of rehabilitation programs through the combination of standard and tailored treatment with a greater intensity, which is possible through technology, with an emphasis to recovering from acquired brain injuries [14].

Sports Training Sports training and activities facilitate improved physical fitness and performance [15]. Therefore, in this section, considering sports as a part of the healthcare sector, we discuss some technological advances in the area. We coarsely categorize technology in sports into VR, sensing technology, internet of things (IoT) or web-based coaching and AI. VR has been widely utilized in sports training and analysis during the past two decades. One of the first digitally-augmented cooperative sports called PingPongPlus was implemented using dynamic graphics and sound-based ball tracking to identify the impact of digital augmentation on gameplay [16]. This endeavour was followed by some of the very first instances of VR integration with ball sports such as handball training [17], analysis of handball kinematics [18] and a virtual bowling game [19]. Apart from ball sports, martial arts has been integrated with virtual elements such as in Kick-Ass Kung-Fu with goals of fitness application and entertainment. In this game, virtual enemies were introduced inside 3D graphics by embedding the player's video image through real-time image processing and computer vision [20]. Several sports evaluation and anticipatory techniques were then developed [21–24]. During the most recent decade, with its rising popularity, a variety of sports were experienced with VR as a skill trainer [25]. A VR-based cricket simulator was developed to investigate changing elements related to action and decision for cricket batsmen [26]. An American football training system was developed using VR and showed 30% average improvement in scores [27]. Another interesting study showed that energy management could be taught to novice rowers through a VR training system [28]. Yamashita et al. proposed an enhanced swimming experience called AquaCAVE [29]. They replaced normal swimming goggles with an immersive stereoscopic projection environment using liquid crystal display (LCD) shutter glasses. In addition, cameras were used to track the swimmer's head position [29]. A mixed reality rock climbing system called VENGA was developed to provide immersive training and a fear-free rock climbing experience [30]. Various innovative wearable and sport equipment sensors have been used in the field of sports recently such as smart fabrics [31–33], accelerometers [34, 35], IMUs [36, 37], multi-sensory force sensors [38], position or monitoring sensors [39–41], body sensor networks (BSN) [42], oral carbohydrate sensors [43] and heartrate sensors [44]. Such sensors have a high significance in the healthcare sector as well. IoT has also been utilized in various sectors of sports such as training [45], analytics [46, 47], monitoring [48, 49], analysis [50], augmentation [51] and safety [52]. Sports also underwent the usage of AI in areas such as training [53, 54], tactics [55], analysis [56, 57], prediction [58] and risk assessment [59].

Telerehabilitation Telerehabilitation is an alternative to conventional rehabilitation approaches to encourage the possibility of conducting rehabilitation sessions at any location irrespective of the physical presence of a therapist. In this section, we discuss some successful remote solutions for rehabilitation purposes that are focused toward the elderly. According to a recent review, telerehabilitation had been used for recovery in the elderly mainly after chronic obstructive pulmonary disease (COPD), total knee replacement, stroke, and in patients suffering from the comorbidity of chronic heart failure (CHF) and COPD [60]. A post-stroke rehabilitation system using a remotely controlled VR program was developed and compared with traditional motor rehabilitation methods and showed potential benefits [61]. A home-based telerehabilitation program was designed for patients suffering from the comorbidity of CHF and COPD. The program contained various exercises and monitoring strategies and was reported as satisfactory by elderly participants [62]. PC-based videoconferencing and motion-analysis tools were used in a telerehabilitation system for recovery after knee replacement surgery [63]. Another interactive virtual telerehabilitation therapeutic system reported for patients who had knee replacement showed no significant recovery when compared to the control group. The system contained sensors for motion analysis and monitoring of the patient's knee [64]. The intervention and control groups for knee replacement recovery through telerehabilitation have not shown any significant differences in recovery until now, considering another study with similar approaches [65]. Robot-assisted telerehabilitation for motor recovery has also been reported in recent years [66]. The primary technologies used for home-based motor recovery include gaming systems, telecommunication, robotic devices, VR, sensors, and portable display units such as tablets and mobile phones. A recent review of this area summarizing related articles of the past decade pointed out significant drawbacks of robotic devices. One of the drawbacks is the requirement of large physical space in the living environment. Another shortcoming is the large forces generated, which may be a safety concern when used unsupervised at home [67].

Wearable Exoskeletons Fast advances in the fields of sensing, computing, actuation and energy sources have led to an increased acceptance of wearable robotics in the areas of assist and rehabilitation in healthcare. Wearable technology is gaining popularity in the past few years due to increased acceptance among people with special needs such as children, motor recovering patients and the elderly. Physical therapy involves extensive repetitive movements and exercises that require physically intensive and psychologically demanding labour from the caregivers [68]. The repetitive behaviour of rehabilitative approaches makes this field a perfect fit for robotics. In addition to rehabilitation, easily approachable robotics systems can also provide assistance in maintaining a healthy lifestyle and performing activities of daily living. Conventional rigid-bodied robotics have faced challenges in realising real-world applications and acceptability by end-users [69]. This setback has resulted in a trend shift from conventional rigid-bodied robotics to a new domain called *soft robotics*. A systematic review of state-of-the-art wearable systems related to upper limb rehabilitation and assistance is presented in [70]. Upper limb rehabilitation mainly constitutes shoulder, elbow, wrist and finger joints. For the lower limb, rehabilitation can be associated with walking, balance, running, lateral stepping, crouching and sit to stand [71]. Soft wearable systems have been implemented using many types of actuation methods such as using Bowden cables and geared motors [72], spring bundles of shape memory alloy (SMA) [73], pneumatic actuation [74, 75], hydraulic actuation [76] and fabric type actuators [77, 78]. The most significant drawback of soft wearable exoskeletons is the absence of an external rigid frame. The whole system depends on the user's skeletal system for mounting, which makes it difficult to install additional components such as sensors, valves and motors and also limits the force that can be transferred from the actuators [79]. Pneumatic actuators, however, are completely soft, low maintenance, lightweight and do not require a frame or skeleton for attachment. The controlling components, such as valves are also lightweight and can be easily accommodated in a portable unit. Soft pneumatic actuators, however, provide a limited amount of force and require a heavyweight compressor for long term operation.

Therefore, in this chapter, we discuss pneumatic gel muscles (PGMs), which can generate large forces even with low air pressure sources. The low air pressure requirement enables these actuators to be used with small portable canisters that do not add much weight to the system. This chapter presents five novel healthcare technologies, out of which four are utilizing the benefits of the soft actuator, PGM:

- a soft exoskeleton jacket for remote human interaction;
- a soft wearable balance exercise device;
- a swing support system using wireless actuation of PGMs;
- a ski exergame for squat training using changeable load with PGMs;
- and an IMU-based assessment of brushed body area.

3 Novel Wearable Healthcare Technologies Using Pneumatic Gel Muscle (PGM)

This section emphasizes the benefits of using a soft, low-pressure pneumatic actuator called pneumatic gel muscle (PGM). The actuator was used in several applications related to healthcare, out of which a chosen few are discussed here. This section also briefly summarizes about the actuation mechanism of the PGM and its force characteristics.

3.1 Pneumatic Gel Muscle (PGM)

The PGM actuator is a specially designed low-pressure artificial muscle capable of generating higher forces at low air pressure when compared to its counterparts. The actuator is a low-pressure type McKibben artificial muscle. Details of the composition and functioning are described in this section [80] (Fig. 1).

3.1.1 Overview

The PGMs were initially developed by DAIYA industry, Japan. Like other pneumatic artificial muscles (PAMs), PGMs also have two layers of materials, namely, an outer mesh and an inner tube. The outer mesh is made of a commercially available plastic mesh while the inner tube is made of a customized styrene-based thermoplastic elastomer. Due to the presence of the customized inner tube, PGMs can generate high forces at very low air pressure values. The inner tube is entirely tied and concealed by the outer mesh. When compressed air is fed to the actuator, the inner tube inflates like a balloon. However, the outer mesh checks this inflation, and the crossed pattern of the mesh results in the PGM shrinking. This shrinking action, in turn, generates a linear force when the endpoints of the PGM are fastened to a base.

Fig. 1 Working mechanism of pneumatic gel muscles (PGMs)

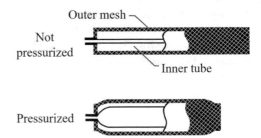

3.1.2 Force Characteristics

The PGM contracts linearly when compressed air is inserted through one of the ends. At zero or very low air pressure, the actuator behaves like a spring. However, the stiffness increases with increased inserted air pressure. Moreover, the force characteristics of PGMs with different lengths can vary significantly. We measured the force characteristics of a 30 cm rest length PGM to show the force characteristics as a function of the input air pressure and displacement. The two ends of the PGM were fixed to a force sensor and metal frame respectively. The force sensor was attached firmly to a linear guide that can be moved vertically, thereby changing the displacement or level of stretch in the PGM. Here, the displacement means the amount of external force applied to the two ends of the actuator. At a fixed value of input air pressure, the displacement was changed from 0 to 3 cm and then back to 0 cm. Figure 2 shows the resultant data of two selected values of air pressure, 0 and 0.2 MPa. In most of the applications, we use the maximum air pressure of 0.2 MPa for the actuated state. Therefore, these two values were chosen for reporting. As can be seen in the force characteristics, the force linearly changes with rising displacement but forms a hysteresis loop.

The speciality of the PGM actuator is that it can generate larger contraction than its commercially available counterpart RF-10, as shown in Fig. 3. In other words, PGMs can generate large forces at very low air pressure values. This property allows

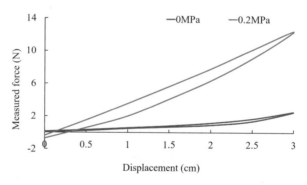

Fig. 2 Force characteristics of a 30 cm pneumatic gel muscle (PGM) at 0 and 0.2 MPa with varying displacement

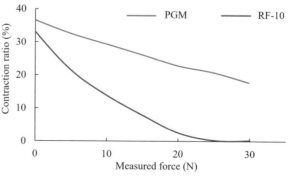

Fig. 3 Comparison of contraction ratios of a pneumatic gel muscle (PGM) with commercially available counterpart RF-10 Here, X-axis represents external load on the actuator in terms of force. [80]

use of this actuator for longer hours with small CO_2 canisters, thereby making the complete system portable.

3.2 A Soft Exoskeleton Jacket for Remote Human Interaction

This section introduces the use of PGMs in designing a wearable human augmentation suit that can be used as a telerehabilitation assistant to generate gestures through force feedback along with visual support in a virtual environment. This jacket was first reported in [81]. Figure 4 illustrates the framework of the proposed system. The motivation behind this concept, system design and assessment are briefly discussed next.

3.2.1 Motivation

Most soft exoskeletons do not use soft materials for the complete design. This system has the potential to be used in telerehabilitation through remote delivery of force feedback on different parts of the body. Conventional methods of physiotherapy involve physically touching the patients to indicate which limb needs to be moved and at what angle. Through wearable force feedback technologies, such as the one proposed here, we will no longer have such requirements and training can be performed remotely. Moreover, the lightweight and flexible characteristics of the prototype enables it to be used by individuals who prefer less obstructive augmentation such as the elderly and individuals with physical impairments.

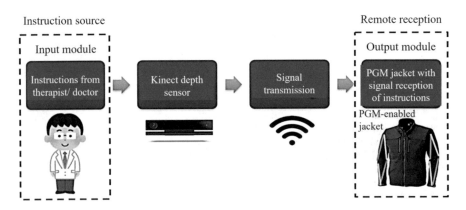

Fig. 4 Integration of different units for the telerehabilitation system [81]

3.2.2   System Description

The system consists of a jacket attached with PGMs on different locations that enable force feedback. A user wearing the jacket can receive remote instructions through a wireless module and receive different motion signals through force feedback delivered by the PGMs [80].

Data Acquisition of the Therapist or Instructor The input module, as shown in Fig. 4, comprises a Kinect V2 sensor to acquire the data of the therapist. An algorithm is used to calculate the angles of the therapist's arms in real-time from the obtained data. These angles are then replicated by an avatar in a VR environment, as shown in Fig. 5, that can be viewed by the instructor. At the same time, with minimum delay, the receiving user can view the same scene of the avatar by wearing a VR headset.

Receiving End The receiving user or the patient wears the exoskeleton jacket shown in Fig. 6 to acquire the force feedback-based instructions from the instructor. A socket type connection implements the wireless transmission and reception of signals. An ESP32 board which has an embedded WiFi module can receive the signals and actuate the PGMs with attached solenoid valves.

The Exoskeleton Jacket The proposed jacket is lightweight and wearable with attached PGMs along the arm as shown in Fig. 6. The current configuration of PGMs support shoulder abduction and elbow flexion motions only. The CO_2 canister required to supply compressed air is enclosed within the jacket. The pneumatic tubing required for the airflow is systematically arranged for not disturbing the natural movements of the user. For shoulder abduction, three PGMs of 42 cm rest length and one PGM of 27 cm rest length are used in straight alignment. For elbow

Fig. 5 Visual information provided to both instructor and receiver or patient through Unity software [81]

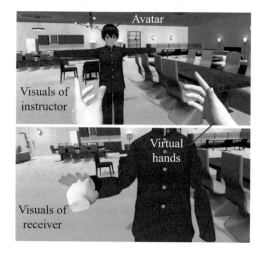

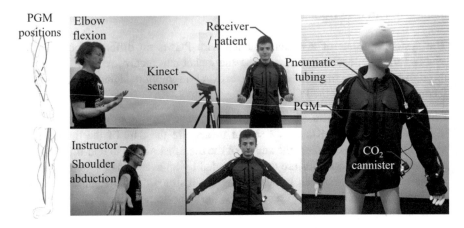

Fig. 6 Positions of the actuators on the jacket for the currently supported degrees of freedom (DOFs), elbow flexion and shoulder abduction, are shown on the left side. The concept of using the soft exoskeleton jacket for telerehabilitation is shown in the center. Components used for the soft pneumatic gel muscle (PGM)-based exoskeleton jacket are shown on the right side [81]

flexion, two PGMs of 42 cm rest length are spirally attached to the arm. Figure 6 indicates the positions and attachment types of PGMs for both motions.

3.2.3 Measurement of Force During Shoulder Abduction and Elbow Flexion

A preliminary assessment was done to measure the force resulting from the PGM actuation. Four males and one female consented for this experiment. The maximum force from the actuation of each set of PGMs was measured. A force transducer (Leptrino PFS080YA501U6) was used for this measurement. For shoulder abduction, the subject stood straight with unfolded arms. The dorsal side of the right hand was placed very close to the sensor such that the palm was parallel to the sensor without physical contact. The sensor was fixed to a metal frame, and its height was adjusted to reach the subject's hand. Figure 7 shows the position of the user and the transducer for measurement of force in both elbow flexion and shoulder abduction cases. The subjects were asked to relax their arms and not oppose the force feedback received from PGM actuation. For elbow flexion, the arm was placed with the palm facing the sensor so that, when the elbow is flexed, the palm hits the force transducer and the force data is recorded. The PGMs were actuated 15 times for each subject, and the average force was calculated from the data representing each DOF.

Figure 8 shows the average physical force measured to identify the PGM force in inducing shoulder abduction and elbow flexion for each subject. The vertical axes represent the force in Newtons, and the horizontal axes represent the different subjects and the overall average. It can be seen that different subjects perceive

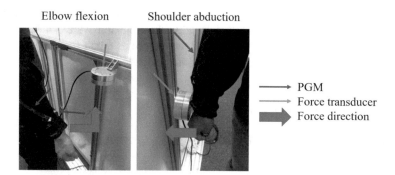

Elbow flexion   Shoulder abduction

→ PGM
→ Force transducer
⇒ Force direction

Fig. 7 Arm positions in alignment to the force transducer for shoulder abduction and elbow flexion force feedback

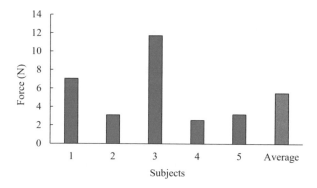

(a) Measured force for shoulder abduction.

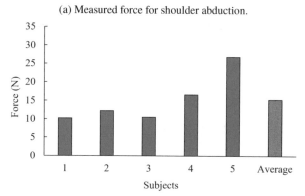

(b) Measured force for elbow flexion.

Fig. 8 Subject wise and average force measurement through pneumatic gel muscle (PGM)-based actuation of the exoskeleton jacket [81]. (**a**) Measured force for shoulder abduction. (**b**) Measured force for elbow flexion

different forces from PGM-based actuation of their arms. The resultant average forces measured for shoulder abduction and elbow flexion were 5.4 N and 15.3 N, respectively. As expected, PGMs could not induce as much force in the case of shoulder abduction compared to elbow flexion due to the weight of the arm involved.

3.2.4 Latency Measurement

The delay of the entire system from Kinect sensing to valve actuation was measured. Latencies include pose estimation (input side), angle calculation (also input side) and finally reception of the data (outside side). These latencies were separately measured and reported. The respective delay components are 602 ms, 55.6 ms and 13.43 ms as shown in Fig. 9, respectively.

3.3   A Soft Wearable Balance Exercise Device

This section describes a wearable exercise device for improving balance among older adults.

3.3.1 Motivation

Older individuals are often associated with the risk of falling due to decreased posture control. Swift reactive posture control in response to small perturbations is highly vital for preventing falls. Therefore, this lightweight balance exercise suit was developed to address the issue of decreased posture control using a form factor that is easy to do in clinical settings [82].

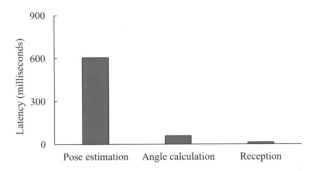

Fig. 9 Measured latency for the exoskeleton jacket actuation [81]

3.3.2 System Description

In this section, we describe the construction of the balance exercise prototype and the different components used. Figure 10 depicts the system with its main constituent parts. The two significant expectations from this prototype while designing it were lightweightedness and low donning time. The total weight is 0.9 kg and it took a person with no domain expertise less than 3 min to do the prototype.

Table 1 details the specifications of the different components used to build the prototype. There are three parts in the prototype, namely wearable, controller and

Fig. 10 Components used for the soft wearable balance exercise suit [82]

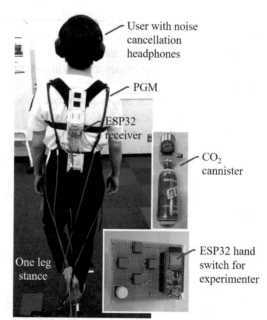

User with noise cancellation headphones
PGM
ESP32 receiver
CO₂ cannister
One leg stance
ESP32 hand switch for experimenter

Table 1 Major components of the soft wearable exercise device. Abbreviations used: Pneumatic gel muscle (PGM), inertial measurement unit (IMU)

Part	Component	Specifications	No. of units
Wearable	Soft supporter	By Babo care for the trunk	1
	Soft supporter	By Zw-3 (NIPPON SIGMAX Co.,Ltd) for the pelvis	1
	PGMs	25 cm natural length	4
Controller	Switches	Push button	5
	Micro-controller	ESP32 (Wifi enabled)	1
Receiver	Micro-controller	ESP32 (Wifi enabled)	1
	Solenoid valves	SMC SYJ312M	4
	CO₂ canister	NTG (Nippon Tansan Gas Co.Ltd) 19 cm long tank	1
	IMU sensor	M5Stack FIRE (MPU 6050)	1
	SD card writer	M5Stack FIRE	1

receiver. The wearable part consists of supporters for the pelvis and trunk portions, which are in turn, used to attach four PGMs. Two PGMs are attached on the front side, and two PGMs are attached on the backside. One end of each PGM was attached to the acromion processes on all sides. The other ends were set near the iliac crest, as shown in Fig. 10. The controller part of the prototype was a wireless module held by the experimenter to induce perturbations in the subject's torso through PGM actuation. The controller had four blue push buttons assigned to four PGMs separately and one yellow push button to start recording IMU data. The instructions were sent wirelessly through an ESP32 board. The receiver part, which was also attached on the subject's body, contains another ESP32 board for receiving the PGM control commands from the controller side. These commands are directed to the individual solenoid valves that can either actuate or deflate each associated PGM. A small CO_2 canister was used to supply compressed air to the input side of the solenoid valves. The final component of the receiver is a M5Stack FIRE IoT development kit that provides an inbuilt IMU sensor and an SD card writer to log the IMU data.

The communication between the controller and the receiver is illustrated in Fig. 11. The experimenter can control the PGM actuation wirelessly using the controller. The actuation of the PGMs on the anterior and posterior sides of the subject's body can induce trunk flexion and extension, respectively, thereby disturbing body balance. The actuation of the PGMs on the left and right sides of the body can also create imbalance, thereby making the subject lean toward the respective side. This mechanism was used to evaluate whether the prototype can help improve balance.

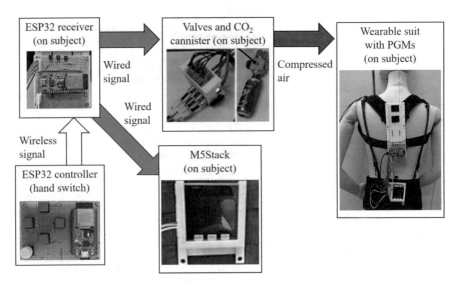

Fig. 11 Control and signal flow used for the actuation of pneumatic gel muscles (PGMs) in the balance exercise suit

3.3.3 Evaluation of the Prototype Through a Single-Leg Stance Test

The single-leg stance is commonly used to assess balance function and fall probability in individuals [83, 84]. The single-leg stance task is also included in clinical balance tests such as the berg balance test and the balance evaluation systems test (BESTest). Therefore, this task was chosen for evaluating the prototype in body balance perspective.

Participants One female and six male participants approved to participate in an experiment to evaluate this prototype. The following are the mean values of various details of the participants:

- Age: 23.9 ± 2.0 years old
- Height: 1.70 ± 0.08 m
- Body weight: 56.0 ± 7.9 kg
- Foot length: 0.26 ± 0.01 m

Participants reported no history of lower limb surgery or gait related pain. Neurological and cardiovascular disorders were also not reported.

Experiment Protocol The single-leg stance was performed by standing on one leg while lifting the other leg and not touching any objects in the vicinity for support. Participants chose their dominant leg by considering which leg they would use for kicking a ball [85]. During all single-leg stance tasks, headphones were worn by subjects to ensure minimal perturbation through channels other than force feedback. There were four sessions in the experimental protocol, the sequence of which were:

- Pre-test
- Reactive postural control assessment
- Exercise
- Post-test

During the pre-test session, subjects performed single-leg stance with their non-dominant leg on the ground. Acceleration data was recorded for 30 s using IMU sensors after 5 s of lifting the non-dominant leg. In the next session, the participants wore the wearable prototype with PGMs attached and started the single-leg stance task again, this time, with PGM-induced perturbations. The experimenter used the controller to introduce force-feedback based perturbations in different directions without warning. This session helped subjects acclimate to the system. During this session, the IMU sensor was not used. The next session was an exercise session. In this session, PGM perturbations were used for four times between 5 and 25 s after the task started. The timing and type of perturbation were randomized. The exercise session was repeated five times. If participants felt tired or stressed, they could take rest. After this session, the final session, identical to the pre-test session, began. Participants performed single-stance without any support for about 30 s. An image taken from the exercise session can be seen in Fig. 10.

Data Analysis The effects of the wearable balance exercise device were identified using acceleration data. Acceleration data was recorded using an M5 Stack IMU sensor that provided data with a sampling frequency of 100 Hz. The IMU sensor was fixed near the fifth lumbar spine (L5) on the posterior trunk as this position is close to our centre of mass (COM). A zero-phase Butterworth filter with a cut off frequency of 8 Hz was used to low pass filter the acceleration data after acquisition.

The peak acceleration values along X, Y and Z axes were identified, where X, Y and Z represent the mediolateral, vertical and anteroposterior directions, respectively. According to previous studies, postural responses can be observed between +100 and +400 ms after a perturbation is introduced [86, 87]. Unexpected perturbations also cause shifting of the COM, which can be closely measured and observed by the acceleration data. Thus, the root mean square (RMS) values of the acceleration, A_x, A_y, and A_z for the pre-test and post-test sessions were calculated and compared. Data of duration 10–20 s were used to calculate the RMS values of acceleration. Normality of the data was checked using the Shapiro Wilk test, and a paired t-test was used to compare the data.

Results The acceleration patterns for X and Y axes of a representative subject is shown in Fig. 12. In these graphs, the origin represents the start point of the perturbation. As can be seen in the graphs, both X and Y axes data show a positive and negative peak, respectively in the post perturbation period of 0 to +400 ms. The data representing the Z-axis was not of much significance because the current configuration of the PGMs cannot create a significant disturbance along the Z-axis. The RMS value of acceleration data showed a significant decrease during the post-test session as compared to the pre-test session for the X-axis, as shown in Fig. 13.

3.4 Swing Support System Using Wireless Actuation of PGMs

Another system using PGMs is described in this section to support the swing motion during walking [88]. This study aimed at reducing the delay involved in the PGM actuation resulting in a failed synchronization between gait and the support given through PGMs.

3.4.1 Motivation

Actuation of assistive support actuators in previous studies is triggered by placing a pressure sensor under the foot of the non-assisted leg [89, 90]. However, there is a significant delay between the trigger point and actuation. This delay may have adverse effects when hemiplegic patients use such assistance. Therefore, eliminating such a delay can help obtain optimum walking support for patients with unique walking parameters.

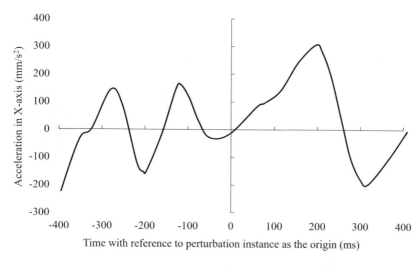

(a)

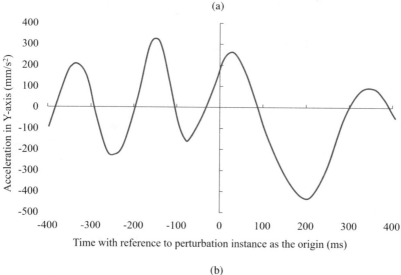

(b)

Fig. 12 Acceleration values measured for all axes during one leg stance exercise [82]. (**a**) Acceleration value in X-axis during one leg stance exercise. (**b**) Acceleration value in Y-axis during one leg stance exercise

3.4.2 System Description

The components used and attached to the wearable part of the walking assist are shown in Fig. 14 and listed in Table 2. The shoe contains a force-sensitive resistor (FSR) sensor and an AD converter module. The module sends the sensor data to a smartphone. The smartphone sends the same to a transistor switching module

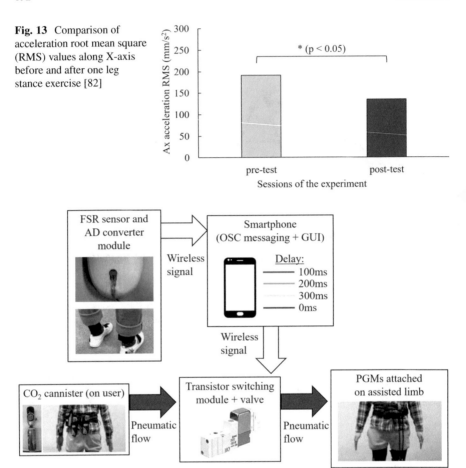

Fig. 13 Comparison of acceleration root mean square (RMS) values along X-axis before and after one leg stance exercise [82]

Fig. 14 Components used for the swing support system

Table 2 Major components of the wireless PGM driver. Abbreviations used: Force sensitive resistor (FSR), analog to digital (AD), open sound control (OSC), graphical user interface (GUI), pneumatic gel muscle (PGM)

Part	Component	Specifications
Shoe	Force sensor	FSR 400 short (Interlink Electronics)
	AD converter	$28.0 \times 39.5 \times 13.2$ mm, 18 g
Smartphone	OSC messaging	Solenoid valve state
	GUI	Adjustable delay with 100 ms increment
PGM part	Transistor switching	$28.0 \times 39.5 \times 13.2$ mm, 18 g
	Solenoid valve	SMC SYJ312M
	CO_2 canister	NTG (Nippon Tansan Gas Co. Ltd) 19 cm long
	PGM	350 mm initial length

through an open sound control (OSC) message. The smartphone is also used to select the desired delay in PGM actuation through a graphical user interface (GUI). According to the OSC message and the selected delay, the solenoid valve is turned on or off. The solenoid valve, in turn, alters the PGM actuation directly without delay. The CO_2 canister output air pressure is fixed at 0.2 MPa. This value of air pressure results in about 30 N force through the PGMs.

3.4.3 Evaluation of the Prototype Through Measurement of Various Lower Limb Parameters

Participants The PGM control system was evaluated using IMU data obtained from three healthy participants. The three participants who gave consent for this experiment were all males aged 22–28 years. The subjects reported no history of trauma, neuromuscular and orthopaedic diseases.

Experiment Protocol Seven IMU sensors (MTw; Xsens) were used at the following positions:

- Sacrum
- Front side of both thighs
- Front side of both shanks
- Bilateral anterior ankle

Two PGMs were attached from the left hip joint to the middle of the thigh using hook and loop fabrics, as shown in Fig. 14. Two CO_2 canisters were placed on the back of the waist using a belt. The waist belt also included the solenoid valves and the transistor module weighing around 1.5 kg. During gait, left hip flexion and right heel contact happen around the same time. Therefore, the FSR sensor was positioned below the right heel to detect ground contact. The AD converter module that processes the FSR sensor data was attached to one side of the shoe.

For all tasks, participants were asked to walk freely through a straight pathway (7 m) inside the laboratory at their preferred walking speed. During the first task, they walked without PGM support but wearing the suit. The next task involved walking with different assist conditions. The delay of PGM actuation after right heel contact was changed from 0 to 300 ms with steps of 100 ms. For each delay condition, the duration of PGM actuation was set to 100, 200, and 300 ms. The sequence of different conditions was randomized for each subject. During all tasks, IMU sensors recorded data at 60 Hz.

Data Analysis An in-house software called DhaibaWorks [91] was used to obtain the concerned joint angles of the lower limb. A plugin called posture reconstruction was used to reconstruct the lower-limb motion [92]. A database containing Japanese body dimensions was used to estimate the body model information from the weight and height of each subject who participated in the experiments [91]. Three gait cycles were selected for data analysis for each subject. First, the data containing angles of knee flexion (KF_θ) and hip flexion (HF_θ) during the swing phase of gait were extracted. The peak values from those data were identified. The standard deviation (SD) and average were also calculated. Following this, the condition of PGM-based assist during which there was a maximum rise in the angle of hip flexion (HF_θ) was identified. This was evidently the most effective assist condition. For this specific condition, the values of % coefficient of variation (CV), hip flexion angular velocity (HF_ω) during swing phase, and peak angle of knee flexion (KF_θ) were determined and compared with the no assist scenario. The %CV was determined using the following equation:

$$\%CV = \frac{SD}{Average} X 100 \tag{1}$$

Results Figure 15 shows the maximum angles of hip flexion (HF_θ) for all walking assist conditions. Subjects A and B did not show consistency in the effectiveness of assisting with PGM actuation. However, subject C showed increased hip flexion for all conditions except one condition, that is, 300 ms delay and 100 ms actuation duration. The maximum increase in hip flexion for subject C was around 7° whereas for subjects A and B the maximum increase was around 2°.

Figure 16 shows additional kinematic data comparing the assist and no assist conditions. For assist, the most effective condition was selected for this comparison. The consistency in the data trend was maintained for all three parameters. The decrease in %CV shows a reduced variability of the angle of hip flexion (HF_θ) under the assist condition. On the other hand, both hip flexion angular velocity (HF_ω) and peak angle of knee flexion (KF_θ) increased for the assisted condition.

4   Stealth Adaptive Exergame Design Framework

One of the most popular recent technological platforms explored for the enrichment of at-home motion training is the exergame [93]. *Exergame* is a term for exercise-based videogames, developed across a variety of platforms. Generally, these games are designed to encourage the user to exercise by requiring regular motion as a driving force for progress and completion of game objectives. The goal of exergames has gradually shifted to at-home rehabilitative training or motion task mediators targeting specific health outcomes. This requires *assessment* of exergames in supervised clinical settings in the presence of therapists and trainers. Despite rapid progress in exergame design, it is not easy to verify the improvement of physical fitness over long-term use [94]. This may at least partially have been due to one aspect of in-person training that was absent in the design of these earlier systems: *adaptation*. While the concept of adaptation has proven to be quite beneficial for effective exergame training in this field [95], exergames implementing dynamic difficulty adaptation have yielded mixed results due to factors such as age in terms of subject performance and engagement in long-term settings [96]. Generally, studies may evaluate exergames through some standardized assessment of motor function

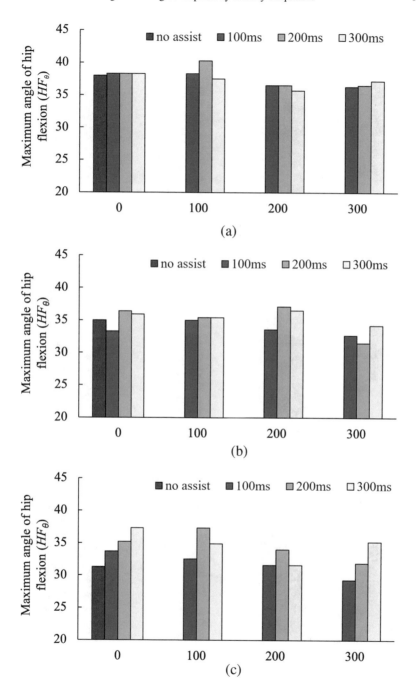

Fig. 15 Maximum values of angles of hip flexion (HF_θ) for no assist and with assist (various values of assist actuation duration) conditions for each subject [88]. (**a**) Maximum values of angles of hip flexion (HF_θ) for no assist and with assist (various values of assist actuation duration) conditions for subject A. (**b**) Maximum values of angles of hip flexion (HF_θ) for no assist and with assist (various values of assist actuation duration) conditions for subject B. (**c**) Maximum values of angles of hip flexion (HF_θ) for no assist and with assist (various values of assist actuation duration) conditions for subject C

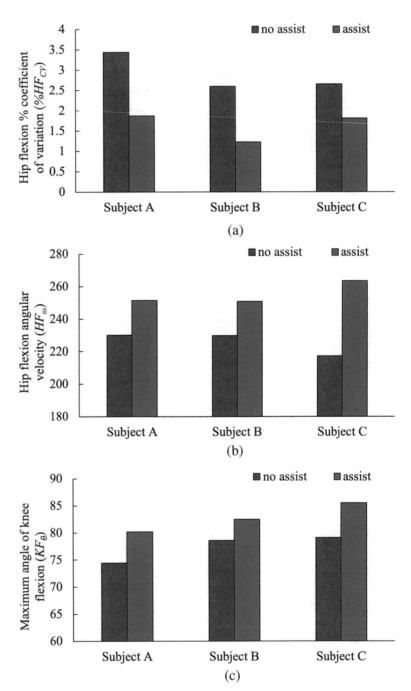

Fig. 16 Different parameters measured for assist and no assist cases for all subjects [88]. (**a**) Change in hip flexion % coefficient of variation ($\%HF_{CV}$) for all subjects. (**b**) Change in hip flexion angular velocity (HF_ω) in all subjects. (**c**) Change in maximum values of angles of knee flexion (KF_θ) for all subjects

to determine whether subjects' performance improved before and after usage of the exergame. However, and quite importantly, it is difficult to determine under such a design whether the functional improvement was directly a result of the exergame itself. This is because game performance cannot be linked as direct evidence for motion task performance in traditional exergame design. A novel approach has been proposed in [97] to address this primary limitation of existing adaptive exergames. Through this approach, rather than treating the motion task and exergame task as loosely similar objectives, the two can be directly mapped to one another by decomposing the motion task into its temporal and spatial characteristics, and then utilizing these characteristics, as well as factors of each individual's preference, to determine a best-matching task abstraction for the task, and then mapping the characteristics of that abstraction directly to the motion task itself. Furthermore, the linkage between the motion task and standardized assessment of motor function should be utilized to drive the adaptation process if it exists, and potentially, be discovered dynamically through AI processes during gameplay if it is not readily known. Under this approach, game task performance serves as evidence for motor task performance, and dynamic difficulty adaptation can utilize this evidence as an input to achieve sensitive and accurate adjustments for each individual and motion task. Such a mechanism for adaptation then allows gameplay to directly drive the success of the individual's functional improvement, allowing the individual to focus on gameplay without awareness of the underlying adaptation mechanism of the game environment. As such, the proposed design framework is entitled the Stealth Adaptive Exergame Design (SAED) framework.

There are five essential steps of the SAED framework of exergame design. The first requirement is that a motion task is determined which has been shown to improve the desired aspect of physical fitness for a particular individual. For elderly users, for example, these may include motor tasks which reduce fall risk and improve mobility. The next step is to determine the appropriate game concept around which the exergame will be built to match the exercise. Through this step, the expectations of the user, the trainer or therapist, and the motion task itself are to be met. If there is no intersection of these requirements, an exergame might not be a viable approach to at-home training for that individual. User preferences for game archetypes or themes can be determined through pre-interviews. The therapist's or trainer's preferences on the complexity of the game, exercise or task duration, and visual assessment of performance should also be considered. Finally, the motion task requires a matching game task which is repetitive and the most natural replication of the task itself. For example, if the task involves rhythmic and circular shoulder movements, a boat rowing game may serve as a natural abstraction. This is followed by the determination of characteristics of motion which can be used to evaluate the performance of the motion task. Three categories can be used to generalize these parameters: posture, corresponding to body position; progression, corresponding to range and precision of motion; and pacing, corresponding to the speed of motion. For example, characteristics of a push-up task include: shoulder/arm alignment, back straightness, core tightening, and hand placement for posture; the vertical degree of motion (how close one can get to the ground while maintaining proper posture) for progression; and the time required to reach the bottom point and return to the initial top point for pacing. This division of any motion task into three categories of performance is referred to as motion task decomposition and encompasses a single repetition or attempt at the motion task. The final step of SAED is the combination of real-time AI and standardized functional assessment to allow for dynamic difficulty adaptation of game parameters. Several parameters related to this adaptation, including frequency of adjustment (how often is the game's difficulty adjusted), tolerance range for error (how far may a subject's performance deviate from the expected level of performance before an adjustment occurs), and other performance factors, are determined in consultation with the trainer or therapist to identify what best suits the exercise or rehabilitation program for each individual. To determine when real-time adjustment is needed, the system must have a mechanism to predict the impact of various levels of difficulty on an individual's performance at standardized assessments of function. Sometimes, these systems are already present, such as the Wolf Motor Function Test (WMFT) used by many rehabilitation programs. In other cases, such as elderly mobility, the relationship between a task and its corresponding standardized motor function assessment are less clear and must be learned by the system. In these cases, a system such as a neural network, Bayes net, or Reinforcement Learning (RL) may be necessary, depending on the nature of the relationship. The learning system utilizes the posture, progression and pacing performance of the subject at the motion task as inputs and then classifies (predicts) the subject's performance at the chosen standard of assessment. This prediction is then used to determine how the corresponding gameplay parameters should be adjusted to match the subject's performance. One key advantage of the decomposition above is that these parameters can be assessed and adjusted independently. For instance, a subject's posture and pacing may meet expected values and only in progression does the subject have weaker performance, in which case only the parameters related to progression should be dynamically adjusted. Two cases of existing work implementing this framework are presented as proofs of concept in the next sections.

4.1 Fruit Slicing Exergame Design

In the first case, detailed in [98], a fruit-slicing exergame was designed to assist a hemiparetic individual in completing bimanual stick swinging exercises at home as a part of that individual's rehabilitative exercise program. The task was provided by the subject's physical trainer: a motion task wherein a stick should be swung in a horizontal arc in a controlled and precise manner. Each repetition of the task involves a single swing of the stick, with postural requirements including that the paretic arm maintains contact with the stick, progression requiring that the stick reach a certain range of motion with as little deviation as possible from the ideal horizontal swing trajectory, and pacing requiring that the swing be completed within a certain time interval. The aforementioned requirements represent those of the trainer. The inclusion of imaginary points in space as 'critical points' in the stick's trajectory resulted in the decision to design a fruit-slicing game wherein fruit objects fall from the sky in waves and each wave requires a single swing of the stick to swing the virtual sword to slice the fruit. Moreover, the individual participant showed a preference to play fruit-slicing games. The virtual sword was held by the subject's paretic arm, requiring that this arm maintains contact to correctly complete a slice. Furthermore, the size and falling rate of the fruit objects determined the precision and speed, respectively, of the swing motion required to slice them.

Having successfully created this mapping, a Bayes net was used to relate the subject's swing performance to an individually tailored functional assessment mechanism designed by the trainer, and parameters were adapted for difficulty based on the system's belief state about the subject after each swing. For example, if the subject's rate of motion fell below the tolerance range of error for pacing set by the trainer, the falling rate of fruit objects would be reduced wave by wave until the subject re-entered this range, and vice versa. In this way, postural, progression and pacing requirements would be individually and independently adapted. As the trainer developed the mechanisms for determining subject performance and assigning exercises, this trainer was utilized to verify the predictions of the Bayes net. The approach was found to match the trainer's performance assessments directly, thereby validating the use of this framework for improving the functional recovery of this individual during rehabilitation.

4.2 Ski Squat Exergame Design

A more recent example detailed in [99] involved the design of an exergame in supporting the at-home reduction of locomotive syndrome risk in the ageing population. The Japanese Orthopaedic Association served as the centre of expertise for functional performance assessment of mobility and recommended exercises in relation to this exergame. A commonly recommended exercise for improving musculoskeletal strength is the squat, with parameters for posture including back straightness, knee shakiness, the position of each knee relative to its corresponding foot, among other parameters. Requirements for progression include that the subject squats as low as possible without falling or causing a knee injury. Finally, the length of time required to reach the fully squatted and fully standing positions constituted requirements in pacing for this exercise. The task of skiing was chosen as a suitable game abstraction since the ski squat is a known standing variant of the squat exercise, and it is a popular activity for all ages in Japan where the study was held. The abstraction utilized a version of skiing wherein gates would appear during the ski course, and the subject would be required to squat under the gates to pass them. The distance between these gates could be mapped directly to the required speed of the squat. In contrast, the height of the top of each gate and their widths (as well as the steadiness of the skiing avatar) corresponded to progression and postural requirements, respectively. These could all be adjusted gate by gate over a virtual ski course.

The Japanese Orthopaedic Association uses a standardized test known as the standard testing battery for the locomotive syndrome (STBLS) [100] for determining one's locomotive risk level. These assessments require three tasks involving standing, walking and providing feedback on one's level of pain at various mobility tasks over the last month. Parameters used to determine squat performance, such as knee bend angle, the centre of mass deviation, and others did not yet have a readily known relationship with the outcomes of the STBLS. Therefore, parameters and outcomes were related through the implementation of a Neural Network trained using labelled data pairing a subject's squat performance with STBLS outcomes. After training, the system was fine-tuned over time by observing the error in its predictions relative to a subject's actual performance. These predictions drove the adaptation mechanism of the system, which not only modified game attributes, but also modified the level of physical support or resistance a subject received, as the system also included a worn soft exoskeletal suit for augmentation [101].

4.2.1   System Description of Ski Exergame

Exosuit Muscular training is highly efficient if an external load activates the muscles. Therefore, in this work, an exosuit was designed to provide an adjustable load to the lower limb muscles externally during squat motion. This exosuit provides an effective training environment through additional load on the lower limb muscles. The components used to build the exosuit are mentioned in Fig. 17. The exosuit

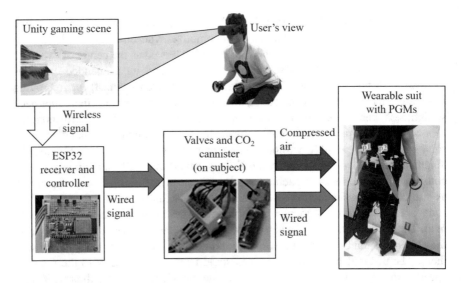

Fig. 17 Control and signal flow for the designed ski exergame

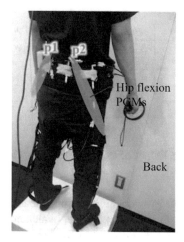
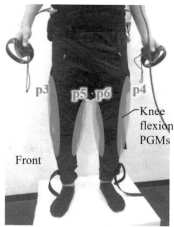

Fig. 18 The pneumatic gel muscle (PGM)-based exosuit designed for lower limbs as a resistive augmentation to the squat motion in a ski exergame [101]

was used while performing squat motions through a ski exergame. The exergame provided an immersive VR experience that could motivate the subjects to continue the exercise for a longer period. An ESP32 micro-controller board enabled with Wi-Fi reception was used to drive the actuation of the PGMs attached to the lower limb exosuit through SMC SYJ312M solenoid valves. The source of compressed air, the CO_2 canister, was placed on the waist of the subject using a belt. A total of three solenoid valves were used to enable individual actuation of the PGMs. The PGMs used for lower limb muscle activation are shown in Fig. 18. Six PGMs were used in total as illustrated (p1 to p6). The PGM pair p1 and p2 were attached from the back of the pelvis to the thighs. These PGMs were designated to oppose hip extension motion. Similarly, p3, p4, p5 and p6 were attached from the thigh to the calf along the medial and lateral sides of both legs to resist knee extension motion. To vary the load on the lower limb muscles, the number of PGMs actuated at different stages were 0, 2, 4 and 6.

Exergame The exergame was used as a motivator to perform squat motions with and without additional load provided by the exosuit. It comprised a skiing scene where the subject had to squat to cross yellow coloured ramps, as shown in Fig. 17. The number of ski ramps was variable according to the decided difficulty level provided to each individual. Table 3 shows the load provided to each individual through a varying number of ramps and actuated PGMs in the ski exergame scene. The risk level defined here was decided according to previous work on the determination of locomotive risk level using neural networks [99].

Table 3 Number of ski ramps and actuated pneumatic gel muscles (PGMs) corresponding to each locomotive risk level [101]

Risk level	Number of ski ramps (N)	Actuated PGMs
1	5	6 (p1, p2, p3, p4, p5, p6)
2	4	4 (p1, p2, p3, p4)
3	3	2 (p1, p2)
4	2	0

4.2.2 sEMG Measurement to Detect the Effect of PGM Based Muscle Loading

Participants The exosuit was intended to provide an additional load to lower extremity muscles while performing squat. Its effectiveness was evaluated through the measurement of surface electromyography (sEMG). Five healthy subjects consented for this experiment. The mean age of the participants was 22.8 ± 1.6. They did not report any history of motor impairment in their lower extremity.

Experiment Protocol This experiment was to evaluate the effects of the exosuit on the lower limb muscles. Therefore, the participants were asked to perform free squat under three conditions:

- without suit;
- with suit and no PGM actuation;
- and with suit and PGM actuation.

The PGM actuation during the third condition was initiated in synchronization with the rising phase of each squat motion. The sequence of the tasks was randomized to avoid any learning effect on the results. The sEMG data were measured on the following lower extremity muscles on the left and right sides:

- Vastus Medialis left and right (VM_L and VM_R);
- Vastus Lateralis left and right (VL_L and VL_R);
- and Rectus Femoris left and right (RF_L and RF_R).

The subjects were instructed to remove body hair if any before the experiment. The sEMG data were recorded using DELSYS Trigno wireless EMG sensors. Before performing the squat, maximum voluntary contraction (MVC) was measured for each muscle to normalize the data later.

Data Analysis The sEMG data obtained for each muscle was normalized using the MVC data to obtain %MVC. The statistical differences were identified among the three conditions using analysis of variance (ANOVA). Holm method was also applied to identify statistical differences between the conditions.

Results The average %MVC of five subjects for three different conditions are illustrated in Fig. 19. ANOVA showed significant differences in the muscle sites of VM_R (F1,3 = 6.08, $p < 0.01$) and RF_L (F1,3 = 3.46, $p < 0.05$). On applying the

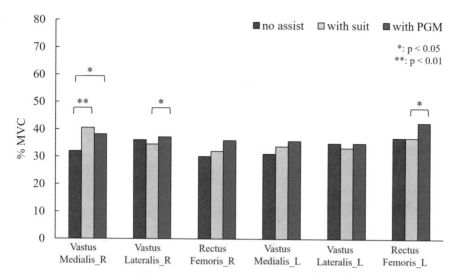

Fig. 19 Results of electromyographical (EMG) data during the ski exergame [101]

Holm method for identifying individual statistical differences, with PGM showed statistically increased %MVC for VL_R and RF_L when compared to with suit case. For VM_R, with suit and with PGM both showed statistically increased %MVC as compared to no suit condition.

5   An IMU-Based Assessment of Brushed Body Area

This section describes a self-assessment technique to evaluate bathing skill. The prototype includes a body brush with an attached IMU sensor. The work is quite significant for the ageing population in terms of self-evaluation, and was first reported in [102].

5.1   *Motivation*

In the medical field in Japan, the Functional Independence Measure (FIM) is used as an index to measure a patient's daily-life performance. The FIM consists of motor items and cognitive items. The motor items include thirteen items related to self-care, excretion, transfer, and movement; the cognitive items include five items concerning social recognition and communication. Self-care items represent the level of independence during eating, dressing, grooming, bathing, and toileting. In the "bathing" category, the experimenter asks the patient to simulate the action of wiping the body in a sitting position. They discern the subject's degree of wiping independence based on observing wiping sites at ten locations on the body, including the chest, right/left upper limb, abdomen, right/left thigh, right/left lower thigh, pudenda, and buttocks. For frail patients, they employ a body brush as an assistance tool. The frailer the patient, the more incomplete the cleansing of each body part, making it difficult to perform a suitable evaluation in terms of a simple number of wiped areas. Consequently, the scoring of bathing is more infeasible than for other items. To address this challenge, a wiping-site assessment system was developed for a quantitative evaluation of "bathing" skill [102].

5.2 System Description

The motion of the brush and whole-body were measured using an IMU-based motion capture system implemented on the DhaibaWorks platform [91]. Dhaiba-Works is a software package for measuring, analyzing, and visualizing human motion using a digital human model. In the IMU-based system, the joint angles of the digital human model are estimated from the orientation data captured by IMUs attached to the subject's body segments. The IMU-based system is applicable for capturing the motion of a hand-held product [92]. In this study, the wiping motion measurement was performed by estimating the posture of the body and body brush based on a contact detection algorithm to quantify the wiped area.

5.3 Calculation of the Contact Area Between Brush and Body Based on Distance Metrics

The mounting position of the IMUs is shown in Fig. 20. The reference points are defined on the surface of the tip of the brush head. The actual contact between the brush and body occurs when the hair of the brush contacts the human body. The threshold for detecting contact is determined accordingly. As shown in Fig. 21a, the normal direction distance $d_n(q_i, v_j, n)$ to a digital human model vertex q_i at a brush reference point v_j is defined in Eq. 2 and the radial distance d_r from the brush mesh to the vertex is defined in Eq. 3.

$$d_n(q_i, v_j, n) = |n(q_i) \cdot (q_i - v_j)| \tag{2}$$

$$d_r = \sqrt{||q_i - v_j||^2 - d_n(q_i, v, n)^2} \tag{3}$$

The contact condition in this algorithm is expressed by the following inequalities:

$$d_n < D_n \tag{4}$$

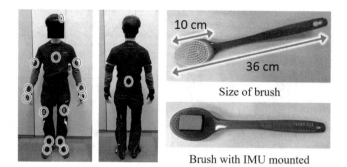

10 cm

36 cm

Size of brush

Brush with IMU mounted

Fig. 20 Mounting positions of the IMU sensors on the user's body and dimensions of the brush used

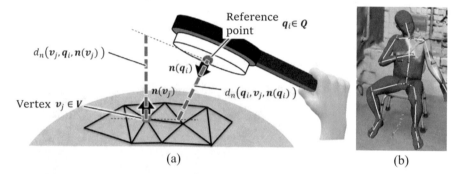

(a)   (b)

Fig. 21 (**a**) Distance calculation between the brush and the human body (**b**) Visualized brushed area on the human model

$$d_r < D_r \tag{5}$$

In Eq. 4, D_n represents the normal direction distance threshold. In Eq. 5, D_r represents the radial distance threshold. At each v_j on the human body, when both Eqs. 4 and 5 are simultaneously satisfied, contact is detected. Figure 21b shows the visualization result. The contact is expressed in colours ranging from red to yellow, green, and blue.

5.4 Comparison of Predicted and Actual Contact Area

The visualization results depend on the values of D_n and D_r. The actual contact area was measured using a paper attached to the front of the body of the subject to verify the accuracy of selected values (Fig. 22). During the experiment, the subject was asked to wipe the paper with a wet brush. The paper colour changed from white to black when it was wiped. The wiped area was detected by image

| Image capture | Trimming | Binarization | Comparison of brushed and unbrushed areas |

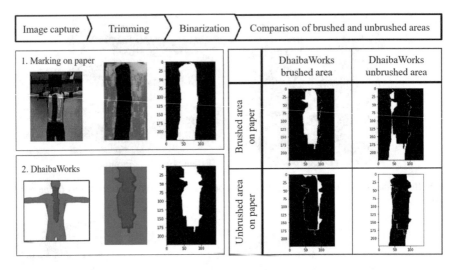

Fig. 22   Overview of the brushed area evaluation experiment

Fig. 23 Evaluation method
of the brushed area

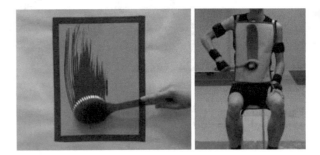

processing. Simultaneously, the wiping movement was measured using the IMUs. The evaluation method is illustrated in Fig. 23.

Table 4 depicts the mean % accuracy of the brushed area in the two brushing motion trials for each threshold. The changes in % accuracy were confirmed by varying the threshold values. When $D_n = 130$ mm and $D_r = 5$ mm, the highest % accuracy (=92%) was achieved. The mean % accuracy for each D_n and D_r values are also depicted in Fig. 24.

6   Conclusion

This chapter described selected state-of-the-art technologies for rehabilitation and assistance with particular emphasis on the elderly. It also provided an extensive review of technologies on personalized rehabilitation, sports training, telerehabilitation and wearable exoskeletons. The actuator called the pneumatic gel muscle

Table 4 Accuracy (%) for different combinations of the values of normal direction distance threshold (D_n) and radial distance threshold (D_r) [102]

Accuracy (%)		D_n (mm)					
		100	110	120	130	140	150
D_r (mm)	1	67.2	68.0	67.2	67.2	67.6	67.7
	2	73.1	72.8	72.3	72.3	72.8	72.3
	3	83.6	84.2	84.5	85.6	85.2	83.6
	4	91.3	91.9	90.7	92.6	92.2	90.8
	5	92.5	92.8	93.6	93.9	92.6	92.6
	6	91.8	92.2	92.2	92.3	92.1	92.3
	7	91.6	91.1	91.1	91.2	91.1	91.9
	8	92.2	93.5	92.8	91.2	91.2	91.2
	9	90.8	92.2	92.3	91.4	92.8	91.2
	10	90.6	90.8	91.0	90.9	91.2	90.7

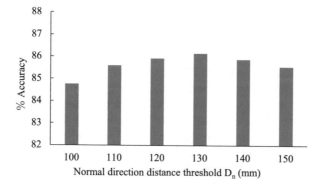

(a) Average % accuracy for different values of normal direction distance threshold (D_n).

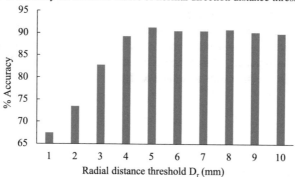

(b) Average % accuracy for different values of radial distance threshold (D_r).

Fig. 24 Average % accuracy for different values of normal direction distance threshold (D_n) and radial distance threshold (D_r) [102]. (**a**) Average % accuracy for different values of normal direction distance threshold (D_n). (**b**) Average % accuracy for different values of radial distance threshold (D_r)

(PGM) that was used for four of the included systems of this chapter was described along with its force characteristics. The customized inner tube of this actuator enables it to actuate and produce larger forces at a significantly low air pressure requirement as compared to commercially available low-pressure soft pneumatic actuators. This low air pressure property of the actuators enables their use for portable applications without the need of a heavyweight compressor. As mentioned in the chapter, small and portable CO_2 canisters were used as a source of compressed air in the four application scenarios. The first was an exoskeleton jacket proposed for remote human interaction. Because of the simplicity, portability and lightweightedness of the system, it holds significant potential to be used in real-world scenarios by people of particular need and the elderly. Moreover, the latency measured in the system was within an acceptable range. The second application scenario was a soft wearable balance exercise device using PGMs. This systems also has immense potential to be used by the elderly because of its lightweight and wearable configuration. The results showed significant stability among subjects after exercising with the system. A wireless swing support system was also developed using PGMs with a unit for delay compensation. The results indicated that leg swing could be assisted more effectively using PGMs using an optimum delay parameter tailored to each user. The importance of exergames in rehabilitation was explained, following which the stealth adaptive exergame design (SAED) framework was elaborated and utilized to design two exergames. A ski exergame for squat training with a changeable load was presented. The game used a PGM-based lower-limb exosuit to provide resistive force while squatting. The results showed significantly increased muscle activity in three measured muscles during the actuated PGM condition. Finally, a novel IMU-based bathing-skill assessment device was presented. An algorithm was discussed to estimate the contact area between the brush and body. The proposed device was validated by comparing the estimated and actual brushed areas.

The aim of this chapter was to highlight novel technological advances in the field of rehabilitation, assistance and daily healthcare. Future work in this area will expand the prospect of such devices being accepted for daily life usage by individuals with special needs and the elderly.

References

1. UN – World Population Ageing (2019). https://www.un.org/en/development/desa/population/publications/pdf/ageing/. Last accessed 2020/09/15
2. Angel, J.L., Mudrazija, S.: Local government efforts to mitigate the novel coronavirus pandemic among older adults. J. Aging Soc. Policy **32**(4–5), 439–449 (2020). https://doi.org/10.1080/08959420.2020.1771240
3. Peek, S.T.M., Luijkx, K.G., Rijnaard, M.D., Nieboer, M.E., van der Voort, C.S., Aarts, S., van Hoof, J., Vrijhoef, H.J.M., Wouters, E.J.M.: Older adults' reasons for using technology while aging in place. Gerontology **62**(2), 226–237 (2015). https://doi.org/10.1159/000430949

4. Agree, E.M.: The potential for technology to enhance independence for those aging with a disability. Disabil. Health J. **7**(1), S33–S39 (2014). https://doi.org/10.1016/j.dhjo.2013.09.004

5. Reeder, B., Meyer, E., Lazar, A., Chaudhuri, S., Thompson, H.J., Demiris, G.: Framing the evidence for health smart homes and home-based consumer health technologies as a public health intervention for independent aging: A systematic review. Int. J. Med. Inform. **82**(7), 565–579 (2013). https://doi.org/10.1016/j.ijmedinf.2013.03.007

6. Nonnekes, J., Nieuwboer, A.: Towards personalized rehabilitation for gait impairments in Parkinson's disease. J. Parkinson's Dis. **8**(s1), S101–S106 (2018). https://doi.org/10.3233/jpd-181464

7. Morita, Y., Nagasaki, M., Ukai, H., Matsui, N., Uchida, M.: Development of rehabilitation training support system of upper limb motor function for personalized rehabilitation. In: 2008 IEEE International Conference on Robotics and Biomimetics, pp. 300–305 (2009). https://doi.org/10.1109/ROBIO.2009.4913020

8. Romano, A.M., Oliva, F., Nastrucci, G., Casillo, P., Di Giunta, A., Susanna, M., Ascione, F.: Reverse shoulder arthroplasty patient personalized rehabilitation protocol. Preliminary results according to prognostic groups. Muscles Ligaments Tendons J., 263–270 (2017). https://doi.org/10.11138/mltj/2017.7.2.263

9. Lee, M.H., Siewiorek, D.P., Smailagic, A., Bernardino, A., Bermúdez i Badia, S.: Interactive hybrid approach to combine machine and human intelligence for personalized rehabilitation assessment. In: Proceedings of the ACM Conference on Health, Inference, and Learning, pp. 160–169. ACM, Toronto (2020). https://doi.org/10.1145/3368555.3384452

10. Klinger, E., Kadri, A., Sorita, E., Le Guiet, J.-L., Coignard, P., Fuchs, P., Leroy, L., du Lac, N., Servant, F., Joseph, P.-A.: AGATHE: A tool for personalized rehabilitation of cognitive functions based on simulated activities of daily living. IRBM **34**(2), 113–118 (2013). https://doi.org/10.1016/j.irbm.2013.01.005

11. González-González, C.S., Toledo-Delgado, P.A., Muñoz-Cruz, V., Torres-Carrion, P.V.: Serious games for rehabilitation: Gestural interaction in personalized gamified exercises through a recommender system. J. Biomed. Inf. **97**, 103266 (2019). https://doi.org/10.1016/j.jbi.2019.103266

12. Kumar, D., González, A., Das, A., Dutta, A., Fraisse, P., Hayashibe, M., Lahiri, U.: Virtual reality-based center of mass-assisted personalized balance training system. Front. Bioeng. Biotechnol. **5**, 85–99 (2018). https://doi.org/10.3389/fbioe.2017.00085

13. Safonicheva, O.G., Ovchinnikova, M.A. New approaches to the development of personalized rehabilitation programs for the children with disabilities, including autism spectrum disorders. In: Autism 360○, pp. 427–475. Academic Press (2020). https://doi.org/10.1016/B978-0-12-818466-0.00022-8

14. Des Roches, C.A., Kiran, S.: Technology-based rehabilitation to improve communication after acquired brain injury. Front. Neurosci. **11**, 382 (2017). https://doi.org/10.3389/fnins.2017.00382

15. Bendíková, E.: Lifestyle, physical and sports education and health benefits of physical activity. Eur. Res. (2–2), 343–348 (2014). https://doi.org/10.13187/issn.2219-8229

16. Ishii, H., Wisneski, C., Orbanes, J., Chun, B., Paradiso, J.: PingPongPlus: design of an athletic-tangible interface for computer-supported cooperative play. In: Proceedings of the SIGCHI Conference on Human Factors in Computing Systems, pp. 394–401 (1999). https://doi.org/10.1145/302979.303115

17. Bideau, B., Kulpa, R., Ménardais, S., Fradet, L., Multon, F., Delamarche, P., Arnaldi, B.: Real handball goalkeeper vs. virtual handball thrower. Presence Teleop. Virt. Environ. **12**(4), 411–421 (2003). https://doi.org/10.1162/105474603322391631

18. Bideau, B., Multon, F., Kulpa, R., Fradet, L., Arnaldi, B., Delamarche, P.: Using virtual reality to analyze links between handball thrower kinematics and goalkeeper's reactions. Neurosci. Lett. **372**(1–2), 119–122 (2004). https://doi.org/10.1016/j.neulet.2004.09.023

19. Pan, Z., Xu, W., Huang, J., Zhang, M., Shi, J.: Easybowling: a small bowling machine based on virtual simulation. Comput. Graph. **27**(2), 231–238 (2003). https://doi.org/10.1016/S0097-8493(02)00280-7

20. Hämäläinen, P., Ilmonen, T., Höysniemi, J., Lindholm, M., Nykänen, A.: Martial arts in artificial reality. In: Proceedings of the SIGCHI Conference on Human Factors in Computing Systems, pp. 781–790 (2005). https://doi.org/10.1145/1054972.1055081

21. Craig, C.M., Berton, E., Rao, G., Fernandez, L., Bootsma, R.J.: Judging where a ball will go: the case of curved free kicks in football. Naturwissenschaften **93**(2), 97–101 (2006). https://doi.org/10.1007/s00114-005-0071-0

22. Bideau, B., Kulpa, R., Vignais, N., Brault, S., Multon, F., Craig, C.: Using virtual reality to analyze sports performance. IEEE Comput. Graph. Appl. **30**(2), 14–21 (2009). https://doi.org/10.1109/MCG.2009.134

23. Fink, P.W., Foo, P.S., Warren, W.H.: Catching fly balls in virtual reality: a critical test of the outfielder problem. J. Vis. **9**(13), 14 (2009). https://doi.org/10.1167/9.13.14

24. Craig, C.M., Goulon, C., Berton, E., Rao, G., Fernandez, L., Bootsma, R.J.: Optic variables used to judge future ball arrival position in expert and novice soccer players. Attention Perception Psychophys. **71**(3), 515–522 (2009). https://doi.org/10.3758/APP.71.3.515

25. Bergamasco, M., Bardy, B., Gopher, D.: Skill training in multimodal virtual environments. CRC Press (2012). https://doi.org/10.1201/b12704

26. Dhawan, A., Cummins, A., Spratford, W., Dessing, J.C., Craig, C.: Development of a novel immersive interactive virtual reality cricket simulator for cricket batting. In: Proceedings of the 10th International Symposium on Computer Science in Sports (ISCSS), pp. 203–210. Springer, Cham (2016). https://doi.org/10.1007/978-3-319-24560-7_26

27. Huang, Y., Churches, L., Reilly, B.: A case study on virtual reality American football training. In: Proceedings of the 2015 Virtual Reality International Conference, pp. 1–5 (2015). https://doi.org/10.1145/2806173.2806178

28. Hoffmann, C.P., Filippeschi, A., Ruffaldi, E., Bardy, B.G.: Energy management using virtual reality improves 2000-m rowing performance. J. Sports Sci. **32**(6), 501–509 (2014). https://doi.org/10.1080/02640414.2013.835435

29. Yamashita, S., Zhang, X., Rekimoto, J.: Aquacave: Augmented swimming environment with immersive surround-screen virtual reality. In: Proceedings of the 29th Annual Symposium on User Interface Software and Technology, pp. 183–184 (2016). https://doi.org/10.1145/2984751.2984760

30. Tiator, M., Geiger, C., Dewitz, B., Fischer, B., Gerhardt, L., Nowottnik, D., Preu, H.: Venga! climbing in mixed reality. In: Proceedings of the First Superhuman Sports Design Challenge: First International Symposium on Amplifying Capabilities and Competing in Mixed Realities, pp. 1–8 (2018). https://doi.org/10.1145/3210299.3210308

31. Scilingo, E.P., Lorussi, F., Mazzoldi, A., De Rossi, D.: Strain-sensing fabrics for wearable kinaesthetic-like systems. IEEE Sensors J. **3**(4), 460–467 (2003). https://doi.org/10.1109/JSEN.2003.815771

32. Chittenden, T.: Skin in the game: the use of sensing smart fabrics in tennis costume as a means of analyzing performance. Fashion Textiles **4**(1), 22 (2017). https://doi.org/10.1186/s40691-017-0107-z

33. Ray, T., Choi, J., Reeder, J., Lee, S.P., Aranyosi, A.J., Ghaffari, R., Rogers, J.A.: Soft, skin-interfaced wearable systems for sports science and analytics. Curr. Opin. Biomed. Eng. **9**, 47–56 (2019). https://doi.org/10.1016/j.cobme.2019.01.003

34. Fong, D.T., Wong, J.C.W., Lam, A.H., Lam, R.H., Li, W.J.: A wireless motion sensing system using ADXL MEMS accelerometers for sports science applications. In: Fifth World Congress on Intelligent Control and Automation (CAT), vol. 6, pp. 5635–5640. IEEE, Piscataway (2004). https://doi.org/10.1109/WCICA.2004.1343815

35. Margarito, J., Helaoui, R., Bianchi, A.M., Sartor, F., Bonomi, A.G.: User-independent recognition of sports activities from a single wrist-worn accelerometer: A template-matching-based approach. IEEE Trans. Biomed. Eng. **63**(4), 788–796 (2015). https://doi.org/10.1109/TBME.2015.2471094

36. Kidman, E.M., D'Souza, M.J., Singh, S.P.: A wearable device with inertial motion tracking and vibro-tactile feedback for aesthetic sport athletes Diving Coach Monitor. In: 2016 10th International Conference on Signal Processing and Communication Systems (ICSPCS), pp. 1–6. IEEE, Piscataway (2016). https://doi.org/10.1109/ICSPCS.2016.7843371
37. Rawashdeh, S.A., Rafeldt, D.A., Uhl, T.L.: Wearable IMU for shoulder injury prevention in overhead sports. Sensors 16(11), 1847 (2016). https://doi.org/10.3390/s16111847
38. Gouwanda, D., Senanayake, S.M.N.A.: Real time multi-sensory force sensing mat for sports biomechanics and human gait analysis. Int. J. Intell. Syst. Technol. 3(3), 149–154 (2008). https://doi.org/10.5281/zenodo.1057839
39. Arumugam, D.D., Sibley, M., Griffin, J.D., Stancil, D.D., Ricketts, D.S.: An active position sensing tag for sports visualization in American football. In: 2013 IEEE International Conference on RFID (RFID), pp. 96–103. IEEE, Piscataway (2013). https://doi.org/10.1109/RFID.2013.6548141
40. Michahelles, F., Schiele, B.: Sensing and monitoring professional skiers. IEEE Pervas. Comput. 4(3), 40–45 (2005). https://doi.org/10.1109/MPRV.2005.66
41. Cummins, C., Orr, R., O'Connor, H., West, C.: Global positioning systems (GPS) and microtechnology sensors in team sports: a systematic review. Sports Med. 43(10), 1025–1042 (2013). https://doi.org/10.1007/s40279-013-0069-2
42. McIlwraith, D., Yang, G.Z.: Body sensor networks for sport, wellbeing and health. In: Sensor Networks, pp. 349–381. Springer, Berlin, Heidelberg (2010). https://doi.org/10.1007/978-3-642-01341-6_13
43. Jeukendrup, A.E., Chambers, E.S.: Oral carbohydrate sensing and exercise performance. Curr. Opin. Clin. Nutr. Metab. Care 13(4), 447–451 (2010). https://doi.org/10.1097/MCO.0b013e328339de83
44. Nenonen, V., Lindblad, A., Häkkinen, V., Laitinen, T., Jouhtio, M., Hämäläinen, P.: Using heart rate to control an interactive game. In: Proceedings of the SIGCHI conference on Human factors in computing systems, pp. 853–856 (2007). https://doi.org/10.1145/1240624.1240752
45. Wang, Y., Chen, M., Wang, X., Chan, R.H., Li, W.J.: IoT for next-generation racket sports training. IEEE Internet Things J. 5(6), 4558–4566 (2018). https://doi.org/10.1109/JIOT.2018.2837347
46. Gowda, M., Dhekne, A., Shen, S., Choudhury, R.R., Yang, L., Golwalkar, S., Essanian, A.: Bringing IoT to sports analytics. In: 14th USENIX Symposium on Networked Systems Design and Implementation (NSDI 17), pp. 499–513 (2017). https://doi.org/10.5555/3154630.3154672
47. Wilkerson, G.B., Gupta, A., Colston, M.A.: Mitigating sports injury risks using internet of things and analytics approaches. Risk Anal. 38(7), 1348–1360 (2018). https://doi.org/10.1111/risa.12984
48. Ikram, M.A., Alshehri, M.D., Hussain, F.K.: Architecture of an IoT-based system for football supervision (IoT Football). In: 2015 IEEE 2nd World Forum on Internet of Things (WF-IoT), pp. 69–74. IEEE, Piscataway (2015). https://doi.org/10.1109/WF-IoT.2015.7389029
49. Rudin, A.R.A., Audah, L., Jamil, A., Abdullah, J.: Occupancy monitoring system for campus sports facilities using the Internet of Things (IoT). In: 2016 IEEE Conference on Wireless Sensors (ICWiSE), pp. 100–105. IEEE, Piscataway (2016). https://doi.org/10.1109/ICWISE.2016.8188550
50. Lee, T.G.: Analysis of golf ball mobility and balancing based on IoT sports environments. Int. J. Adv. Smart Convergence 8(3), 78–86 (2019). https://doi.org/10.7236/IJASC.2019.8.3.78
51. Kim, J., Kim, S.: Development of wearable sports helmet model using IoT server technology. In: Information Science and Applications, pp. 691–695. Springer, Singapore (2020). https://doi.org/10.1007/978-981-15-1465-4_69
52. Catarinucci, L., De Donno, D., Mainetti, L., Patrono, L., Stefanizzi, M.L., Tarricone, L.: An IoT-aware architecture to improve safety in sports environments. J. Commun. Softw. Syst. 13(2), 44–52 (2017). https://doi.org/10.24138/jcomss.v13i2.372

53. Novatchkov, H., Baca, A.: Fuzzy logic in sports: a review and an illustrative case study in the field of strength training. Int. J. Comput. Appl. **71**(6), 8–14 (2013). https://doi.org/10.5120/12360-8675

54. Vales-Alonso, J., Chaves-Diéguez, D., López-Matencio, P., Alcaraz, J.J., Parrado-Garcia, F.J., Gonzalez-Castano, F. J.: SAETA: A smart coaching assistant for professional volleyball training. IEEE Trans. Syst. Man Cybern. Syst. **45**(8), 1138–1150 (2015). https://doi.org/10.1109/TSMC.2015.2391258

55. Brault, S., Bideau, B., Craig, C., Kulpa, R.: Balancing deceit and disguise: How to successfully fool the defender in a 1 vs. 1 situation in rugby. Hum. Mov. Sci. **29**(3), 412–425 (2010). https://doi.org/10.1016/j.humov.2009.12.004

56. Fok, W.W., Chan, L.C., Chen, C.: Artificial intelligence for sport actions and performance analysis using recurrent neural network (RNN) with long short-term memory (LSTM). In: Proceedings of the 2018 4th International Conference on Robotics and Artificial Intelligence, pp. 40–44 (2018). https://doi.org/10.1145/3297097.3297115

57. Farley, O.R., Abbiss, C.R., Sheppard, J.M.: Performance analysis of surfing: a review. J. Strength Cond. Res. **31**(1), 260–271 (2017). https://doi.org/10.1519/JSC.0000000000001442

58. Bunker, R.P., Thabtah, F.: A machine learning framework for sport result prediction. Applied Comput. Inf. **15**(1), 27–33 (2019). https://doi.org/10.1016/j.aci.2017.09.005

59. Claudino, J.G., de Oliveira Capanema, D., de Souza, T.V., Serrão, J.C., Pereira, A.C.M., Nassis, G.P.: Current approaches to the use of artificial intelligence for injury risk assessment and performance prediction in team sports: a systematic review. Sports Med. Open **5**(1), 28 (2019). https://doi.org/10.1186/s40798-019-0202-3

60. Velayati, F., Ayatollahi, H., Hemmat, M.: A systematic review of the effectiveness of telerehabilitation interventions for therapeutic purposes in the elderly. Methods Inf. Med. **2020**(01) (2020). https://doi.org/10.1055/s-0040-1713398

61. Piron, L., Turolla, A., Agostini, M., Zucconi, C., Cortese, F., Zampolini, M., Tonin, P.: Exercises for paretic upper limb after stroke: a combined virtual-reality and telemedicine approach. J. Rehabil. Med. **41**(12), 1016–1020 (2009). https://doi.org/10.2340/16501977-0459

62. Bernocchi, P., Vitacca, M., La Rovere, M. T., Volterrani, M., Galli, T., Baratti, D., Paneroni, M., Campolongo, G., Sposato, B., Scalvini, S.: Home-based telerehabilitation in older patients with chronic obstructive pulmonary disease and heart failure: a randomised controlled trial. Age Ageing **47**(1), 82–88 (2018). https://doi.org/10.1093/ageing/afx146

63. Russell, T.G., Buttrum, P., Wootton, R., Jull, G.A.: Low-bandwidth telerehabilitation for patients who have undergone total knee replacement: preliminary results. J. Telemed. Telecare **9**(2_suppl), 44–47 (2003). https://doi.org/10.1258%2F135763303322596246

64. Piqueras, M., Marco, E., Coll, M., Escalada, F., Ballester, A., Cinca, C., Belmonte, R., Muniesa, J.M.: Effectiveness of an interactive virtual telerehabilitation system in patients after total knee arthroplasty: a randomized controlled trial. J. Rehabil. Med. **45**(4), 392–396 (2013). https://doi.org/10.2340/16501977-1119

65. Bini, S.A., Mahajan, J.: Clinical outcomes of remote asynchronous telerehabilitation are equivalent to traditional therapy following total knee arthroplasty: a randomized control study. J. Telemed. Telecare **23**(2), 239–247 (2017). https://doi.org/10.1177/2F1357633X16634518

66. Linder, S.M., Reiss, A., Buchanan, S., Sahu, K., Rosenfeldt, A.B., Clark, C., Wolf, S.L., Alberts, J.L.: Incorporating robotic-assisted telerehabilitation in a home program to improve arm function following stroke: a case study. J. Neurol. Phys. Ther. JNPT **37**(3), 125–132 (2013). https://dx.doi.org/10.1097%2FNPT.0b013e31829fa808

67. Chen, Y., Abel, K.T., Janecek, J.T., Chen, Y., Zheng, K., Cramer, S.C.: Home-based technologies for stroke rehabilitation: a systematic review. Int. J. Med. Inform. **123**, 11–22 (2019). https://doi.org/10.1016/j.ijmedinf.2018.12.001

68. Heo, P., Gu, G.M., Lee, S.J., Rhee, K., Kim, J.: Current hand exoskeleton technologies for rehabilitation and assistive engineering. Int. J. Precis. Eng. Manuf. **13**(5), 807–824 (2012). https://doi.org/10.1007/s12541-012-0107-2

69. Bogue, R.: Exoskeletons and robotic prosthetics: a review of recent developments. Ind. Robot. Int. J. **36**(5), 421–427 (2009). https://doi.org/10.1108/01439910910980141

70. Varghese, R.J., Freer, D., Deligianni, F., Liu, J., Yang, G.Z., Tong, R.: Wearable robotics for upper-limb rehabilitation and assistance: A review of the state-of-the-art challenges and future research. In: Wearable Technology in Medicine and Health Care, pp. 23–69. Elsevier (2018). https://doi.org/10.1016/B978-0-12-811810-8.00003-8

71. Pons, J.L.: A review of performance metrics for lower limb wearable robots: preliminary results. In: Wearable Robotics: Challenges and Trends: Proceedings of the 4th International Symposium on Wearable Robotics (WeRob2018). Pisa, vol. 22, pp. 147–151. Springer (2018). https://doi.org/10.1007/978-3-030-01887-0_29

72. Asbeck, A.T., Dyer, R.J., Larusson, A.F., Walsh, C.J.: Biologically-inspired soft exosuit. In: 2013 IEEE 13th International Conference on Rehabilitation Robotics (ICORR), pp. 1–8. IEEE, Piscataway (2013). https://doi.org/10.1109/ICORR.2013.6650455

73. Park, S.J., Park, C.H.: Suit-type wearable robot powered by shape-memory-alloy-based fabric muscle. Sci. Rep. **9**(1), 1–8 (2019). https://doi.org/10.1038/s41598-019-45722-x

74. Polygerinos, P., Lyne, S., Wang, Z., Nicolini, L.F., Mosadegh, B., Whitesides, G.M., Walsh, C.J.: Towards a soft pneumatic glove for hand rehabilitation. In: 2013 IEEE/RSJ International Conference on Intelligent Robots and Systems, pp. 1512–1517. IEEE, Piscataway (2013). https://doi.org/10.1109/IROS.2013.6696549

75. Oguntosin, V.W., Mori, Y., Kim, H., Nasuto, S.J., Kawamura, S., Hayashi, Y.: Design and validation of exoskeleton actuated by soft modules toward neurorehabilitation–vision-based control for precise reaching motion of upper limb. Front. Neurosci. **11**, 352 (2017). https://doi.org/10.3389/fnins.2017.00352

76. Polygerinos, P., Wang, Z., Galloway, K.C., Wood, R.J., Walsh, C.J.: Soft robotic glove for combined assistance and at-home rehabilitation. Robot. Auton. Syst. **73**, 135-143 (2015). https://doi.org/10.1016/j.robot.2014.08.014

77. Payne, C.J., Hevia, E.G., Phipps, N., Atalay, A., Atalay, O., Seo, B.R., Walsh, C.J.: Force control of textile-based soft wearable robots for mechanotherapy. In: 2018 IEEE International Conference on Robotics and Automation (ICRA), pp. 1–7. IEEE, Piscataway (2018). https://doi.org/10.1109/ICRA.2018.8461059

78. Guo, J., Xiang, C., Helps, T., Taghavi, M., Rossiter, J.: Electroactive textile actuators for wearable and soft robots. In: 2018 IEEE International Conference on Soft Robotics (RoboSoft), pp. 339–343. IEEE, Piscataway (2018). https://doi.org/10.1109/ROBOSOFT.2018.8404942

79. Satoh, H., Kawabata, T., Sankai, Y.: Bathing care assistance with robot suit HAL. In: 2009 IEEE International Conference on Robotics and Biomimetics (ROBIO), pp. 498–503. IEEE, Piscataway (2009). https://doi.org/10.1109/ROBIO.2009.5420697

80. Ogawa, K., Thakur, C., Ikeda, T., Tsuji, T., Kurita, Y.: Development of a pneumatic artificial muscle driven by low pressure and its application to the unplugged powered suit. Adv. Robot. **31**(21), 1135–1143 (2017). https://doi.org/10.1080/01691864.2017.1392345

81. Ramirez, A.V., Kurita, Y.: A soft exoskeleton jacket with pneumatic gel muscles for human motion interaction. In: International Conference on Human-Computer Interaction, pp. 587–603. Springer, Cham (2019). https://doi.org/10.1007/978-3-030-23563-5_46

82. Yamamoto, M., Kishishita, Y., Shimatani, K., Kurita, Y.: Development of new soft wearable balance exercise device using pneumatic gel muscles. Appl. Sci. **9**(15), 3108 (2019). https://doi.org/10.3390/app9153108

83. MacRae, P.G., Lacourse, M., Moldavon, R.: Physical performance measures that predict faller status in community-dwelling older adults. J. Orthop. Sports Phys. Ther. **16**(3), 123–128 (1992). https://www.jospt.org/doi/10.2519/jospt.1992.16.3.123

84. Michikawa, T., Nishiwaki, Y., Takebayashi, T., Toyama, Y.: One-leg standing test for elderly populations. J. Orthop. Sci. **14**(5), 675–685 (2009). https://doi.org/10.1007/s00776-009-1371-6

85. Dingenen, B., Staes, F.F., Janssens, L.: A new method to analyze postural stability during a transition task from double-leg stance to single-leg stance. J. Biomech. **46**(13), 2213–2219 (2013). https://doi.org/10.1016/j.jbiomech.2013.06.026

86. Cavanagh, P.R., Komi, P.V.: Electromechanical delay in human skeletal muscle under concentric and eccentric contractions. Eur. J. Appl. Physiol. Occup. Physiol. **42**(3), 159–163 (1979). https://doi.org/10.1007/BF00431022

87. Santos, M.J., Kanekar, N., Aruin, A.S.: The role of anticipatory postural adjustments in compensatory control of posture: 2. Biomechanical analysis. J. Electromyogr. Kinesiol. **20**(3), 398–405 (2010). https://doi.org/10.1016/j.jelekin.2010.01.002

88. Toda, H., Tada, M., Maruyama, T., Kurita, Y.: Effect of contraction parameters on swing support during walking using wireless pneumatic artificial muscle driver: a preliminary study. In: 2019 58th Annual Conference of the Society of Instrument and Control Engineers of Japan (SICE), pp. 727–732. IEEE, Piscataway (2019). https://doi.org/10.23919/SICE.2019.8859803

89. Thakur, C., Ogawa, K., Tsuji, T., Kurita, Y.: Soft wearable augmented walking suit with pneumatic gel muscles and stance phase detection system to assist gait. IEEE Robot. Autom. Lett. **3**(4), 4257–4264 (2018). https://doi.org/10.1109/LRA.2018.2864355

90. Park, Y.L., Chen, B.R., Pérez-Arancibia, N.O., Young, D., Stirling, L., Wood, R.J., Goldfield, U.C., Nagpal, R.: Design and control of a bio-inspired soft wearable robotic device for ankle–foot rehabilitation. Bioinspir. Biomim. **9**(1), 016007 (2014). https://doi.org/10.1088/1748-3182/9/1/016007

91. Endo, Y., Tada, M., Mochimaru, M.: Dhaiba: development of virtual ergonomic assessment system with human models. In: Proceedings of the 3rd International Digital Human Modeling Symposium, 58 (2014). http://www.dhm2014.org/program.html. Last accessed 2020/09/15

92. Maruyama, T., Tada, M., Sawatome, A., Endo, Y. Constraint-based real-time full-body motion-capture using inertial measurement units. In: 2018 IEEE International Conference on Systems, Man, and Cybernetics (SMC), pp. 4298–4303. IEEE, Piscataway (2018). https://doi.org/10.1109/SMC.2018.00727

93. Sween, J., Wallington, S.F., Sheppard, V., Taylor, T., Llanos, A.A., Adams-Campbell, L.L.: The role of exergaming in improving physical activity: a review. J. Phys. Activity Health **11**(4), 864–870 (2014). https://doi.org/10.1123/jpah.2011-0425

94. Kari, T.: Can exergaming promote physical fitness and physical activity?: A systematic review of systematic reviews. Int. J. Gaming Comput. Mediated Simul. (IJGCMS) **6**(4), 59–77 (2014). https://doi.org/10.4018/ijgcms.2014100105

95. Kaplan, O., Yamamoto, G., Taketomi, T., Plopski, A., Sandor, C., Kato, H.: Exergame experience of young and old individuals under different difficulty adjustment methods. Computers **7**(4), 59 (2018). https://doi.org/10.3390/computers7040059

96. Muñoz, J.E., Cameirão, M., Bermúdez i Badia, S., Gouveia, E.R.: Closing the loop in exergaming-health benefits of biocybernetic adaptation in senior adults. In: Proceedings of the 2018 Annual Symposium on Computer-Human Interaction in Play, pp. 329–339 (2018). https://doi.org/10.1145/3242671.3242673

97. Tadayon, R., Sakoda, W., Kurita, Y.: Stealth-adaptive exergame design framework for elderly and rehabilitative users. In: International Conference on Human-Computer Interaction, pp. 419–434. Springer, Cham (2020). https://doi.org/10.1007/978-3-030-50249-2_30

98. Tadayon, R., Amresh, A., McDaniel, T., Panchanathan, S.: Real-time stealth intervention for motor learning using player flow-state. In: 2018 IEEE 6th International Conference on Serious Games and Applications for Health (SeGAH), pp. 1–8. IEEE, Piscataway (2018). https://doi.org/10.1109/SeGAH.2018.8401360

99. Tadayon, R., Ramirez, A.V., Das, S., Kishishita, Y., Yamamoto, M., Kurita, Y.: Automatic exercise assistance for the elderly using real-time adaptation to performance and affect. In: International Conference on Human-Computer Interaction, pp. 556–574. Springer, Cham (2019). https://doi.org/10.1007/978-3-030-23563-5_44

100. Yoshimura, N., Muraki, S., Oka, H., Tanaka, S., Ogata, T., Kawaguchi, H., Akune, T., Nakamura, K.: Association between new indices in the locomotive syndrome risk test and

decline in mobility: third survey of the ROAD study. J. Orthop. Sci. **20**(5), 896–905 (2015). https://doi.org/10.1007/s00776-015-0741-5

101. Sakoda, W., Tadayon, R., Kishishita, Y., Yamamoto, M., Kurita, Y.: Ski exergame for squat training to change load based on predicted Locomotive risk level. In: 2020 IEEE/SICE International Symposium on System Integration (SII), pp. 289–294. IEEE, Piscataway (2020). https://doi.org/10.1109/SII46433.2020.9026280

102. Minakata, M., Maruyama, T., Tada, M., Toda, H., Kurita, Y.: Quantitative assessment of brushed bodily area by measuring of brush motion using IMUs and its accuracy evaluation. In: 2019 58th Annual Conference of the Society of Instrument and Control Engineers of Japan (SICE), pp. 723–726. IEEE, Piscataway (2019). https://controls.papercept.net/conferences/conferences/SICE19/program/SICE19_ContentListWeb_3.html. Last accessed 2020/09/15

Haptic Mediators for Remote Interpersonal Communication

Troy McDaniel and Ramin Tadayon

Abstract The advent of smart and connected societies has led to increased prevalence of remote communication worldwide. However, these traditionally audio-visual communication environments can often lack the same richness of expressive information and feedback present in face-to-face interactions. Haptic mediators have emerged as a novel solution to bridge this gap across multiple dynamics of interpersonal communication. This chapter reviews the state of the art of this steadily emerging field of research under three primary categories of communication: social touch, nonvisual and visual information. The implications of existing solutions and evaluations are provided along with directions for future development.

Keywords Haptics · Haptic mediators · Social touch · Nonverbal communication · Verbal communication · Human-computer interaction · Robotics

1 Introduction

As we transition toward the era of smart cities, with infrastructures that facilitate multimodal technology in nearly every aspect of our lives, human beings are leading increasingly mobile and remotely connected lifestyles. Workplaces infused with technology allow colleagues to collaborate remotely and an increasing number support employees who work from remote locations [1]. Families, friends and romantic couples communicate remotely at an increasing frequency, and stay connected even when separated by their respective careers or living situations [2]. Teleconferencing, tele-presence, virtual communication, instant messaging and other forms of distant socialization have become commonplace among the global

T. McDaniel (✉) · R. Tadayon
Arizona State University, Mesa, AZ, USA
e-mail: troy.mcdaniel@asu.edu; rtadayon@asu.edu
https://cubic.asu.edu

© The Author(s), under exclusive license to Springer Nature Switzerland AG 2021
T. McDaniel, X. Liu (eds.), *Multimedia for Accessible Human Computer Interfaces*,
https://doi.org/10.1007/978-3-030-70716-3_8

217

population, fueled by the presence of ubiquitous technology such as smart phones and the increasing strength and availability of internet connectivity worldwide. Truly, we have ushered in a new standard of interpersonal communication across all dynamics of human relationships.

Yet, in their current forms, these mediums of expression and interaction, when consisting primarily of a camera, screen, speaker and/or keyboard, hold significant limitations in comparison to traditional face-to-face communication. As one consideration, people cannot touch one another in remote communication as they regularly and mutually do in physical interactions, including handshakes, hugs and other forms of what is known as social touch. Often in addition to social touch, nonverbal information is limited or missing (such as, for example, seeing a conversation partner's face, body movements or hand gestures in a phone call or text). Furthermore, verbal information can often be limited in remote interactions, particularly when text is used, since characteristics of speech such as intonation and emphasis are missing in these mediums.

As a growing and evolving body of recent research reveals, haptics, or the science of touch, may provide a solution to these challenges. We experience the world significantly through touch in addition to hearing, vision and our other senses [3]. Touch can affect us physically and emotionally, and combined with visual and audio cues it can help us to understand others in social settings [4]. Concepts can, in some cases, be communicated more clearly by adding this modality [5]. Recent research has therefore attempted to bridge the gap between face-to-face and remote interpersonal communication by leveraging haptics technology. Research into the development of the tactile internet [6], wherein touch information is encoded in exchanges over the internet, serves as further encouragement for the inclusion of this modality into daily remote interactions.

This chapter explores the body of work focused upon the introduction of touch interaction to mediators, or the technology and platforms through which remote interpersonal communication occur, and identifies the key advantages provided by these mediators through notable examples in literature. Three categories of touch mediation are reviewed: haptics for remote social touch, haptic communication of nonverbal cues and information, and haptic augmentation of verbal information. The most popular application contexts in each category, such as haptic instant messaging, are presented along with the various roles that touch plays or might conceivably play in enhancing them. The chapter concludes with a consideration for the directions of future expansion of the field along with insights for design.

2 Social Touch

While there are a wide variety of haptic mediation techniques designed to facilitate various forms of nonverbal communication (as discussed in the next section), social touch is of particular interest in this chapter as it encompasses physical contact in social settings, which is a natural haptic exchange. Therefore, unlike other applications of haptic mediators, sensory substitution is unnecessary, and instead, solutions seek to mimic social contact as naturally and realistically as possible in remote exchanges. The primary categories of social touch discussed in this work are hugs, handshakes, pats/taps, and massages, each of which have their own meanings and contexts within interpersonal communication.

The significance of social touch in interpersonal communication has been well established in research. When social touch is included in communication, particularly when the communicators are family members or are in a romantic relationship, both parties benefit in their emotional and physical health and well-being [7]. Furthermore, the presence of touch also strengthens these relationships and improves both members' sense of connection and bonding. Haans and IJsselsteijn [8] further find in their own review that even in less intimate relationships, such as those between colleagues, friends, acquaintances and competitors, haptic mediation of social touch, when designed appropriately, can build a sense of trust, strengthen both cooperation and competition, and improve the impression of one party toward the other.

An important phenomenon observed by several studies of mediated social touch, as detailed in a review by Huisman [9] is the Midas touch effect [10] in which the addition of touch into a mediated social interaction increases the likelihood of favorable outcomes such as compliance with requests or assistance with tasks. As authors are careful to note, however, the presence of the Midas touch effect relies heavily on both the context in which social touch is applied as well as the quality and characteristics of the touch delivery mechanism. Therefore, careful design of haptics is essential for successful facilitation of social touch in remote interpersonal communication.

2.1 Hugging

Hugging has been extensively studied as a form of mediated social touch in remote settings due to the well-established positive physical [11] and psychological [12] effects of frequent hugging. Robotic mediation is perhaps the most explored form of remote hugging as robots provide the type of full-body interaction with the most close resemblance to a natural hug between individuals. Hugs both direct and are directed by heightened emotions in social interactions, and personal, emotional and contextual characteristics of interaction participants result in biases and motor tendencies in hugs [13]. These properties, in addition to the universality and widespread significance of hugging among the different forms and dynamics of dyadic relationships, cement the hug as one of the most significant manifestations of social touch in any form of human communication.

The mediation of hugging through robot agents has been in study for decades, with early examples including DiSalvo et al. [14] who explored the significance of capturing the form of a hug—holding and squeezing with the arms, stroking the back, and verbal exchange among others. According to this study, the creation of a rich medium of interaction assists in successfully eliciting a positive and natural emotional response.

Mueller et al.'s Hug Over a Distance [15] combines the usage of robotic mediation and wearable technology to facilitate remote hugging. A stuffed koala with an interactive screen is used as an input mechanism, allowing the sender to initiate a hug interaction through simple touches, while the receiver feels a hug through a worn vest which, upon receiving the remote signal, inflates using air pressure to simulate the upper body squeezing sensation of a hug.

The HugMe system by Cha et al. [16] improves upon the realism of remote interactions by synchronizing the hug feedback directly with a hugging gesture by the sender. In this case, a depth camera and positional tracking technology are used to allow the sender to imitate hugging the receiver in real-time over a teleconferencing audio-visual medium, and the hug is then felt by the receiver through tactile actuators on a worn jacket which accurately represent points of virtual contact between the two.

Tsetserukou automates the interaction further in the design of the HaptiHug system [17], wherein a wearable strap simulates a hug by tightening using automatically modulated belt tension. In this case, the cue for a hug is automatically recognized from text exchanges or virtual interactions in an existing remote interaction between individuals in an online platform (Second Life). The implementation of hugging in this context was shown to successfully improve social immersion and the sensation of a real hug in virtual interaction.

Yonezawa and Yamazoe's [18] wearable partner agent, a small robotic stuffed toy animal which can be attached to the arm, shoulder, thigh or flank, as conveyed in Fig. 1, indicates that while the positive benefits of a mediated hug do not necessarily require fully-human-sized mediators, a system which accounts for the user's body context can be applicable in a wide variety of situations for communication. For instance, their robot is able to determine when an individual is in motion while the

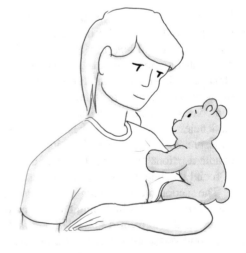

Fig. 1 Artist's rendition of a wearable agent, capable of emotional support and affection through hugs and eye contact

remote interaction is occurring, in which case the robot simply clings to the body of the subject. Furthermore, the thickness of the clothing of an individual can be detected, and determines the strength of haptic force applied during a hug.

More recent implementations of remote hugging include the Huggy Pajama by Cheok and Zhang [19] which focuses on parent-child interaction. This system is similar to Hug Over a Distance in the sense that remote hugging is mediated by a stuffed animal input and air pressurized wearable output. However, in this case, the hug input involves directly hugging the stuffed animal input, a more realistic input mechanism similar to HugMe which provides greater immersion and emotional elicitation to the sender, while the wearable pajamas on the receiver end include thermal stimulation in addition to the squeezing sensation by air pressure to create an even more realistic and comforting experience. The evolution of these interfaces indicates that haptic hug research is constantly pushing the boundaries of realism in social touch simulation.

2.2 Handshaking

Handshakes are another form of social touch perhaps most prevalent in professional interactions, as a gesture indicating a sense of trust, agreement, commitment or initiation and continuation of partnerships. They are also popularly used as a greeting and introduction mechanism, making them useful even when individuals are unfamiliar with one another in a communication environment. Dolcos et al. [20] have explored the power of a handshake in professional social contexts and found that it improves individuals' positive evaluations and diminishes negative evaluations of social interactions in these settings, including approach and avoidance scenarios.

Early implementations of remote handshakes such as Alhalabi and Horiguchi's Tele-Handshake [21] utilize force stimulation interfaces such as the Phantom device to allow two humans to feel the force feedback of a handshake while simultaneously sending their own force input to reciprocate. Of particular importance to the design of these systems is that the handshake is a bilateral exchange wherein both partners are sending and receiving touch information simultaneously. This challenges researchers to develop mediators which facilitate this bilateral exchange remotely, such as the system of Pedemonte et al. [22].

Nakanishi et al. developed a remote handshake system [23] in which a robotic arm is combined with one-on-one video telecommunication to mediate handshakes in such a way that the input action of the sender is made invisible to the receiver of the handshake (see Fig. 2). In other words, the only visual reference of the receiver is the movement of the robotic arm to initiate and complete a handshake. This mechanism was found to successfully improve the receiver's feeling of closeness to the handshake sender, though it requires that the sender always initiate the handshake process, which could prove to be limited in some applications. Perhaps one reasonable explanation for the implementation of this mechanism is that it

Fig. 2 Artist's sketch of a
robotic platform to support
remote handshaking for
enhanced social telepresence

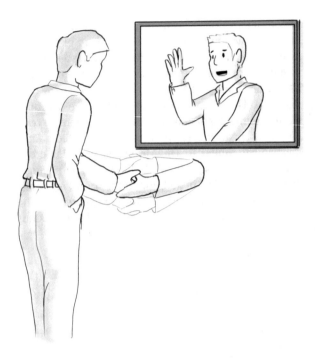

visually embodies a realistic handshake through relative positioning of the robotic
arm and face. Similar mechanisms such as that of Park et al. [24] further explore
this idea by incorporating a full-body mannequin with a robotic arm for handshakes
and a head replaced by a video feed of the remote partner's face.

2.3 Patting, Tapping, and Stroking

Touch gestures such as pats, tabs, and strokes are also of significance in social
settings as they can be used to direct attention to the sender, comfort the receiver,
or even communicate more complex meanings and expressions. These gestures are
also professionally applied by therapists during touch therapy, and can be utilized
as a part of telemedicine due to their physically calming and emotionally supportive
effects as well [25]. As such, these gestures merit inclusion in remote interactive
environments to strengthen interpersonal communication. While implementations
of these gestures often have a particular application domain in mind, many of the
designs can apply across these domains so long as the method of interaction is
intuitive, easily understood and integrates well into a variety of communicative
environments.

As an implementation of wearable touch therapy, Bonanni et al.'s TapTap system
presents an interesting format of touch therapy delivery through asynchronous

exchange [26]. The advantage of asynchronicity in touch is that it provides for mass distribution on a large scale of effective touch patterns to reach a large group of recipients without having to individually manage each interaction. The TapTap system allows for such an interaction, wherein a therapist inputs a therapeutic touch pattern and then distributes that exchange to all applicable patients, who receive the gesture via a wearable scarf interface. While this approach requires offline input, by utilizing the notion that a common set of socially recognizable patterns for pats and taps (for example. three taps on the shoulder) exist, one can design a real-time application in which these common gestures are pre-programmed into the device and then called on-demand in live exchanges.

The therapeutic effects of remotely delivered touching, patting, tapping, stroking, and similar gestures may even have an advantage over real physical contact in some cases. For instance in Autism Spectrum Disorder (ASD), one potential symptom is a hypersensitivity to physical contact by others. Tang et al. [27] designed a haptic sleeve to provide therapy which can help alleviate this sensitivity over time by turning taps, pats and other contacts on an avatar's arm during virtual reality interactions into physical sensations delivered through tactile actuation to the receiver. This design not only facilitates remote delivery of these forms of social touch, but also gives greater purpose to the implementation of remote touch communication in general. A key factor in this dynamic is the notion that the recipient in remote environments has full control over the delivery of a touch interaction, as the touch stimuli can be turned on or off at will.

In an attempt to incorporate multiple touch gestures including pats, taps and rubs into a single interface for mediated social touch, Huisman et al. designed the Tactile Sleeve for Social Touch, or TaSSt [28]. This forearm-worn sleeve used tactile stimulation to project various touch gestures between remote subjects in an attempt to increase the degrees of freedom (DoF) of interaction over previous designs. One noteworthy outcome of its evaluation is that dynamic gestures such as stroking and rubbing are more difficult to simulate in worn tactile designs than simpler gestures such as pokes, as they require an input mechanism which is sensitive to more delicate surface-tracing patterns.

Morikawa's HyperMirror [29] is exemplary of the importance of integration when introducing tactile stimuli into existing remote social environments. The HyperMirror environment includes shoulder-worn vibration motors which actuate when a tapping motion is sensed on video in a remote teleconferencing environment. These shoulder pats express the shoulder tapping motion to gain the attention of an individual toward the remote sender in the teleconference. It was found in evaluation that when the tactile stimuli of these sensors was combined with a video interface wherein the receiver could see the face of the sender seeking their attention, the interaction was much more naturally received than when tactile information was used alone or when video information (such as waving to the camera to gain attention as is popularly done in current remote interaction setups) was used without any additional tactile interface. Many of these touch gestures in natural environments are accompanied by visual confirmation for their meaning to be successfully registered.

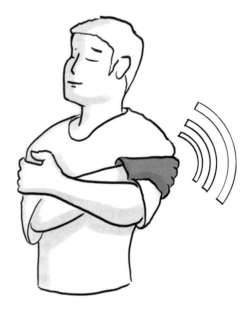

Fig. 3 Drawing of a vibrotactile glove to enable physical touch from a distance to support remote couples

Finally, the Flex-N-Feel system by Singhal et al. [30] presents an interesting form of affective touch that does not necessarily relate to instances of real physical contact but rather augments the emotional effect of an affective gesture using touch as a medium. Two types of gloves are used in this system: an input glove worn by the sensor transmits signals whenever the sender flexes his or her fingers, while an output glove worn by the receiver is equipped with vibrotactile motors (three along each finger on the palmar side) which vibrate when the corresponding finger of the input glove is flexed. The receiver's interface is depicted in Fig. 3. The prototype is intended for use by romantic couples in long distance relationships and presents two compelling design considerations for the domain of social touch: portability and flexibility of surface application. In the case of Flex-N-Feel, as it does not rely on a static object such as a robotic hand, mirror or other mechanism, the device need not be limited to indoor or static use and is portable enough to be utilized on-the-go, which opens the way for a variety of contexts in which remote interaction can occur. Furthermore, the receiver glove emits haptic signals on its surface to reflect the flexing of the senders fingers. This allows for the receiver to touch any surface of his or her body including the shoulder, arm, and other areas, and feel the touch sensation at the point of contact of his or her choosing, thus giving the receiver more freedom and control over the interaction. This can be of critical importance in social touch as context and interpersonal variation can change the effective surfaces and manifestations of these interactions.

2.4   Massaging

A final form of social therapeutic touch, perhaps most useful when applied between family, romantic couples, or therapist and client, is the massage. Massages have proven to be a highly effective method of mutual care between couples and can improve mental well being and perceived stress levels [31]. When applied by professional therapists, massage therapy has also been shown to provide a plethora of positive mental, emotional and physical effects [32]. A review of some of the most renowned implementations of massage touch reinforce these benefits and establish its continued significance as a form of complex social touch with medical, rehabilitative and relationship-building applications.

As an early implementation of remote mediated massage, Chung et al.'s Stress Outsourced (SOS) [33] presents an interesting alternative to the one-on-one high-familiarity context of the typical massage and instead frames the interaction as an anonymized, distributed, peer-to-peer remote therapy mechanism. The prototype includes a worn array of tactors which can be distributed in a variety of orientations along the body. When feeling stressed, an individual can press one of these worn modules to alert peers within the network of the individual's need for massage. These individuals can then deliver the therapy by pressing their own modules, which are then sent to the receiver as vibrotactile signals. The pattern can be composed of touch signals from multiple peers or a single peer, providing high flexibility and scalability of design. The inclusion of anonymity in the exchange also removes the stigma of receiving therapeutic intervention from a stranger, thereby paving the way for a high degree of applicability.

When massages are implemented, as they are a form of therapy, feedback from the recipient is critical and can help the sender or therapist determine what points of contact are effective and which areas require the most attention and care. As such, interfaces designed for professional delivery of rehabilitative or therapeutic massage may consider how feedback is presented to the therapist. One such system is GoodVybesConnect by Ramírez-Fernández et al. [34], which utilizes the Vybe gaming pad, a device which covers the surface area of the back, in addition with an audio-visual virtual environment, to allow therapists to connect with clients and deliver massage therapy. In this system, as the therapist utilizes a virtual back avatar to deliver remote massage via vibrotactile stimulation, the Emotiv brain-computer interface is calibrated and then used in real-time to evaluate the subject's response to the therapy, presenting interesting implications for the design of a feedback loop. Furthermore, massage patterns can be saved and later used offline by the client, once again indicating the benefits of an asynchronous style of delivery.

A recent implementation of massage by Haritaipan et al. [35] utilizes shoulder delivery for massage between individuals in close relationships. A sender device models a set of human shoulders with input sensors for each finger on both shoulders, and a receiver device implements two robotic arms, secured to the recipient's shoulders with a strap, whose digits react to the input pressure from the sender's remote shoulder device. This apparatus allows the sender to remotely

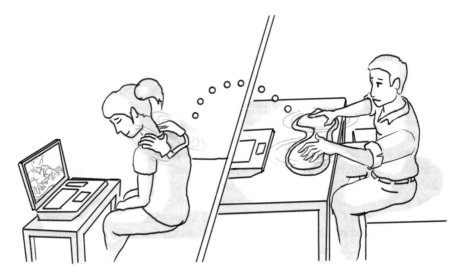

Fig. 4 Artist's rendition of a vibrotactile massage device to enable therapeutic touch from a distance for remote couples

massage the shoulders of the recipient during a video call to augment the interaction, as illustrated in Fig. 4. During evaluation, it was noted that a purpose for the addition and integration of massage into these interactions is that it communicates empathy, support and encouragement in ways that facial expressions and the voice alone cannot effectively accomplish in these settings.

In a later implementation by Ramírez-Fernández et al. [36], the RehWave system implements in design the idea that modern massage therapy includes, in addition to touch and pressure, thermal and audio stimulation for enhanced effect. In this full-body system, a series of heating pads and vibration motors are distributed along the neck, shoulders, upper back, lower back, and legs, in addition to two speakers (one by each ear) and combined to deliver a variety of telerehabilitative massage treatments which can include heat application and relaxing music in addition to massage vibration to assist in the therapy. This work draws upon many of the successes of previous implementations and combines them to indicate the true potential for remote delivery and mediation of massages.

3 Non-verbal Communication

An important category of information toward the accessibility of remote communication is non-verbal cues. This includes all forms of communicative expression outside of speech and social touch. It has been established in research, for example, that facial expressions comprise at least 55% of communication [37]. Non-verbal cues also include posture, physical mannerisms and gestures. The environment has an effect on the usage of nonverbal expressions in communications, including familiarity with the conversation partner, privacy, formality and warmth [38]. The significance of non-verbal expression in interpersonal communication is quite evident, as often it is the channel through which we convey emotions, intentions and priorities in ways that spoken words and intonation alone cannot adequately express [39].

In teleconferencing and video calls, non-verbal information is often available through visual feeds including live camera video. However, there are several forms of remote communication in which this visual information is not available. For example, a significant amount of remote conversation occurs over phone calls, wherein no video display is present. Furthermore, one or more of the participants may be blind or visually impaired, resulting in the need to present visual information through a different channel. Finally, even in video calls where no participant has a visual disability, limitations of the video display, occlusions and noise can cause non-verbal data to be difficult or impossible to depict visually. Under these circumstances, haptic information may serve as an effective medium for non-verbal communication.

This section explores the design of haptic mediators for non-verbal cues. The primary categories of nonverbal information included in this review are facial features, emotions, body movements and gestures (excluding social touch). A variety of approaches and designs for haptic mediation are described, including those whose primary purpose are for mediation of remote communication and those created for some other purpose but which can readily be applied within this domain. Evaluations of these systems provide insights and guidelines into the future of development for haptics within this field in an area where more and more of our daily conversations occur outside of face-to-face contexts, and over 285 million individuals around the world lack access to visual information during conversation due to visual impairment [40].

3.1 Facial Features and Emotions

The facial features of an individual can be an invaluable asset in interpersonal communication. As one simple example, eye gaze and head orientation, in combination with one another, are a primary indicator of the focus of an individual's attention, particularly in social settings [41]. Furthermore, emotion is an important aspect of communication which can determine how we interact, and can often not be conveyed completely through our voice [42]. Emotion and facial features can go hand-in-hand; our feelings during conversation can often be conveyed through expressions in our face [43]. Consequently, having access to information about an individual's facial features, and enabling individuals to convey emotion in other ways, helps those conversing with them to direct the flow of conversation accordingly. For example, if an individual notices that his or her remote conversation partner is bored during the conversation, he or she may choose to switch topics to something more exciting to re-engage the partner in a more stimulating discussion. While it may be argued that haptics is not the only modality which can be used to depict these attributes, it is perhaps the most useful in cases wherein one or both individuals in the conversation have visual impairment or are conversing while on the ago, as in such cases the audio and visual channels are preoccupied [44]. Here a series of designs for the transmission of facial features, as well as the manual expression of emotion between individuals in remote interpersonal communication, are presented and interpreted in context.

In the context of social interaction for individuals who are blind and visually impaired, haptics has proven particularly useful as a modality for the communication of nonverbal information. Research in this area was inspired by the fact that the lack of access to visual, non-verbal cues sometimes leads to miscommunications and misunderstandings, which can strain relationships and lead to social avoidance and isolation [45]. To address this, Panchanathan et al. developed the Social Interaction Assistant [46], a system designed to detect the facial features of a conversation partner through a mounted camera and convey this information using haptics, either through direct expression of facial features, or through emotion classified through machine learning, to individuals who are blind or individually impaired.

In the latter case, emotions are classified and then conveyed through patterns in various representations. Two primary mediums were developed to present emotions mapped to vibrotactile representations: a glove equipped with an array of vibrotactile motors along the back of the hand [47] and a chair equipped with an array of actuators along the back [48]. As the surface of the hand limits the number of motors that can be used, emotions were expressed as emojis through spatio-temporal patterns in the VibroGlove device. For example, happiness could be expressed as a set of actuations moving in an arc along the back of the hand to represent a smiling mouth. In the case of the Haptic Chair, more complex patterns, such as a spiral motion, or slithering snake motion, or up and down vibration along the spine, can be used to represent various emotions. Both cases represent a mapping from facial features to emotion to haptic expression during social interaction.

In the former case, facial features can be directly conveyed to the user without attempting to automatically interpret the emotion of an individual beforehand. This approach has several advantages: it avoids the potential error of classification by a machine when interpreting emotion, and it empowers the human to make decisions on the partner's emotions from visual features just as sighted individuals do in face-to-face conversation. However, for haptics to convey facial features, it is necessary to determine which facial elements form the building blocks of emotional expression. This was achieved by Friesen and Ekman in 1978 [49] and then later mapped to tactile facial action units in [48] and [50]. One can then imagine the utilization of this technology for remote interactions even with sighted individuals, such as phone conversations wherein the face of the partner cannot be seen. In this case, a local camera can detect the subject's facial features, extract the necessary facial action units, and convey them remotely through the chair or worn glove of the individual on the other end of the conversation.

The sharing of emotion need not be limited to situations in which individuals are in direct conversation with one another. Interpersonal communication includes shared experiences as well, wherein spoken dialog is absent. In these cases, emotions can be shared by one individual to describe his or her experience to another individual. An example of such an approach is AWElectric by Neidlinget et al. [51]. The primary purpose of the AWElectric system is to detect when an individual expresses a feeling of awe, and subsequently use electrical stimulation to reproduce this sensation to an individual in a remote location wearing a tech-embedded fabric. Potential extension of this approach toward other emotional responses, including laughter and joy, may allow for a rich and intimate language of expression in the future.

Affective communication need not be as complex as facial feature mapping or involve automatic detection of emotion on the sender's side. Research has indicated that even with very simple touch interfaces, a variety of basic emotions can be communicated manually and remotely between individuals. Two noteworthy examples include the knob manipulated remote affective display by Smith and MacLean [52] and the LumiTouch remote lightning picture frame by Chang et al. [53]. Both technologies present a simple, easily interpreted interface for synchronous symbolic augmentation of affect. In the case of the knob manipulation display, a sender interacts by turning a knob, resulting in a rotational force sent to the knob of the recipient. An evaluation indicated promising results in the ability of the recipient to comprehend the intended emotion conveyed by the sender based only on this interaction and on their closeness with one another. The LumiTouch provides an even simpler, 1-bit interaction: each remote participant in a dyadic interaction has a picture frame equipped with lights and a touch mechanism. When the sender wishes to convey warm thoughts toward the recipient, he or she touches the sending frame and the remotely located receiving frame lights up to signal the partner. This provides a simple mechanism by which family members, close friends, romantic partners and others may interact when apart.

More complex representations of affect may choose to represent it as a multi-dimensional construct. One such representation which is often used in subjective evaluations of affect in research is the PAD emotional state model of Mehrabian and Russell [54], which classifies emotion in the dimensions of pleasure, arousal and dominance. This model is employed by Tsalamlal et al. [55] in the design of a system which uses pressure from an air jet with a moving nozzle (see Fig. 5) to convey various emotional states to remote recipients. Properties of the stimulus including the degree of air flow, the continuity of air flow, and the rate of movement of the nozzle are modified to influence the subject's perception of the pleasure, arousal and dominance of an expressed emotion. In some cases, dominance is removed and valence (pleasure) and arousal are left to express emotions, as in the case of Rantala et al.'s system [56] which conveys these dimensions through touch and squeeze gestures. When represented this way, subjects can assess a partner's emotional output either in simple terms through analysis on a single dimension (high versus low pleasure, for example), or through multiple dimensions in conjunction with one another, allowing for a high range of possible expressions.

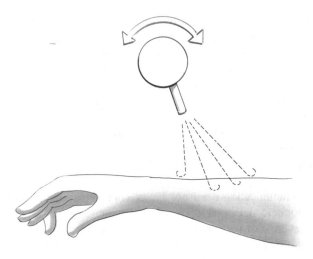

Fig. 5 Drawing of apparatus for evaluating the affective response to mobile air jet stimulation

Most approaches to remote haptic representation of emotion lack a key feature that would broaden accessibility and application: the ability of a user to create his or her own language for symbolic affect. Indeed, many of the emoticons present in text interactions were the creations of individuals utilizing text to communicate remotely. As such, the ability to create one's own expression results in a more flexible medium which accounts for the notion that interpersonal variation exists in interactions with technology, as emphasized by the person-centric multimedia computing paradigm [57]. As an example, Shin et al. [58] designed an interface for the expression of haptic emoticons which includes an authoring interface allowing for any individual to create his or her own touch emoticons, or TCONs. The haptic display for these TCONS contains a pair of hands and mouth which are augmented through actuation.

Finally, eye gaze is of importance in expression as well, as it provides another category of information related to affective state: attention. During a conversation, eye gaze is a useful indicator of attention and interest. Technologies originally intending to make eye gaze information available to individuals who are blind or visually impaired can be adapted to this scope of application quite readily. For example, Qiu et al. [59] designed a vibrotactile headband which would actuate when the gaze of a conversation partner is focused on the wearer of the headband, as depicted in Fig. 6.

Fig. 6 Artist's depiction of a
Tactile Band that
communicates gaze
information (glance versus
stare) of an interaction
partner

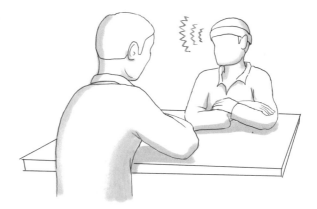

3.2 *Body Movements and Gestures*

While the face is a significant source for nonverbal information during social interaction, it is not the only important source for these cues. Indeed, motions of the entire body can help guide interactions, particularly when those interactions involve a shared motion task such as exercise. In-depth examinations of body language have revealed that motions such as hand movements convey thoughts which are absent in verbal expression or augment spoken intentions and goals [60]. These body movements and gestures may occur unknowingly or unknowingly, depending on context. For example, we may often make hand gestures during phone conversations even though we are aware that the other individual is not physically present to see them, sometimes as a form of self-demonstration or by habit [61]. Due to their role in enhancing the manner by which a remote participant's thoughts are externally understood [62, 63], recent research, as shown here, has focused upon making gestural information, particularly involving the hands, and whole body movement, particularly in remote collaborative motion, more accessible through haptics.

One potential solution for the projection of gestures and motions is the manipulation of mediator objects, or artifacts. A review of artifact-based gestural mediation of remote communication by Van Den Hoven and Ali [64] reveals that these artifacts can be used not only as input mechanisms or sensing mechanisms for gestural interaction, but also as mediums for enhancing these gestures as manifestations of the motion being demonstrated, projections of the intent behind the gestures, augmentations of the body or concept, and more. As in other forms of haptic communication, these gestures can be symbolic as well, such as a forward-backward spatial gesture indicating agreement [65]. The definition of artifacts in this respect is quite broad; they need not be restricted to handheld objects such as pens, small robots and manipulables. These artifacts can include surfaces and larger objects like vehicles. In this broad context, a plethora of research solutions have been explored in recent work.

Fig. 7 Artist's drawing of
The Hover, a device that
augments telecommunication
by conveying activity and
presence of remote partners

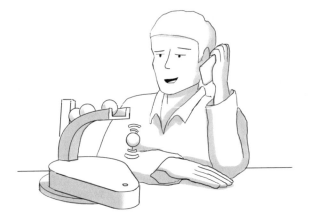

Perhaps the simplest example of gestural detection is to detect whether an individual is still or in motion, and to convey this through an artifact. This basic information is the core inspiration for the Hover haptic telephone device by Maynes-Aminzade et al. [66]. This device, as shown in Fig. 7, utilizes a hovering ball as the mechanism for a remote partner's motion during telephone conversation, but also utilizes interaction with the ball as an artifact to facilitate the initiation and answering of calls. When an individual wishes to call a contact, he or she places the sphere corresponding to that contact on the ramp of the device. That individual will then receive a call and the sphere corresponding to the caller floats in the air, which can be placed in turn on the receiver's ramp. Then on each user's phone, the ball hovers in the air. An external camera tracks the motion of each user and transmits the level of motion remotely to the other end, wherein the floating ball moves up and down in the air to signify the movement occurring. If a user is still, their sphere on the other end hovers in place. Knowing a conversation partner's level of motion can help an individual understand the level of energy and excitedness of that individual, or to determine their focus on the conversation at hand.

Taking this remote phone metaphor a step further in complexity, Sekiguchi et al.'s RobotPhone [67] serves as a manipulable phone-conversation-based artifact for remote communication of body movements. The premise of the system is simple: each partner in a dyadic remote interaction uses a small robot, prototyped in this case as a stuffed animal, which can be manipulated by its owner. Whenever one of these two robots is manipulated, usually by changing the orientation of its arms, legs or other movable joints, the other remote robot automatically adjusts its body orientation to match. Under this approach, each robot in RobotPhone serves as both input and output, allowing two individuals to express basic motion-based gestures and body positions. The limitations of this approach include the degrees of freedom of the robot as well as potential conflicts which can occur when robots on both ends are manipulated, which require a resolution approach to ensure synchronicity of orientation. One simple solution is to use a turn-taking mechanism to swap roles of the two devices between sender and receiver.

An application of gestural communication quite useful in social bonding and relationship building is that of play. Some artifacts for remote communication are designed with interpersonal entertainment in mind. Among these is the HandJive device by Fogg et al. [68]. The Handjive is a manipulable consisting of two spheres connected to a central pivot with two degrees of motion: forward/backward and side-to-side. Two of these devices can remotely interact with one another in synchronicity, with each user controlling one of the axes of motion. For example, a user could utilize forward and backward motions while the other user controlled side to side motions. Similar to the RobotPhone, the pair of devices match their movements. Under this separation of movement axes, both users can provide input and receive output on their devices, which allows for a variety of games and patterns of interaction. The device was designed with the intent that users should have the freedom to invent their own methods of play and interaction, which helps to validate these form factors as mediums for expression through haptics.

Collaborative tasks, perhaps more than any other application context, benefit greatly from haptic representation of gestures and body motions as the medium can be used to encode body positioning and body motions more effectively than utilizing visual or audio feedback alone [69]. Leveraging this advantage, several researchers have developed haptic systems designed to convey the relative motions and positions of others during a shared task. In one instance, de Jesus Oliveira et al. [70] modified the headset of a VR system, enabling hand gesture input on the back of one's own headset to communicate information about surroundings such as object locations. Swipes and taps are used as input to a smartphone attached to the back of the head and allow collaborative information sharing about one's surroundings to other remote participants in virtual environments. When an individual inputs a gesture on the device, collaborators feel the gesture on the surface of their own headsets through actuation of co-located vibrotactile motors. This mechanism could also conceivably be used for real objects through a head mounted device without VR display.

Training is another form of collaboration which can be facilitated through haptics. In particular, motor skill training requires an individual to be aware of not only his or her own motions and orientation, but the spatial and temporal differences between a trainer's positions and motions and their own. Several research developments have been dedicated to achieving this task in a variety of training contexts. Perhaps one of the simplest examples is that of a 1-DOF movement task, wherein a trainer moves a point along a single axis to various positions and the learner must attempt to match this trainer's motion as closely as possible. To facilitate this in remote interaction, Simard and Ammi [71] designed a system using a combination of spring force, viscosity, and vibrotactile cueing to convey the current distance from the learner to the trainer, the difference in movement speed between the two, and a warning to the learner when the trainer changes direction, respectively. Vibrotactile cues have also been used to encode relative positioning of others to a subject, in addition to distance, in the Haptic Belt by McDaniel et al. [72]. In this approach, a body-worn camera senses faces of others and a belt equipped with vibrotactile motors along the waist then vibrates the motor located in the direction of interaction partners around the user, with frequency denoting the distance. This allows the user to then turn toward the individual of interest until the vibration moves to the center of the waist, denoting that the two are facing one another. This technology, while it was applied in this research toward face-to-face use for individuals who are blind or visually impaired, may also find application in remote settings where a shared collaborative task requires multiple individuals to synchronize their orientations.

This intuition applies to guided remote physical exercise and rehabilitation as well. The CASPER system by Kadomura et al. [73] utilizes air pressure from an externally positioned air cannon as a form of haptic confirmation to alert the trainee when he or she has completed a motion in accordance with the guidance of a trainer, who the trainee can view in a visual display along with his or her own reflection to determine deviations in performance. A similar strategy is adopted by the Autonomous Training Assistant of Tadayon et al. [74], in which a subject completes motor tasks using a smart rod-shaped exercise device, the Intelligent Stick, equipped with motion sensing and tactile feedback capabilities. The subject can view an avatar which reflects his or her own motion using motion tracking, and compare it in real-time with the avatar demonstrating a motion pre-recorded by a trainer. Tactile cues delivered through the stick represent confirmation that the subject has reached an endpoint of the task. The difference in this case is that the training is asynchronous (the trainer records and uploads the example motion from a remote location beforehand rather than communicating directly with the subject in real-time).

When designed to build upon existing cognitive structures for spatial and temporal orientation, synchronized well with visual and audio feedback, and constructed with context-aware input and output mechanisms, haptic mediators may facilitate increasingly complex forms of collaborative interpersonal communication in the future. For example, large synchronous group actions such as orchestra performances and choreographed dance routines serve as extremely complex forms of interaction challenging the limits of haptic representation in remote settings. Based on the progress of current work, the role of touch within these interactions seems critical and shows promise for growth.

4   Verbal Communication

Finally, we arrive at haptic mediation for remote verbal communication. The role of haptics within this realm is perhaps not immediately apparent, as most remote communication already involves verbal information in some form or another. An immediate conclusion might be, therefore, that we may mediate verbal aspects of communication with haptics in cases where participants are deaf to speech or blind to text. However, as shown in the examples within this chapter, the benefits of haptics, even in verbal context, need not restrict themselves to applications of sensory substitution or accessibility of verbal content. Rather, in many cases, it is not the words themselves but the characteristics of their delivery which are lacking in remote contexts. For example, when we speak, we tend to emphasize words or parts of our speech we find important, and vary our intonation as indications of this emphasis as well as emotion, confidence and other forms of self-expression [75].

There are two primary contexts of verbal cue augmentation reviewed in this chapter. The first, as implied above, is the augmentation of verbal information for emphasis, attention and turn taking. Tonality and other modulations of speech audio are lost in many cases, whether it be due to attributes of the verbal information (delivered as text, for example, which has some attributes to establish emphasis such as the use of bold text or all-caps, but often does not contain these modifications as they would be too time-consuming to use in real-time conversation) or attributes of the speaker or listener (hearing impairment or speech impairment that would impair the delivery or production of varying tone, emphasis or verbal cues). Second, the concept of haptic instant messaging, or the use of haptics to replace or enhance text-based instant messaging exchanges, is discussed along with advantages and limitations of current approaches. While it is often the case that the applications of research solutions presented in this chapter overlap (in other words, tools developed for haptic instant messaging may also be adopted for use in emphasis or turn taking when combined with a different channel for verbal communication), they are categorized here according to the scope of application to which they can be most readily applied, either through the intention and evaluations presented by their respective authors or by observation.

4.1 *Emphasis, Attention and Turn Taking*

As noted above, verbal intonation allows speakers to establish importance and attention in various subjects and topics while speaking. Capturing these attributes within verbal information can help the listener establish the purposes and meanings within communicated sentences, which in turn help drive the course of discussion to a mutually beneficial conclusion. In other words, intonation can be viewed as a tool through which to establish emphasis during speech, and through this technique, various outcomes may be achieved. Schaffer [76] established that intonation, for example, may play a role in turn taking when multiple speakers engage in a conversation. In conference presentations among academics, Guest [77] determined that proper intonation plays a significant role in engaging the audience and bringing attention to the key points of the presentation. Furthermore, loudness of speech can be used to grab attention, and verbal cues may be used to take turns when more than two speakers are present. Given that their presence in communication is of such great importance, these elements of verbal expression can be considered vital in many cases. Yet, these attributes generally present in clear, intelligible, face-to-face discussion between individuals are frequently lost or more difficult to include when spoken word is no longer the format of this discussion or one or more participants have difficulty in hearing or speaking.

Without speech or audio communication of words and sentences, tonality is no longer inherently present or is more difficult to discern in traditional communication channels. Furthermore, even if speech with varying tonality is used, without physical presence, it may be difficult for intonation alone to achieve the desired level of emphasis in speech. Recent solutions have therefore turned to haptics to produce emphasis, capture attention and cue speakers in remote communication, with the understanding that tactile cues can gather our attention when applied at precise points during speech or text. This section observes a few key examples of how this technique has been successfully applied and evaluated. In some cases, while the primary purpose of the research was not to develop a means for achieving the above effects, it is interpreted here through an interpersonal communication lens with discussion on the elements of the work which show promise if adapted to the targeted context. To realize these adaptations, future work could modify the frameworks and prototypes developed to fit the purpose of remote exchange, and therefore determine to what extent they help augment verbal information.

As an initial example of conceptual adaptation for emphasis, consider Lahtinen and Palmer's [78] structured framework for the formation of haptic communication. Messages in the haptic channel are deconstructed into a simple two-degree grammar: haptices and haptemes. Haptices are full haptic messages and parallel the role of sentences in verbal communication. These messages are comprised of haptemes, or simple haptic patterns serving as building blocks in a manner similar to words. The original purpose of this deconstruction was to formalize an understanding of the role of haptics in social communication, forming what is termed *social-haptic* communication. The authors do not necessarily restrict this concept to the scope of remote haptic interpersonal communication; nevertheless, it is critically useful to perform this deconstruction as these authors and others [79] have done, as it provides a platform through which to differentiate haptic patterns for emphasis (for example, an alternate characteristic of haptemes such as increased signal amplitude for emphasis) from the others present in haptic messages (haptices).

When associated with the characteristics of audio, haptic signals hold similarities which can be very useful in establishing emphasis or tonality. For example, frequency and amplitude can be used to describe a haptic signal as well. Enriquez et al. [80] utilize these characteristics in their own deconstruction of haptic signals to form a language. The building blocks they develop are called haptic phonemes in parallel to the speech equivalent. Twelve distinct stimuli are identified in their study by modulation of frequency and amplitude characteristics of signals, and under this context, a natural connection to the formation of haptic intonation can potentially be realized as similar modulations are used for intonation in spoken communication. Future work could further evaluate the effectiveness for establishing tonality or emphasis within haptic language, particularly when transmitted through remote interfaces.

While the approaches above seek to provide full expressions of information through haptics, in some cases it is sufficient only to use haptic cues for a very precise purpose within the communication, such as emphasizing a word during a live conversation or quickly grabbing a listener's attention. Several approaches have adapted tactile cueing to achieve this limited augmentation as a part of a multimodal environment of communication. Some simple yet effective examples are noted within this work. One such case in earlier work is the ComTouch system by Chang et al. [81], a worn vibrotactile glove which facilitates emphasis during telephone conversation by applying pressure to send a vibrotactile signal. ComTouch assumes the existence of audio and/or video and provides tactile augmentation as a means to enrich expression. It also serves as a form of accessibility of information, rather than simple enhancement, when audio or visual disability is involved, as noted by the authors, since haptic information is universally perceived across both these forms of sensory impairment. The advantage of the simple mapping of ComTouch was the speed by which users were able to learn the mapping of touch to vibrations as determined in their preliminary study.

Another take on the remote haptic signal approach, but with a slight variation on the conceptualization of the application, is the Pressages system by Hoggan et al. [82]. In pressages, the user also applies pressure to a touch interface to send a vibrotactile signal, or pressage, to the other party at a remote location. Pressages, however, was designed without a specific usage case in mind. Rather, the applications of Pressages were left to users during testing. Subjects were given the system and told how to operate it but without being given a pre-determined purpose by which to use the system when making calls and conversing with others. At the conclusion of the study, subjects were asked to report on the ways in which they applied pressages during its duration. One of the most reported applications for use, as implied in this chapter, was for emphasis during conversation. Other purposes included expressions of affection, alerting of presence and elicitation of surprise reactions in conversation partners. It was also determined through evaluation that subjects quickly and readily adapted the use of pressages into their regular conversations, which indicates that an intuitive and practical interface can readily be adopted into existing remote communication mediums in practice.

One particularly interesting and highly relevant domain for the establishment of emphasis is music. Musical scores often contain high points reached by gradually increasing sound called crescendos and high points reached by sudden increases called sforzandos. In one perspective, these crescendos and sforzandos could be considered as points of emphasis within the music. While music is not speech in a literal sense, it is a useful metaphor as a form of artistic expression drawing many parallels to spoken dialog. The characteristics of music were utilized by Brown et al. [83] in the formation of tactons—building blocks of tactile expression similar in nature to the haptices and haptic phonemes described above—with variation in vibrotactile characteristics to form distinct tactile crescendos and sforzandos. An evaluation yielded recognition rates between 92 and 100%, which indicates that these tactons could be highly useful if applied as an augmentation mechanism toward emphatic points during remote conversation.

Suhonen et al.'s [84] study of remote haptic interpersonal communication closely matches the scope of this chapter, as it provides an evaluation directly comparing the application of two different types of haptic mediation (squeezing and thermal input) to traditional remote communication between subjects. The mediators in this

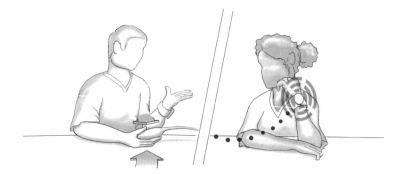

Fig. 8 Artist's rendition of a wearable technology for augmenting remote interpersonal communication through touch-based devices

study are illustrated in Fig. 8. In contrast to Brown et al., some basic instruction for the application of these mediators was given to subjects prior to participation in the study, such as using the device during the conversation to emphasize emotions or emphasize one's messages. However, the exact timings and details of usage for these mediators were determined by subjects and revealed to the researchers over the course of the study. Worn straps conveyed these two signals as remote output: a strap which would tighten when a squeeze signal was sent and a thermal strap which would adjust its temperature according to the input. Of the two, the squeeze interface was reported as being the most frequently used and provided emphasis for a variety of expressions such as sympathy. Thermal modulation related more closely to the level of positivity (warm) or negativity (cold) of the conversation.

One particular situation in which the augmentation of verbal cues can be extremely beneficial in remote conversation occurs when more than two subjects are involved in a conversation. When a large group of individuals communicate simultaneously, particularly in remote environments, speech can overlap and make it difficult for a listener to direct his or her attention. Haptics, as several researchers of related work have demonstrated, may play a role in resolving this issue if used as a cueing mechanism to direct attention, cue a speaker and organize the progression of turns for speech. Several solutions toward this goal have been tested in recent studies. One such implementation occurs within a study of multimodal exchange in synchronous distributed communication environments by Ho and Sarter [85]. In this case, a distributed military operation was utilized as a context of application, with multiple mediations of exchange including radio, text, drawing or tactile buzzing. Among the other modalities of exchange, the tactile buzz was used most naturally for drawing attention, with other modalities like radio communication following suit to disambiguate the object of attention and provide further elaboration or instruction.

Turn taking allows participants to organize the control over a conversation among multiple participants to prevent chaos and disruption during exchange. A haptic mediation solution specifically focused on turn taking during these situations was developed by Chan et al. [86]. In this study, tactons were developed to express requests for control of an application at varying levels of urgency. This allows for easier conflict resolution when multiple participants request control within the group. One important requirement for these tactons as identified by the researchers in this study is that they must be clearly identifiable even in the midst of high cognitive load due to the context in which they are used (multiple subjects collaborating on a task and communicating with one another in real-time during task performance). The tactons were delivered through a mouse equipped with vibrotactile motors, and represented combinations of various control dynamics, such as control attainment (gaining and losing control) and control request (gentle request, urgent request, takeover). While in this case, the control mechanism referred specifically to control over a shared online application, a clear parallel is drawn toward control over a social conversation as well, which follows a similar dynamic.

Cao et al. [87] observed an interesting acceleration phenomenon related to the application of haptics toward turn taking in remote verbal communication. In their applications, tactile displays were used to send and receive signals relating to requests for control and transfer of control to various individuals within a conversation during a shared task. In this case, distinct tactons were developed to signify both the requests and releases of control and who initiated each message, which would allow all participants to determine the flow of conversation directly from tactile mediation. This was designed for a three-way conversation among users, which made it easy to convey individuality within the display. However, it would have difficulties in scalability, as exponentially more distinct tactons would be required as the number of participants increases. The primary finding in this work was that, when tactile exchange was used in contrast to remote conversations without, the delay in time between a request for control of the conversation by an individual and the release of that control by the current speaker was significantly reduced. This indicates that in longer conversations, the use of tactile exchange for this purpose can shorten delays and produce a smoother discussion.

One final implementation for consideration in the subject of turn taking is the Contact IM device by Oakley and O'Modhrain [88]. This device differs from the previous approaches in that the targeted domain was asynchronous exchange of a haptic instant message. This example provides a suitable transition into the next section on Haptic Messaging; however, it is described instead here due to a simple yet significant relationship with turn-taking: one common practice in face-to-face communications among multiple nearby individuals in a closed setting is the use of an object such as a ball to establish a speaker in control of the conversation. When a speaker is finished with his or her message, the ball is then passed to another individual as a symbolic transfer of control. This action is represented in Fig. 9. This physical artifact provides visual and tactile confirmation of control and facilitates turn taking in a simple yet highly effective manner. Contact IM uses a force feedback mechanism and visual display to provide haptic messaging capability under the metaphor of passing a ball. A ball, hand and court are visually displayed, and when a message arrives, the ball appears on the recipient's side of the court. This individual can then pick up the ball with the hand, which is felt through force feedback with an

Fig. 9 Artist's sketch of platform for sending haptic instant messages by swinging and throwing a tethered ball

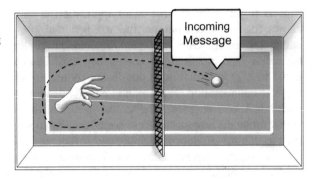

interface such as the Phantom device. To send a message the user then throws the ball to the other side of the court, where it disappears on his or her display to indicate successful transmission. Consider the application of this approach in conversational turn taking, wherein the active speaker has control of the ball, with multiple targets to which to toss the ball, each representing a participant in the conversation, and what results is an intriguing conversational haptic mediation mechanism.

4.2 Haptic Messaging

As a final purpose for haptic mediation, we consider the realm of instant messaging, an ever-popular method of remote communication due to its flexibility toward both synchronous and asynchronous use, its lack of usage of audio which allows for portable use and some degree of privacy and discretion in public environments. Instant messages represent perhaps the most successful transition of verbal remote communication from traditional audio transmission in phone conversations. Here the function of haptics within this space is explored. Haptic exchanges also have the benefit of being discreet, and perhaps even more so, as a haptic message is felt only by its intended recipient, as opposed to visual and audio messages which can be seen and heard by others. Furthermore, tactile messages are perhaps even more advantageous in the wild as our visual and auditory channels are generally preoccupied during daily activity. It should be noted that with these advantages come potential limitations; tactile reading, for example, has been shown in some studies to be significantly slower (roughly three times) than visual reading [89]. Clever design of tactile representation, however, may help in addressing this challenge.

As perhaps one of the earliest demonstrations of this concept, consider the InTouch system by Brave and Dehley [90]. The transmission of haptic signals in InTouch is facilitated through the manipulation of rollers at two remote locations. Three rollers on each communication device allows for a surprisingly high degree of complexity in communication (each roll can vary in both in direction and length) while maintaining compactness of design to facilitate single-handed use. Technological restrictions at the time of implementation limited the ability of InTouch to be deployed in a remote setting with electronic transmission, which resulted in a prototype of mechanically connected rollers.

Several approaches take the route of augmentation rather than replacement. In these cases, haptics is used in conjunction with text messages to transmit some aspect of the message. One frequently chosen component of instant messaging is the emoticon, or an expression of the sender's emotion generally conveyed symbollicaly through text. Haptic emoticons have been explored to a growing extent due to the effectiveness by which haptics conveys and elicits emotions as previously described. One example is the Haptic Instant Messenger (HIM) system by Rovers and Van Essen [91]. This framework proposes the development of hapticons for expression of various emoticons with the idea that they are utilized during synchronous instant messaging sessions under a direct transmission strategy. It is an open framework without concrete implementation of these hapticons and only basic guiding discussion about the implementation of input/output devices for the haptic exchange (that they should allow for single-handed and minimally-intrusive use to free the hands for keyboard use).

In later work [92, 93], the authors adapted this framework in the development of a foot-worn interaction device entitled FootIO for transmission of the hapticons. Careful consideration of tactor placement is critical in using this surface since, as the authors showed through a progression of prototype iterations and evaluations, sensitivity to contact varies across the bottom of the foot and proper contact at each point is crucial when multi-tactor spatiotemporal patterns are presented. Furthermore, while the foot may be a suitable device for output, it is more difficult to manipulate the digits and other anatomy of the feet as opposed to the hands, making input more limited. To resolve this, a setup in which a keyboard is used for input of the emoticons which are then converted to haptic output via the foot-worn device shown in Fig. 10 is proposed.

Fig. 10 Sketch of apparatus for investigating vibrotactile stimulation in haptic interpersonal communication using the foot

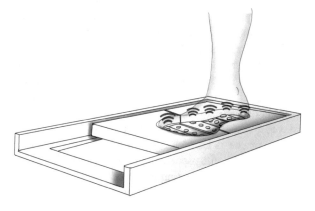

As Tsetserukou et al. indicate, this transition from text input to haptic output can be fully automated, allowing for a seamless interchange between the two modalities. Their HaptiHug system described in the Social Touch section above was utilized, in combination with other haptic output devices, in the iFeel_IM! system [94], wherein emotions are automatically detected by software within text instant messages, and on detection, the associated emotion (among nine distinct emotions of surprise, fear, interest, joy, disgust, shame, sadness, guilt and anger) is transmitted to an appropriate haptic output device (for example, joy presented as a hug through the HaptiHug). Automatic detection of emotion within text has the drawbacks of being subject to errors in classification as well as the limitations of the set of emotions within its library (in reality, we can express a much broader range of emotions of varying complexity). However, for the sake of simplicity, one might consider the range of commonly used emoticons, establish a predominant emotion to each, and use this set to form the full range of emotions to detect within text. Modern machine learning approaches may assist as well in improving detection accuracy.

Another approach to automation of input when dealing with text exchange is the direct translation from text to haptics. Perhaps the most commonly used haptic language for readers is Braille. Therefore, an approach in which text is automatically converted to Braille representation and then transmitted through a Braille display has the benefit of making text accessible to individuals with visual impairments who also know Braille. One could imagine text-to-Braille exchanges among the broad population, but learning Braille is nontrivial, which presents a potential barrier for widespread adoption. This automated translation is implemented by Choudhary et al. [95] and transmission is facilitated through a smart glove wearable device. One side of the glove's surface allows for the user to input braille expressions which are converted to text and then output through an instant messaging application, and the other side outputs Braille symbols through vibrotactile motors when receiving a message. This mechanism has uses beyond making text accessible—it can also facilitate, as implied above, message exchange as a secondary task when vision and hearing are focused on a primary task like walking in a crowded environment.

While haptics alone can be richly expressive in the delivery of messages, what if more complex expressions could be more clearly conveyed when it is combined with another modality? This intuition is utilized by Brown et al. [96] in development of Shake2Talk, an alternative to haptic mediation in remote messaging. Shake2Talk uses messages consisting of a combination of audio and haptic signals, which interact to convey deeper meaning than either modality alone. Gestural input is used to construct these messages, which are then output through a mobile phone with vibrotactile actuator attachments. The phone provides the audio while the tactors convey the tactile portion of the message. As an example, an individual indicates that he or she is home through a key turning gesture, which is then conveyed via mixed audio/tactile representation of a key lock sensation. This combination serves the advantage of providing a redundancy in the case that one or the other channels of information cannot be transmitted to the recipient due to a disability or other condition.

As a final consideration, haptic messages have been demonstrated through multiple implementations to facilitate a range of complexities of communication. In some instances, the messages being sent should be quite simple, or the mechanism could be simple enough to cover a variety of usage scenarios. The simplest case is one-bit exchange, wherein an on/off mechanism is utilized to simplify the interface. Examples of this include Mole Messenger [97] wherein a model of a mole acts as a large pushable button. When the mole is pushed in, the corresponding mole on the other end pops out to signify a message delivery. This is a very basic interaction intended for children, but multiple mole messengers can be used, increasing the bits of interaction and allowing for more complex messages to be shared. Another such example is the FeelLight device [98], which consists of a single pushable button which also lights up in various colors to act as a tactile input and visual output. When one user presses the button, the color changes, and the corresponding color on the light of the other side changes to match, enabling the communication of simple one- or two-bit messages. In other cases, more complex vocabularies are required, as demonstrated by the TAPS Tactile Phonemic Sleeve system of Tan et al. [99] which found through evaluation that 500 English words could be represented and learned at a reasonable rate by users of the technology. Whether it uses simple or complex vocabularies, haptics has clearly established potential for use in instant messaging.

5   Conclusions and Future Directions

While the examples of remote haptic mediation detailed in this chapter are not exhaustive, they are fairly representative of the many forms of potential held by this modality for improving remote communication. An increasing variety of such devices are being developed every day, but more extensive longitudinal research can evaluate how effectively each implementation improves communication in practice. This is one of the most severe limitations of the research within this space; while haptic mediation as a concept, through sensory substitution and other strategies, has been well-validated in face-to-face interpersonal communication contexts, particularly involving communicators with visual or auditory disabilities, its application in remote environments requires more extensive testing across a broader variety of users to help shape its role within the space. Many of the applications above were tested in limited, controlled environments with a very specific target audience, and limited steps to generalize to the broader population.

The addition of haptics, if not completed under consideration of existing communication interfaces, may introduce excess complication in interaction and cognitive load, particularly for elderly users and when the haptic feedback is not synergistic to the information being communicated. Furthermore, the addition of haptics hardware can often be inconvenient, particularly when the communication occurs on the go. Many of the applications presented were not tested in these environments, which may contribute to reductions in weight, volume, complexity, and the overhead associated with setup and usage between users. Effectively, this application scenario presents one of the greatest challenges and limitations on the design space for these mediators as it involves a context in which vision and hearing are often preoccupied, requiring haptics to carry more of the burden in communication capacity and information transmission.

Several insights can be drawn from observation of these mediators as a whole. One is that intuitiveness of design, human factors considerations, and usability prevail. Implementations which take into account the existence of other modalities which together contribute toward increased cognitive load, the context of use which may include secondary tasks that distract attention such as walking on the street during a phone conversation, and interpersonal and intrapersonal variations in goals, lifestyles, ability and disability among users have proven more effective during evaluation. Another is that the disability space provides clear insights into what aspects of communication can become inaccessible and how haptics can serve to make them more accessible. Several of the approaches were inspired by improving the accessibility of communication for individuals with complete loss or impairment of vision or hearing. These solutions naturally apply within the remote communication environment since it provides a context by which the individuals communicating encounter an impairment: in a text conversation, we cannot see or hear our conversation partner, for example.

Finally, it can be observed that often individuals define their own usage of haptic mediators both in purpose and operation. This creativity has been observed in many of the designs discussed here, as often the authors chose an experimental setup which allowed subjects the freedom to choose how they apply the observed prototype within the conversation. While it is uncertain exactly how people across populations, societies, settings and cultures will choose to apply these haptic mediators, designs which allow for such individually variant input and customization are beneficial. Future work may accommodate this process through participatory design; by involving the target audience in the process of prototyping and refinement, and carefully extracting subjective feedback on usage throughout, new ideas for interface customization may emerge.

Acknowledgments The authors thank Josh Chang for his assistance with designing the graphics contained within this chapter. The authors thank Arizona State University and the National Science Foundation for their funding support. The preparation of this chapter was supported by the National Science Foundation under Grant No. 1828010.

References

1. U.S. Bureau of Labor Statistics: Table 6. Employed persons working at home, workplace, and time spent working at each location by full- and part-time status and sex, jobholding status, and educational attainment, 2018 annual averages. https://www.bls.gov/news.release/atus.t06.htm. Last accessed 2020/05/03
2. Pew Research Center, Inquiries, D. 20036USA202-419-4300 | M.-857-8562 | F.-419-4372 | M.: Global Digital Communication: Texting, Social Networking Popular World-

wide. https://www.pewresearch.org/global/2011/12/20/global-digital-communication-texting-social-networking-popular-worldwide/. Last accessed 2020/05/03

3. Gibson, J.J.: The Senses Considered as Perceptual Systems. Houghton Mifflin, Oxford (1966)
4. Cascio, C.J., Moore, D., McGlone, F.: Social touch and human development. Dev. Cogn. Neurosci. **35**, 5–11 (2019). https://doi.org/10.1016/j.dcn.2018.04.009
5. Richards, A.: Teaching mechanics using kinesthetic learning activities. Phys. Teacher **57**, 35–38 (2018). https://doi.org/10.1119/1.5084926
6. Aijaz, A., Dohler, M., Aghvami, A.H., Friderikos, V., Frodigh, M.: Realizing the tactile internet: haptic communications over next generation 5G cellular networks. IEEE Wirel. Commun. **24**, 82–89 (2017). https://doi.org/10.1109/MWC.2016.1500157RP
7. Field, T.: Touch for socioemotional and physical well-being: a review. Dev. Rev. **30**, 367–383 (2010). https://doi.org/10.1016/j.dr.2011.01.001
8. Haans, A., IJsselsteijn, W.: Mediated social touch: a review of current research and future directions. Virtual Reality **9**, 149–159 (2006). https://doi.org/10.1007/s10055-005-0014-2
9. Huisman, G.: Social touch technology: a survey of haptic technology for social touch. IEEE Trans. Haptics **10**, 391–408 (2017). https://doi.org/10.1109/TOH.2017.2650221
10. Haans, A., IJsselsteijn, W.A.: The virtual midas touch: helping behavior after a mediated social touch. IEEE Trans. Haptics **2**, 136–140 (2009). https://doi.org/10.1109/TOH.2009.20
11. Light, K.C., Grewen, K.M., Amico, J.A.: More frequent partner hugs and higher oxytocin levels are linked to lower blood pressure and heart rate in premenopausal women. Biol Psychol. **69**, 5–21 (2005). https://doi.org/10.1016/j.biopsycho.2004.11.002
12. Shiomi, M., Nakata, A., Kanbara, M., Hagita, N.: A hug from a robot encourages prosocial behavior. In: 2017 26th IEEE International Symposium on Robot and Human Interactive Communication (RO-MAN), pp. 418–423 (2017). https://doi.org/10.1109/ROMAN.2017.8172336
13. Ocklenburg, S., Packheiser, J., Schmitz, J., Rook, N., Güntürkün, O., Peterburs, J., Grimshaw, G.M.: Hugs and kisses – The role of motor preferences and emotional lateralization for hemispheric asymmetries in human social touch. Neurosci. Biobehav. Rev. **95**, 353–360 (2018). https://doi.org/10.1016/j.neubiorev.2018.10.007
14. DiSalvo, C., Gemperle, F., Forlizzi, J., Montgomery, E.: The Hug: an exploration of robotic form for intimate communication. In: The 12th IEEE International Workshop on Robot and Human Interactive Communication, 2003. Proceedings. ROMAN 2003, pp. 403–408 (2003). https://doi.org/10.1109/ROMAN.2003.1251879
15. Mueller, F.F., Vetere, F., Gibbs, M.R., Kjeldskov, J., Pedell, S., Howard, S.: Hug over a Distance. In: CHI '05 Extended Abstracts on Human Factors in Computing Systems, pp. 1673–1676. ACM, New York (2005). https://doi.org/10.1145/1056808.1056994
16. Cha, J., Eid, M., Rahal, L., Saddik, A.E.: HugMe: An interpersonal haptic communication system. In: 2008 IEEE International Workshop on Haptic Audio visual Environments and Games, pp. 99–102 (2008). https://doi.org/10.1109/HAVE.2008.4685306
17. Tsetserukou, D.: HaptiHug: A novel haptic display for communication of hug over a distance. In: Kappers, A.M.L., van Erp, J.B.F., Bergmann Tiest, W.M., van der Helm, F.C.T. (eds.) Haptics: Generating and Perceiving Tangible Sensations, pp. 340–347. Springer Berlin Heidelberg, Berlin (2010)
18. Yonezawa, T., Yamazoe, H.: Wearable partner agent with anthropomorphic physical contact with awareness of user's clothing and posture. In: Proceedings of the 2013 International Symposium on Wearable Computers, pp. 77–80. Association for Computing Machinery, Zurich (2013). https://doi.org/10.1145/2493988.2494347
19. Cheok, A.D., Zhang, E.Y.: Huggy Pajama: remote hug system for family communication. In: Cheok, A.D. and Zhang, E.Y. (eds.) Human–Robot Intimate Relationships, pp. 33–75. Springer International Publishing, Cham (2019). https://doi.org/10.1007/978-3-319-94730-3_3
20. Dolcos, S., Sung, K., Argo, J.J., Flor-Henry, S., Dolcos, F.: The power of a handshake: neural correlates of evaluative judgments in observed social interactions. J. Cogn. Neurosci. **24**, 2292–2305 (2012). https://doi.org/10.1162/jocn_a_00295
21. Alhalabi, M.O., Horiguchi, S.: Tele-handshake: a cooperative shared haptic virtual environment. In: Proceedings of Eurohaptics, pp. 60–64. University of Birmingham Press (2001)

22. Pedemonte, N., Laliberté, T., Gosselin, C.: A haptic bilateral system for the remote human–human handshake. J. Dyn. Syst. Meas. Control. **139** (2017). https://doi.org/10.1115/1.4035171
23. Nakanishi, H., Tanaka, K., Wada, Y.: Remote handshaking: touch enhances video-mediated social telepresence. In: Proceedings of the SIGCHI Conference on Human Factors in Computing Systems. pp. 2143–2152. Association for Computing Machinery, Toronto, Ontario (2014). https://doi.org/10.1145/2556288.2557169
24. Park, S., Park, S., Baek, S.-Y., Ryu, J.: A human-like bilateral tele-handshake system: preliminary development. In: Auvray, M., Duriez, C. (eds.) Haptics: Neuroscience, Devices, Modeling, and Applications, pp. 184–190. Springer, Berlin, Heidelberg (2014). https://doi.org/10.1007/978-3-662-44196-1_23
25. Maratos, F.A., Duarte, J., Barnes, C., McEwan, K., Sheffield, D., Gilbert, P.: The physiological and emotional effects of touch: Assessing a hand-massage intervention with high self-critics. Psychiatry Res. **250**, 221–227 (2017). https://doi.org/10.1016/j.psychres.2017.01.066
26. Bonanni, L., Vaucelle, C., Lieberman, J., Zuckerman, O.: TapTap: a haptic wearable for asynchronous distributed touch therapy. In: CHI '06 Extended Abstracts on Human Factors in Computing Systems, pp. 580–585. ACM, New York (2006). https://doi.org/10.1145/1125451.1125573
27. Tang, F., McMahan, R.P., Allen, T.T.: Development of a low-cost tactile sleeve for autism intervention. In: 2014 IEEE International Symposium on Haptic, Audio and Visual Environments and Games (HAVE) Proceedings, pp. 35–40 (2014). https://doi.org/10.1109/HAVE.2014.6954328
28. Huisman, G., Frederiks, A.D., Dijk, B.V., Hevlen, D., Kröse, B.: The TaSSt: Tactile sleeve for social touch. In: 2013 World Haptics Conference (WHC), pp. 211–216 (2013). https://doi.org/10.1109/WHC.2013.6548410
29. Morikawa, O.: Shoulder tapping illusion by vibrator in HyperMirror. ICCS/JCSS99. 382–387 (1999)
30. Singhal, S., Neustaedter, C., Antle, A.N., Matkin, B.: Flex-N-Feel: emotive gloves for physical touch over distance. In: Companion of the 2017 ACM Conference on Computer Supported Cooperative Work and Social Computing, pp. 37–40. Association for Computing Machinery, Portland, Oregon (2017). https://doi.org/10.1145/3022198.3023273
31. Naruse, S.M., Moss, M.: Effects of couples positive massage programme on wellbeing, perceived stress and coping, and relation satisfaction. Health Psychol. Behav. Med. **7**, 328–347 (2019). https://doi.org/10.1080/21642850.2019.1682586
32. Field, T.M.: Massage therapy effects. Am. Psychol. **53**, 1270–1281 (1998). https://doi.org/10.1037/0003-066X.53.12.1270
33. Chung, K., Chiu, C., Xiao, X., Chi, P.-Y. (Peggy): Stress Outsourced: a haptic social network via crowdsourcing. In: CHI '09 Extended Abstracts on Human Factors in Computing Systems, pp. 2439–2448. ACM, New York (2009). https://doi.org/10.1145/1520340.1520346
34. Ramírez-Fernández, C., García-Canseco, E., Morán, A.L., Pabloff, O., Bonilla, D., Green, N., Meza-Kubo, V.: GoodVybesConnect: a real-time haptic enhanced tele-rehabilitation system for massage therapy. In: García, C.R., Caballero-Gil, P., Burmester, M., Quesada-Arencibia, A. (eds.) Ubiquitous Computing and Ambient Intelligence, pp. 487–496. Springer International Publishing, Cham (2016). https://doi.org/10.1007/978-3-319-48746-5_50
35. Haritaipan, L., Hayashi, M., Mougenot, C.: Design of a massage-inspired haptic device for interpersonal connection in long-distance communication. Adv. Hum. Comput. Interaction **2018**, 5853474 (2018). https://doi.org/10.1155/2018/5853474
36. Ramírez-Fernández, C., Hernández-Capuchin, I., Meza-Sánchez, M., Clemente, E., Pérez-López, N.-D., Abundiz, E., Campos-García, J.: RehWave: a real-time tele-rehabilitation haptic device for massage therapy. In: Proceedings of the 7th Mexican Conference on Human-Computer Interaction, pp. 1–4. Association for Computing Machinery, Merida (2018). https://doi.org/10.1145/3293578.3293581
37. Mehrabian, A., Ferris, S.R.: Inference of attitudes from nonverbal communication in two channels. J. Consult. Psychol. **31**, 248 (1967)

38. Knapp, M.L., Hall, J.A., Horgan, T.G.: Nonverbal Communication in Human Interaction. Cengage Learning (2013)
39. Hans, A., Hans, E.: Kinesics, haptics and proxemics: aspects of non-verbal communication. IOSR J. Humanit. Soc. Sci. (IOSR-JHSS) **20**, 47–52 (2015)
40. WHO|Global data on visual impairment (2010). http://www.who.int/blindness/publications/globaldata/en/. Last accessed 2020/04/21
41. Langton, S.R.H., Watt, R.J., Bruce, V.: Do the eyes have it? Cues to the direction of social attention. Trends Cogn. Sci. **4**, 50–59 (2000). https://doi.org/10.1016/S1364-6613(99)01436-9
42. Schirmer, A., Adolphs, R.: Emotion perception from face, voice, and touch: comparisons and convergence. Trends Cogn. Sci. **21**, 216–228 (2017). https://doi.org/10.1016/j.tics.2017.01.001
43. Adolphs, R.: Recognizing emotion from facial expressions: psychological and neurological mechanisms. Behav. Cogn. Neurosci. Rev. **1**, 21–62 (2002). https://doi.org/10.1177/1534582302001001003
44. Neider, M.B., McCarley, J.S., Crowell, J.A., Kaczmarski, H., Kramer, A.F.: Pedestrians, vehicles, and cell phones. Accid. Anal. Prev. **42**, 589–594 (2010). https://doi.org/10.1016/j.aap.2009.10.004
45. Segrin, C., Flora, J.: Poor social skills are a vulnerability factor in the development of psychosocial problems. Hum. Commun. Res. **26**, 489–514 (2000). https://doi.org/10.1111/j.1468-2958.2000.tb00766.x
46. Panchanathan, S., Chakraborty, S., McDaniel, T.: Social interaction assistant: a person-centered approach to enrich social interactions for individuals with visual impairments. IEEE J. Sel. Top. Signal Process. **10**, 942–951 (2016). https://doi.org/10.1109/JSTSP.2016.2543681
47. Krishna, S., Bala, S., McDaniel, T., McGuire, S., Panchanathan, S.: VibroGlove: An assistive technology aid for conveying facial expressions. In: CHI '10 Extended Abstracts on Human Factors in Computing Systems. pp. 3637–3642. ACM, New York (2010). https://doi.org/10.1145/1753846.1754031
48. Bala, S., McDaniel, T., Panchanathan, S.: Visual-to-tactile mapping of facial movements for enriched social interactions. In: 2014 IEEE International Symposium on Haptic, Audio and Visual Environments and Games (HAVE) Proceedings, pp. 82–87 (2014). https://doi.org/10.1109/HAVE.2014.6954336
49. Friesen, E., Ekman, P.: Facial action coding system: a technique for the measurement of facial movement. Palo Alto **3**, 5 (1978)
50. McDaniel, T., Devkota, S., Tadayon, R., Duarte, B., Fakhri, B., Panchanathan, S.: Tactile facial action units toward enriching social interactions for individuals who are blind. In: Basu, A., Berretti, S. (eds.) Smart Multimedia, pp. 3–14. Springer International Publishing, Cham (2018)
51. Neidlinger, K., Truong, K.P., Telfair, C., Feijs, L., Dertien, E., Evers, V.: AWElectric: that gave me goosebumps, did you feel it too? In: Proceedings of the Eleventh International Conference on Tangible, Embedded, and Embodied Interaction, pp. 315–324. ACM, New York (2017). https://doi.org/10.1145/3024969.3025004
52. Smith, J., MacLean, K.: Communicating emotion through a haptic link: Design space and methodology. Int. J. Hum. Comput. Stud. **65**, 376–387 (2007). https://doi.org/10.1016/j.ijhcs.2006.11.006
53. Chang, A., Resner, B., Koerner, B., Wang, X., Ishii, H.: LumiTouch: An emotional communication device. In: CHI '01 Extended Abstracts on Human Factors in Computing Systems, pp. 313–314. ACM, New York (2001). https://doi.org/10.1145/634067.634252
54. Mehrabian, A., Russell, J.A.: An Approach to Environmental Psychology. The MIT Press, Cambridge (1974)
55. Tsalamlal, M.Y., Ouarti, N., Martin, J.-C., Ammi, M.: Haptic communication of dimensions of emotions using air jet based tactile stimulation. J Multimod. User Interfaces **9**, 69–77 (2015). https://doi.org/10.1007/s12193-014-0162-3
56. Rantala, J., Salminen, K., Raisamo, R., Surakka, V.: Touch gestures in communicating emotional intention via vibrotactile stimulation. Int. J. Hum. Comput. Stud. **71**, 679–690 (2013). https://doi.org/10.1016/j.ijhcs.2013.02.004

57. Panchanathan, S., Chakraborty, S., McDaniel, T., Tadayon, R.: Person-centered multimedia computing: a new paradigm inspired by assistive and rehabilitative applications. IEEE MultiMedia **23**, 12–19 (2016). https://doi.org/10.1109/MMUL.2016.51
58. Shin, H., Lee, J., Park, J., Kim, Y., Oh, H., Lee, T.: A tactile emotional interface for instant messenger chat. In: Smith, M.J., Salvendy, G. (eds.) Human Interface and the Management of Information. Interacting in Information Environments, pp. 166–175. Springer Berlin Heidelberg, Berlin (2007)
59. Qiu, S., Rauterberg, M., Hu, J.: Designing and evaluating a wearable device for accessing gaze signals from the sighted. In: Antona, M., Stephanidis, C. (eds.) Universal Access in Human-Computer Interaction. Methods, Techniques, and Best Practices, pp. 454–464. Springer International Publishing, Cham (2016)
60. Beattie, G.: Rethinking Body Language: How Hand Movements Reveal Hidden Thoughts. Psychology Press, New York (2016)
61. Bavelas, J., Gerwing, J., Sutton, C., Prevost, D.: Gesturing on the telephone: Independent effects of dialogue and visibility. J. Mem. Lang. **58**, 495–520 (2008). https://doi.org/10.1016/j.jml.2007.02.004
62. McNeill, D.: Hand and Mind: What Gestures Reveal about Thought. University of Chicago Press, Chicago (1992)
63. Bekker, M.M., Olson, J.S., Olson, G.M.: Analysis of gestures in face-to-face design teams provides guidance for how to use groupware in design. In: Proceedings of the 1st Conference on Designing Interactive Systems: Processes, Practices, Methods, & Techniques, pp. 157–166 (1995)
64. Van Den Hoven, E., Mazalek, A.: Grasping gestures: Gesturing with physical artifacts. AI EDAM **25**, 255–271 (2011). https://doi.org/10.1017/S0890060411000072
65. Heikkinen, J., Rantala, J., Olsson, T., Raisamo, R., Lylykangas, J., Raisamo, J., Surakka, V., Ahmaniemi, T.: Enhancing personal communication with spatial haptics: Two scenario-based experiments on gestural interaction. J. Vis. Lang. Comput. **20**, 287–304 (2009). https://doi.org/10.1016/j.jvlc.2009.07.007
66. Maynes-Aminzade, D., Tan, B.-K., Goulding, K., Vaucelle, C.: Hover: conveying remote presence. In: ACM SIGGRAPH 2002 Conference Abstracts and Applications, pp. 194–194. ACM, New York (2002). https://doi.org/10.1145/1242073.1242207
67. Sekiguchi, D., Inami, M., Tachi, S.: RobotPHONE: RUI for interpersonal communication. In: CHI '01 Extended Abstracts on Human Factors in Computing Systems, pp. 277–278. ACM, New York (2001). https://doi.org/10.1145/634067.634231
68. Fogg, B., Cutler, L.D., Arnold, P., Eisbach, C.: HandJive: A device for interpersonal haptic entertainment. In: Proceedings of the SIGCHI Conference on Human Factors in Computing Systems, pp. 57–64. ACM Press/Addison-Wesley Publishing Co., New York (1998). https://doi.org/10.1145/274644.274653
69. Lin, C.-L., Shaw, F.-Z., Young, K.-Y., Lin, C.-T., Jung, T.-P.: EEG correlates of haptic feedback in a visuomotor tracking task. NeuroImage **60**, 2258–2273 (2012). https://doi.org/10.1016/j.neuroimage.2012.02.008
70. de Jesus Oliveira, V.A., Nedel, L., Maciel, A.: Assessment of an articulatory interface for tactile intercommunication in immersive virtual environments. Comput. Graph. **76**, 18–28 (2018). https://doi.org/10.1016/j.cag.2018.07.007
71. Simard, J., Ammi, M.: Gesture coordination in collaborative tasks through augmented feedthrough. In: Joint Virtual Reality Conference of EGVE - EuroVR - VEC, 8 pp. The Eurographics Association (2010). https://doi.org/10.2312/EGVE/JVRC10/043-050
72. McDaniel, T., Krishna, S., Balasubramanian, V., Colbry, D., Panchanathan, S.: Using a haptic belt to convey non-verbal communication cues during social interactions to individuals who are blind. In: 2008 IEEE International Workshop on Haptic Audio visual Environments and Games, pp. 13–18 (2008). https://doi.org/10.1109/HAVE.2008.4685291

73. Kadomura, A., Matsuda, A., Rekimoto, J.: CASPER: a haptic enhanced telepresence exercise system for elderly people. In: Proceedings of the 7th Augmented Human International Conference 2016, pp. 1–8. Association for Computing Machinery, Geneva (2016). https://doi.org/10.1145/2875194.2875197

74. Tadayon, R., McDaniel, T., Goldberg, M., Robles-Franco, P.M., Zia, J., Laff, M., Geng, M., Panchanathan, S.: Interactive motor learning with the autonomous training assistant: a case study. In: Kurosu, M. (ed.) Human-Computer Interaction: Interaction Technologies, pp. 495–506. Springer International Publishing, Cham (2015). https://doi.org/10.1007/978-3-319-20916-6_46

75. Coleman, H.O.: Intonation and emphasis. Le Maître Phonétique **3**(40), 6–26 (1925)

76. Schaffer, D.: The role of intonation as a cue to turn taking in conversation. J. Phonetics **11**, 243–257 (1983). https://doi.org/10.1016/S0095-4470(19)30825-3

77. Guest, M.: Intonation, visuals, text, and narrative. In: Guest, M. (ed.) Conferencing and Presentation English for Young Academics, pp. 181–187. Springer, Singapore (2018). https://doi.org/10.1007/978-981-13-2475-8_18

78. Lahtinen, R., Palmer, R.: Haptices and Haptemes–environmental information through touch. In: 3rd International Haptic and Auditory Interaction Design Workshop. Citeseer (2008)

79. McDaniel, T.L.: Somatic ABC's: A theoretical framework for designing, developing and evaluating the building blocks of touch-based information delivery. PhD Thesis, Arizona State University, Tempe, Arizona, United States (2012)

80. Enriquez, M., MacLean, K., Chita, C.: Haptic phonemes: basic building blocks of haptic communication. In: Proceedings of the 8th International Conference on Multimodal Interfaces, pp. 302–309. Association for Computing Machinery, Banff, Alberta (2006). https://doi.org/10.1145/1180995.1181053

81. Chang, A., O'Modhrain, S., Jacob, R., Gunther, E., Ishii, H.: ComTouch: Design of a vibrotactile communication device. In: Proceedings of the 4th Conference on Designing Interactive Systems: Processes, Practices, Methods, and Techniques, pp. 312–320. ACM, New York (2002). https://doi.org/10.1145/778712.778755

82. Hoggan, E., Stewart, C., Haverinen, L., Jacucci, G., Lantz, V.: Pressages: augmenting phone calls with non-verbal messages. In: Proceedings of the 25th Annual ACM Symposium on User Interface Software and Technology, pp. 555–562 (2012)

83. Brown, L.M., Brewster, S.A., Purchase, H.C.: Tactile crescendos and sforzandos: applying musical techniques to tactile icon design. In: CHI '06 Extended Abstracts on Human Factors in Computing Systems, pp. 610–615. Association for Computing Machinery, Montréal, Québec (2006). https://doi.org/10.1145/1125451.1125578

84. Suhonen, K., Müller, S., Rantala, J., Väänänen-Vainio-Mattila, K., Raisamo, R., Lantz, V.: Haptically augmented remote speech communication: a study of user practices and experiences. In: Proceedings of the 7th Nordic Conference on Human-Computer Interaction: Making Sense Through Design, pp. 361–369. Association for Computing Machinery, Copenhagen (2012). https://doi.org/10.1145/2399016.2399073

85. Ho, C.-Y., Sarter, N.B.: Supporting synchronous distributed communication and coordination through multimodal information exchange. In: Proceedings of the Human Factors and Ergonomics Society Annual Meeting, vol. 48, pp. 426–430 (2004). https://doi.org/10.1177/154193120404800332

86. Chan, A., MacLean, K., McGrenere, J.: Designing haptic icons to support collaborative turn-taking. Int. J. Hum. Comput. Stud. **66**, 333–355 (2008). https://doi.org/10.1016/j.ijhcs.2007.11.002

87. Cao, H., Gapenne, O., Aubert, D.: Accelerative effect of tactile feedback on turn-taking control in remote verbal-communication. In: CHI '13 Extended Abstracts on Human Factors in Computing Systems, pp. 1581–1586. Association for Computing Machinery, Paris (2013). https://doi.org/10.1145/2468356.2468639

88. Oakley, I., O'Modhrain, S.: Contact IM: Exploring asynchronous touch over distance. In: Proceedings of CSCW, pp. 16–20 (2002)
89. Mohammed, Z., Omar, R.: Comparison of reading performance between visually impaired and normally sighted students in Malaysia. Br. J. Vis. Impairment **29**, 196–207 (2011). https://doi.org/10.1177/0264619611415004
90. Brave, S., Dahley, A.: inTouch: A medium for haptic interpersonal communication. In: CHI '97 Extended Abstracts on Human Factors in Computing Systems, pp. 363–364. ACM, New York (1997). https://doi.org/10.1145/1120212.1120435
91. Rovers, A.F., van Essen, H.A.: HIM: A framework for haptic instant messaging. In: CHI '04 Extended Abstracts on Human Factors in Computing Systems, pp. 1313–1316. ACM, New York (2004). https://doi.org/10.1145/985921.986052
92. Rovers, A.F., van Essen, H.A.: FootIO: design and evaluation of a device to enable foot interaction over a computer network. In: Proceedings of the First Joint Eurohaptics Conference and Symposium on Haptic Interfaces for Virtual Environment and Teleoperator Systems, pp. 521–522. IEEE Computer Society, Washinton D.C. (2005). https://doi.org/10.1109/WHC.2005.56
93. Rovers, A.F., van Essen, H.A.: Guidelines for haptic interpersonal communication applications: an exploration of foot interaction styles. Virtual Reality **9**, 177–191 (2006). https://doi.org/10.1007/s10055-005-0016-0
94. Tsetserukou, D., Neviarouskaya, A.: iFeel_IM!: Augmenting emotions during online communication. IEEE Comput. Graph. Appl. **30**, 72–80 (2010). https://doi.org/10.1109/MCG.2010.88
95. Choudhary, T., Kulkarni, S., Reddy, P.: A Braille-based mobile communication and translation glove for deaf-blind people. In: 2015 International Conference on Pervasive Computing (ICPC), pp. 1–4 (2015). https://doi.org/10.1109/PERVASIVE.2015.7087033
96. Brown, L.M., Williamson, J.: Shake2Talk: multimodal messaging for interpersonal communication. In: Oakley, I., Brewster, S. (eds.) Haptic and Audio Interaction Design, pp. 44–55. Springer Berlin Heidelberg, Berlin (2007)
97. Shen, X., George, M., Hernandez, S., Park, A., Liu, Y., Ishii, H.: Mole messenger: pushable interfaces for connecting family at a distance. In: Proceedings of the Thirteenth International Conference on Tangible, Embedded, and Embodied Interaction, pp. 269–274. ACM, New York (2019). https://doi.org/10.1145/3294109.3300990
98. Suzuki, K., Hashimoto, S.: Feellight: A communication device for distant nonverbal exchange. In: Proceedings of the 2004 ACM SIGMM Workshop on Effective Telepresence, pp. 40–44. ACM, New York (2004). https://doi.org/10.1145/1026776.1026786
99. Tan, H.Z., Reed, C.M., Jiao, Y., Perez, Z.D., Wilson, E.C., Jung, J., Martinez, J.S., Severgnini, F.M.: Acquisition of 500 English Words through a TActile Phonemic Sleeve (TAPS). IEEE Trans. Haptics, 1 (2020). https://doi.org/10.1109/TOH.2020.2973135

Part IV
Multimodal Technologies for Accessible Human Computer Interfaces

Human-Machine Interfaces for Socially Connected Devices: From Smart Households to Smart Cities

Juana Isabel Méndez, Pedro Ponce, Adán Medina, Alan Meier, Therese Peffer, Troy McDaniel, and Arturo Molina

Abstract This chapter defines a smart community as a set of smart homes, commercial buildings, public spaces, and transportation with boundaries based on walking distance, located in a physical region. This smart community uses social products and provides community public services, smart water management, smart mobility management to promote social interaction. The communication uses a tailored Human Machine Interface (HMI) within a gamification structure that provides feedback and adjustments based on user profiles and behavior to teach, motivate, and engage end-users in achieving specific goals, such as energy reduction. Hence, gamification builds strategies to make engaging applications by triggering internal and external motivations in end-users. A smart home gathers and analyzes data from its sensors, then delivers analytics and predictions to end-users and service provides as well as strives to improve the management of its various subsystems through social products. In that regard, the multi-sensor system allows experts to know more about the needs of homes to propose actions that reduce energy consumption and improve the home and community quality of life by galvanizing individuals to read, analyze, and act upon their energy consumption through sensor profile patterns. Thus, this chapter discusses the use of an adaptive neural network fuzzy inference and a fuzzy logic decision system to evaluate the level of energy consumption in households and the type of environmental home.

J. I. Méndez · P. Ponce (✉) · A. Medina · A. Molina
School of Engineering and Sciences, Tecnológico de Monterrey, México City, Mexico
e-mail: A01165549@itesm.mx; pedro.ponce@tec.mx; A01331840@itesm.mx; armolina@tec.mx

A. Meier
Lawrence Berkeley National Laboratory, University of California, Berkeley, CA, USA
e-mail: akmeier@ucdavis.edu

T. Peffer
Institute for Energy and Environment, University of California, Berkeley, CA, USA
e-mail: tpeffer@berkeley.edu

T. McDaniel
Arizona State University, Mesa, AZ, USA
e-mail: troy.mcdaniel@asu.edu

© The Author(s), under exclusive license to Springer Nature Switzerland AG 2021
T. McDaniel, X. Liu (eds.), *Multimedia for Accessible Human Computer Interfaces*,
https://doi.org/10.1007/978-3-030-70716-3_9

253

These decision systems give insights to propose an interactive and tailored HMI for each kind of home and community interaction. Finally, this chapter discusses improving the quality of life of people who are elderly using connected devices that transmit and receive information inside households or public spaces via an HMI.

Keywords Smart community · Smart home · Social products · Socially connected products · Multi-sensor system · ANFIS · Gamification · HMI

1 Introduction

This chapter introduces a multi-sensor system for use in a smart community environment composed of a set of smart homes, commercial buildings, public spaces, and transportation with boundaries based on the walking distance, located in the same geographical space. This multi-sensor system enables connectivity of sensors in a smart home toward understanding the neighborhoods' requirements, specifically, for promoting pro-environmental attitudes among neighbors to achieve a reduction in energy consumption and improve quality of life.

Figure 1 shows the proposed multi-sensor structure focused on decision fusion where the home behavior (local point of view) and the community behavior (global point of view) provide information into the system throughout the social products. The adaptive neural network fuzzy inference (ANFIS) analyzes and evaluates this information to propose actions to perform regarding energy, quality of life, and the

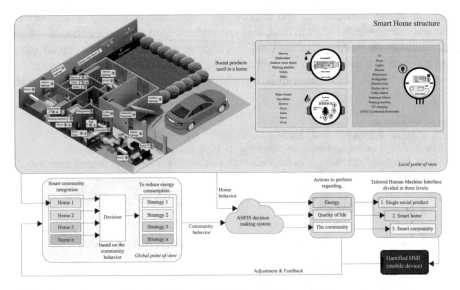

Fig. 1 General proposal for data fusion and HMI in smart homes and the smart community

community. Finally, a Human Machine Interface (HMI) uses a gamification strategy with a fuzzy logic decision system to run on a tailored interface in three levels:

1. A single social product, for instance, a connected thermostat,
2. The smart home, which is the set of social products within the home,
3. The smart community.

1.1 Smart Community

Although the concept of a smart community is nascent, it is still not yet well defined as there is no clear separation between a smart community and a smart city. This section considers that it is necessary to determine the single concept of a community first without considering its smartness. Thus, in [24], Łucka believes that a community should have these characteristics:

- Be self-sustaining and dense to enable residents short commutes by bicycle or walking rather than by automobile.
- Layout should support a normal walking distance, which is typically a radius of 0.25–0.5 miles.
- Be organized around public transportation.
- Promote social relationships by interconnected networks of streets and public spaces.
- Be safe by making strangers fell noticed and potentially unwelcomed if they plan to commit a crime. This safety is provided by promoting "eyes on the street" in the neighborhoods.
- Besides housing, there are places of work, leisure, and shopping near the community.

Thus, a community in terms of energy is composed of not only residential sectors, but also industrial, commercial, and transport sectors. Figure 2 depicts the total energy consumption by sector in the U.S. from January 2019 to February 2020 obtained from the database *Energy consumption estimates by sector* of the U.S. Energy Information Administration [11]. According to this information, residential buildings, commercial sectors, and transportation represent 21.69%, 18.22%, and 27.84%, respectively. Communities therefore belong to 67.75% of the total U.S energy consumption in the last year. An essential task for communities is to promote a reduction in energy consumption without being obtrusive or losing the quality of life by transitioning the community into a smart community. An essential task for smart communities is to promote pro-environmental attitudes.

Several authors have defined their concept of the Smart Community. Li et al. [21] describe it as a set of smart homes, amenities, and green areas where residents have social interaction and relationships with their neighborhoods. Homes are virtually connected in the same geographic region by powerline communication, wireless

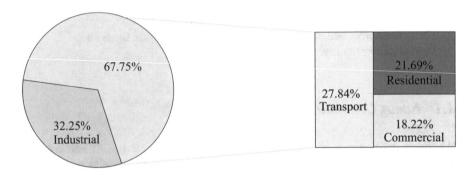

Fig. 2 Total energy consumed by industrial, transportation, residential and commercial sector in percentage from January 2019 to February 2020 [11]

communication, such as Bluetooth or Wi-Fi, phone line communication, and/or technologies that require dedicated wiring such as Ethernet.

Eltoweissy et al. [12], indicate that a smart community has four key characteristics:

- Sustainability: the community is self-sufficient regarding services offered and the resources needed to enable those services.
- Resilience: the community changes dynamically; for instance, the smart community can react in a precise and timely way in response to incipient emergencies.
- Empathy-driven proactive intelligence: the community can predict future needs using artificial intelligence algorithms within smart products.
- Emergent behavior: the community evolves based on current needs as profiled by smart products.

Wang [48] emphasizes that the smart community should use smart products, a management method, and a community philosophy featured with multinetwork integration. He mentions that there is a lack of standardization due to a miss in the unified local region. This author describes three development stages for a smart community:

- Initial stage: community uses smart products and provides management, e-commerce services, and health services within the smart community and the smart home.
- Development stage: A smart platform application reaches the community. This application gathers multiple mobile apps to enhance the community.
- Improvement stage: A standardized service system should be initiated for the smart community. This stage focuses on continuous improvement and development.

London [49], Oslo [52], and Copenhagen [16] have launched smart community initiatives where there is a continuous interaction between the citizen and the communities (government, agency, company, and institutions) and user-centered designs by encouraging the digital engagement of the populace. A key component for a smart community is the smart home. There is an interaction between the building, user, and the software and hardware technology within the smart home through smart household appliances, or social products. Ponce et al. [40] define a social product as a product that modifies the behavior of the end-user by observing, registering, and analyzing her or his consumption patterns. This product can adapt its characteristics online or offline to improve its performance and acceptability. Thus, a smart product, or an intelligent household appliance, can be considered a social product for tracking and understanding users [8, 14, 29].

Social interaction plays a primary role in understanding users' patterns [30, 31]. A way to shape occupants' habits is by sending stimuli through gamification strategies [29–32, 39, 40]. Gamification, in this context, is defined as a process to improve services through gameful experiences to augment value creation for users [15].

We therefore define smart community as a creative community located in a physical region by a set of smart homes, commercial buildings, public spaces, and transportation with boundaries based on walking distance. A smart community uses social products to provide community public services, smart water management, and smart mobility management to promote social interaction. Communication uses a tailored HMI within a gamification structure that includes feedback and adjustments based on user profiles and behavior to teach, motivate, and engage end-users to perform specific tasks and achieve certain goals, as energy reduction (Fig. 3). For this chapter, the set of homes is used as a fundamental part of smart community integration.

Currently, the *IESE Cities in Motion Index* [5] presented a report on 147 cities' smartness. Figure 4 shows the top 10 smart cities around the world based on nine dimensions described below. Note that each of the top cities has strengths and weakness based on these dimensions.

- Economy: this dimension measures 13 indicators that promote the economic development of a territory: productivity, the time required to start a business, ease of starting a business, headquarters, motivation to start early-stage entrepreneurial activity, estimated annual GDP growth, GDP in millions of dol-

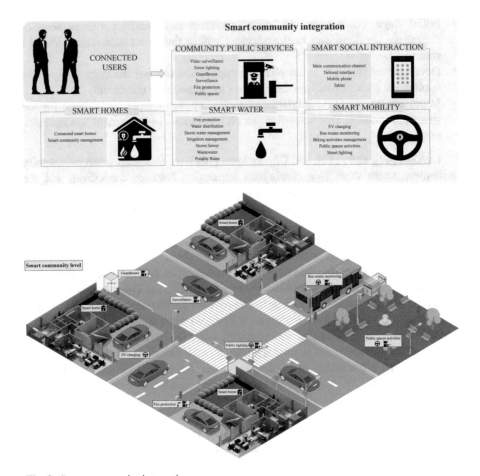

Fig. 3 Smart community integration

lars, GDP per capita, mortgage, Glovo and Uber services, salary, and purchasing power.
- Human capital: this dimension measures 10 indicators to promote education accessibility at different levels, as well as promote arts and recreation activities.
- Social cohesion: this dimension measures 16 indicators to determine how happy citizens are and how much equality exists among city's population; also how other factors may alter these levels, such as crime, death, homicide, terrorism, and suicide rates.
- Environment: this dimension measures 11 indicators that take into account the amount of pollution a city produces, such as air pollution, garbage or emissions, as well as environmental performance, future climate estimations, and public water access.

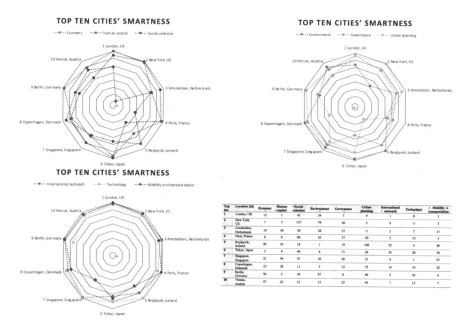

Top ten	Location [18]	Economy	Human capital	Social cohesion	Environment	Governance	Urban planning	International outreach	Technology	Mobility & transportation
1	London, UK	12	1	45	34	7	9	1	8	3
2	New York, US	1	3	137	78	26	2	8	11	5
3	Amsterdam, Netherlands	10	36	38	28	27	11	2	7	11
4	Paris, France	8	6	86	54	37	50	3	15	4
5	Reykjavik, Iceland	90	53	18	1	19	108	22	4	46
6	Tokyo, Japan	3	9	49	6	71	24	35	20	29
7	Singapore, Singapore	21	44	47	10	20	31	4	1	67
8	Copenhagen, Denmark	25	28	11	3	12	75	16	10	25
9	Berlin, Germany	50	5	39	47	6	40	5	32	6
10	Vienna, Austria	57	23	31	15	25	45	7	13	7

Fig. 4 Top 10 smart cities around the world and their place regarding each dimension [5]

- Governance: this dimension measures 12 indicators to determine how well prepared a city is to confront economic problems, incentivize investments, legal strength, international presence, democracy, corruption rankings, and how inclusive a government is to its citizens.
- Urban planning: this dimension measures five indicators that take into account the number of bicycle rental or sharing points, percentage of urban population with access to private sanitation services, number of people per household, percentage of high rise buildings, and number of completed buildings, including high rises.
- International outreach: this dimension measures six indicators to assess how prepared a city is to receive outside visitors; this means the number of passengers per airport, number of hotels and restaurants, and how attractive a city is, taking into account the number of international businesses implemented in the city, and the number of photos taken in city locations.
- Technology: this dimension measures 11 indicators to assess how proficient the population is with technology by use of the internet and social networks, also internet quality, and cell phone accessibility.
- Mobility and transportation: this dimension measures 10 indicators that determine the efficiency of the city by means of transportation, either private cars or public transportation, as well as bicycle accessibility.

1.2   Smart Home

A smart home gathers and analyzes data from its sensors, then delivers analytics and predictions to end-users and service provides as well as strives to improve the management of its various subsystems through social products [2]. The system controls home electronics and appliances such as HVAC, telecommunications, A/V, security, lighting, and sprinklers, and provides residents with analytics such as how much electricity they have consumed on specific appliances or system. Moreover, utilities are capability of reading meters from a distance [14]. Furthermore, a smart home interface with a gamification structure provides interactions that make users feel comfortable; for instance, in [29], a gamified smart home structure was proposed that uses social products to promote ecological-saving and money-saving activities to promote energy-saving behavior in end-users (Fig. 5).

Also, a smart home requires an Energy Management System between the home and the household products to track and monitor users' activities to generate profiles [6]. Artificial intelligence enables communication between homes by monitoring and enriching services to end-users, from entertainment, to security, to lighting and temperature access and optimization [44].

There are four categories of smart homes based on the types of services they offer [27]:

1. Assistive homes: this home assists occupants based on their daily actions, providing care for everyone from children to the elderly. These homes are mostly used for healthcare.
2. Detection and multimedia information gathering: this home collects photos and videos of the occupants.
3. Surveillance home: This home processes data that alert users of upcoming natural disasters or invasions of security.
4. Ecological home: this type of home promotes environmental sustainability by providing occupants with capabilities to manage energy supply versus demand.

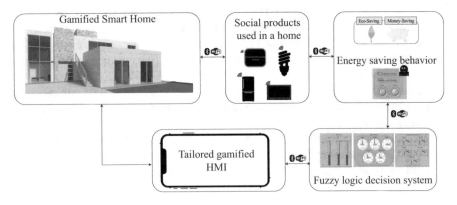

Fig. 5 Examples of a gamified smart home structure presented in [29]

Smart home services can be added to homes by transitioning from a traditional home to a smart home. Thus, smart homes have the potential to improve the quality of living for many families.

1.3 Socially Connected Products

In [34], the S^3 product development reference framework was proposed to implement sensing, smart, and sustainable products:

- *Sensing* is the ability of a system to detect events, obtain information, and measure changes utilizing sensors for observing physical and/or environmental conditions.
- *Smart* is the complementary consolidation of physical parts, components, and connectivity to make a product intelligent and accessible to interface with other gadgets.
- *Sustainable* incorporates social, environmental, and economic elements to produce balanced and optimized performance.

Social products can be promoted by knowing the types of behavior and usability problems in the use of connected devices and involving residential energy users in planning, implementing, and monitoring energy usage.

Figure 6 displays the social products of a smart home, divided by the type of utility consumption (water, gas, and electricity) and needs to be satisfied within the smart community environment to provide safety, transportation, and healthcare. Those elements working together provide a more in-depth insight into the improvement of energy behavior. For instance, if the homeowner knows the weather, the individual could determine the type of clothes to wear; hence, when he or she returns home, with the appropriate outfit, the individual would not need

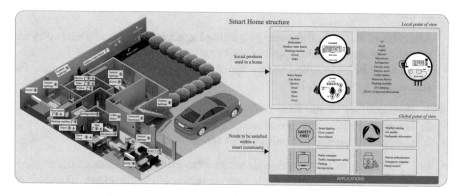

Fig. 6 Social products divided by the type of utility

to increase or decrease the indoor temperature. Thus, the individual could avoid consuming extra electricity as she or he is thermally comfortable.

Social products acceptability has the following characteristics [13]:

- Users know that when they buy a connected product, they can exploit advantages.
- Products fit with the user's current and changing lifestyles.
- Appliances and devices are quick and cheap to obtain.
- Products demonstrate reduced or eliminated physical demands in operation.
- Neither a high degree of background knowledge, nor routine interventions by professionals, is needed for installation, use, and/or maintenance.
- The usability of the product considers end-user skills; the product does not fail or act unpredictability.
- Products interpret user requirements.
- Products have privacy and security features, so users' information is secure and safe.

1.4 Gamification

Several authors have defined gamification:

- For Terrill [50], gamification takes game mechanics and uses them in web properties to increase engagement.
- For Huotari and Hamari [15], gamification is a process to improve services through gameful experiences to augment value creation for users.
- For Deterding et al. [9], it is the employment of game design and elements within non-gaming contexts.
- For Chou [7], it is the art of designing fun, engaging elements found traditionally in games, and employing these features in real-world activities.

For environmental purposes, gamification has the following addresses and considerations:

- Albertalli et al. [1], defined energy gamified applications as traditional software targeting an environmental goal using serious game features.
- An analysis of 25 gamified energy applications suggests three best practices for sustainable applications [43]:

  1. Sustainability should be rewarding and fun.
  2. Leverage positive peer pressure.
  3. Use gamification to galvanize useful action.

- In [3], a variety of game design elements were explored to enhance the engagement of end-users in energy saving and optimization applications. Examples of game design elements ranged from incentives such as discounts and prizes, to competitive aspects such as leaderboards and badges.

1.4.1   Energy Adapted Octalysis Framework

The Octalysis framework proposed by Chou [7] analyzes and builds strategies to make engaging applications. This framework considers extrinsic and intrinsic motivations, among other elements:

- Extrinsic motivation: motivation stems from the desire to attain something for outer recognition or monetary prizes. Encompasses a variety of factors from identification to external regulation.
- Intrinsic motivation: motivation stemming from a source that is rewarding or of value wholly on its own in the absence of a particular objective to accomplish. Following [19], this motivation considers three elements applicable for an energy purpose:

    - Autonomy through customization and independence including control of goals and tasks. Contributes to familiar routines, improved performance, reinforced success, responsibility, and internalized rewards.
    - Competence can relate to task complexity/understanding, execution challenge, and memory, and may be categorized as performance, achievement or engagement based.
    - Relatedness pertains to preferences, sharing, relationships and their interactions. Contributes to forging social relationships, disseminating achievements and milestones, sharing experiences, enhancing empathy, setting examples, exchanging suggestions and feedback, and validation.

In previous research [39], an adaptation for the Octalysis framework was proposed. This adaptation includes the game design elements offered in [3], the Hexad gamified user, the role player, and the end-user in the energy segment and the target group proposed in [4, 7, 26, 36, 38, 45]. Table 1 shows the extrinsic and intrinsic motivations regarding energy applications [3].

Table 1 Gamification elements for extrinsic and intrinsic motivations

Extrinsic motivation	Intrinsic motivation
Offers, coupons	Notifications
Bill discounts	Messages
Challenges	Tips
Levels	Energy community
Dashboard	Collaboration
Statistics	Control over peers
Degree of control	Social comparison
Points, badges, leaderboard	Competition

2   Multisystem: Data Fusion

When multiple sensors collect information, data fusion is often useful for making more robust inferences compared to single modalities, especially when a reference framework is utilized to map attribute or property values to quantitative measurements in a way that is both predictable and consistent. The utility of a multi-sensor data fusion framework is attractive for its functions of information processing, integration, communication, and compensation [18, 23, 47].

Multi-sensor data fusion is a concept based on animals' and humans' fundamental ability to integrate redundant and complementary information across modalities to improve the chance of survival. The primary functions are:

- Compensation: diagnose, calibrate, and adapt in response to environmental variations.
- Information processing: attention, event recognition, and decision-making.
- Communication: standard inference protocol for conveying perceptions and interpretations of sensor data to the external world.
- Integration: seamlessly coupled sensing, processing, and actuator subsystems.
- Decision-making: analyze and make predictions from sensed data to inform decisions.

While data fusion is not novel, we are now able to realize higher performance and more robost systems for data fusion through advancements in sensors, artificial intelligence, digital systems, information processing techniques, and embedded systems.

2.1   ANFIS: Adaptive Neuro-Fuzzy Inference Systems

In the presence of uncertain or vague information, conventional modeling techniques may face challenges. The IF-THEN linguistic rules of fuzzy systems employ human-like reasoning without complete or precise information. The issue arises in transferring human knowledge to that of fuzzy logic systems, and tuning these systems. Many approaches have been proposed, including of fusing fuzzy systems with artificial neural networks (ANNs), which can adapt and learn based on experience. One example is the adaptive neuro-fuzzy inference system (ANFIS) by Jang [18], which automatically produces fuzzy membership functions and IF-THEN rule bases. ANFIS uses adaptive networks, which are a superset of the feed-forward type ANNs [18, 37], in a directionally-connected topology of nodes. Learning takes place through rules that minimize an error criterion as connection parameters are updated. A common learning rule is gradient descent although Jang introduced a hybrid learning rule using least squares estimation. The ANFIS topology [18] is depicted in Fig. 7.

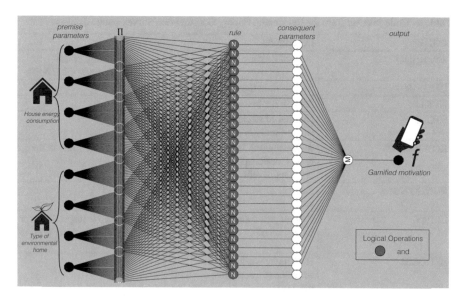

Fig. 7 ANFIS topology

2.2 Topology Proposed: Detection of Gamified Motivation at Home for Saving Energy

The proposed system is based on two elements: the level of household energy consumption and the type of ecological behavior.

2.3 Input 1: Level of Energy Consumption

The level of energy consumption was obtained from the 2015 Residential Energy Consumption Survey public database [10]. Table 2 depicts the code and characteristics selected to meet the following criteria:

- Single-family house detached from any other home.
- No basement in the housing unit.
- No attic in the housing unit.
- One story.
- Owned by someone in the household.
- 10–15 windows in heated areas.
- Household is responsible for paying incurred electricity costs.
- Members of household are home most weekdays.
- Square footage ranges from 1100 sq. ft. to 1800 sq. ft.
- Located in the Bay Area (California).

Table 2 Code selected from the Residential Energy Consumption Survey public database [10]

CODE	Description	Information
TYPEHUQ	Type of housing unit	2 – single-family house detached from any other house
CELLAR	Basement in the housing unit	0 – no
ATTIC	Attic in the housing unit	0 – no
STORIES	Number of stories in a single-family home	10 – one story
KOWNRENT	A housing unit is owned, rented, or occupied without payment of rent	1 – owned by someone in the household
WINDOWS	Number of windows in heated areas	41 – 10 to 15
ELPAY	Who pays the electricity used in the home?	1 – household is responsible for paying for all electricity used in this home
ATHOME	How many weekdays is someone at home most or all of the day?	5 – 5 days
TOTSQFT_EN	Total square footage (includes heated/cooled garages, all basements, and finished/heated/cooled attics). Used for EIA data tables	The range used between 1100 sq. ft. and 1800 sq. ft.
CLIMATE_REGION_PUB	Building America Climate Region (collapsed for public file)	5 – marine
IECC_CLIMATE_PUB	International Energy Conservation Code (IECC) climate zone (collapsed for public file)	3C IECCC climate zone 3C (California, Bay Area)

Once the kWh energy consumption is obtained during the year, we may estimate the 30-day energy consumption from each type of home to profile the households using (1),

$$Monthly\ house\ energy\ consumption \left(\frac{kWh}{month}\right)$$
$$= \frac{kWh}{year} \bullet \frac{year}{8760\ hours} \bullet \frac{24\ hours}{1\ day} \bullet \frac{30\ days}{1\ month} \tag{1}$$

The house is then profiled, and a 30-day table is generated with random values where the limit value is the monthly house energy consumption. As the database does not present information about months, this calculation has the premise that the total monthly hours should be at least under the monthly average of the household energy consumption reference. Next, from the 30-day table, the following data is obtained:

- The complete set of types of homes.
- The minimum value of the set.
- The maximum value of the set.
- Mean.
- Standard Deviation.
- House low consumption: Mean – Standard Deviation.
- House high consumption: Mean + Standard Deviation.

Finally, these values are normalized using (2),

$$X1 = \frac{X - (Min_{set} - 5)}{(Max_{set} + 5) - (Min_{set} - 5)} \tag{2}$$

where,

$X1$ = normalized value.
X = value to be normalized.
Min_{set} = Minimum value of the set.
Max_{set} = Maximum value of the set.
$+/-5$ = This value is used to avoid having a maximum normalized number of 1 and a minimum normalized number of 0.

2.4   Input 2: Type of Environmental Home

The type of pro-environmental user is related to the level of energy consumption: *It is assumed that based on the criteria selected from* Table 2, *there is similar home behavior. Hence, there is a lower limit for a home that consumes less energy than the other houses, an average energy consumption, and an upper limit for a home that consumes more power than the other houses.*

A pro-environmental home can be designed a lower limit home as this type of house demonstrates awareness for energy consumption; an average environmental home can be designated for average energy consumption; and a disengaged-environmental home can be designated an upper limit energy consumer, i.e., a lack of awareness for energy consumption. Thus, each type of home is associated with a value from 0 to 1:

- Pro-environmental home: 0.2
- Average environmental home: 0.4
- Disengaged-environmental home: 0.6

A new database was created and associated with the type of pro-environmental home by considering these premises (3),

$$Type\ of\ home \begin{cases} \dfrac{x}{0.20} & if\ x2 > x \quad \rightarrow\ pro-environmental\ home \\[2mm] \dfrac{x}{0.60} & if\ x3 < x \quad \rightarrow\ disengaged-environmental\ home \\[2mm] \dfrac{x}{0.40} & if\ x2 > x < x3. \quad \rightarrow\ Average\ environmental\ home \end{cases}$$

(3)

Finally, these values are normalized using (2).

2.5 Output: Gamified Motivation (Local Point of View)

Gamified motivation considers intrinsic and/or extrinsic motivators: *The disengaged-environmental home and the home that consumes more kWh requires extrinsic motivation as they are moved by outer recognition and external rewards. The pro-environmental home and the home that consumes less kWh can be related to intrinsic motivation as the house is using less kWh than others in similar conditions due to this activity being rewarding on its own. On the other hand, the average home in either environmental type and kWh consumed use both motivations as this type of home may be motivated by external recognition or by autonomy, competence, and relatedness elements.*

Thus, a Sugeno Fuzzy Inference System is employed where the input variables are Input 1: Level of energy consumption and Input 2: Type of environmental home, and the output values are the gamified motivators (see Fig. 8).

2.5.1 Community Gamified motivation's Detection (Global Point of View)

Obtaining the output values for each type of home, we may then calculate the mean value of the four output values from each household to get the average. Then, these values are used to create the ANFIS system using backpropagation as an optimization method and subclustering to generate the Fuzzy Inference System.

3 Proposal

From a representational sample of 118,208,250 households around the country, 55,727 houses represented in four groups met the criteria established in Table 2. Table 3 depicts the four types of homes with their characteristics and their household appliances, according to [10]. The ranges of energy consumption are from a house the consumed 4159 kWh to a house that consumed 10,674 kWh. Surprisingly, the second biggest home (home type 3) consumed the most energy during the year,

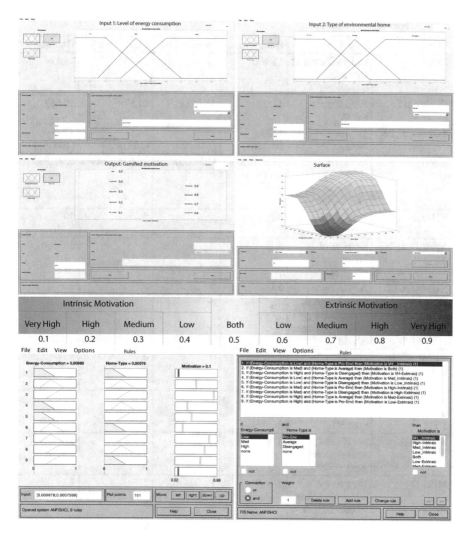

Fig. 8 Sugeno fuzzy logic inference system

likely due to the number of refrigerators (three), and that this home, when compared to home type 4, does not have a smart meter.

3.1 Input 1: Level of Energy Consumption

Based on (1), Table 4 shows the daily kWh consumption per home, and Table 5 depicts the estimated 30-day kWh consumption per household and their normalized values.

Table 3 Four types of households

CODE	Description	Home type 1	Home type 2	Home type 3	Home type 4
DOEID	Unique identifier for each respondent	11,106	12,192	12,834	15,114
NWEIGHT	Final simple weight	17,076	13,385	11,678	13,588
TOTSQFT_EN	Total square footage	1125 (104 m^2)	1550 (144 m^2)	1652 (153 m^2)	1793 (166 m^2)
KWH	Total site electricity usage per household over a year	4159.13 kWh	8920.06 kWh	10,674.33 kWh	6371.80 kWh
HHAGE	Age of the survey responder	36	76	50	79
NHSLDMEM	Number of household members	3	2	4	6
NUMADULT 18 years or older	A housing unit is owned, rented, or occupied without payment of rent	2	2	4	4
NUMCHILD 0–17 years old	Number of windows in heated areas	1	0	0	2
SMARTMETER 0 No 1 Yes	Does your home have a "smart meter"?	1	1	0	1
NUMFRIG	Number of refrigerators used	1	2	3	1
MICRO	How many microwaves are in your home?	1	1	2	1
TOAST 0 No 1 Yes	Is the toaster used at least once a week in your home?	1	1	0	1
COFFEE 0 No 1 Yes	Coffee maker used	1	1	0	1
DISHWASH 0 No 1 Yes	Dishwasher used	1	1	1	0
CWASHER 0 No 1 Yes	Clothes washer used in home	1	1	1	1
DRYER 0 No 1 Yes	Clothes dryer used in home	1	1	1	1
TVCOLOR	Number of televisions used	5	3	1	3

Table 4 Daily energy consumption per house

Home	kWh/year	Year/8760 h	24 h/day
Home type 1	4159.13	0.47	11.39
Home type 2	8920.06	1.02	24.44
Home type 3	10,674.33	1.22	29.24
Home type 4	6371.80	0.73	17.46
Average	7531.33	0.86	20.63

Table 5 Estimated monthly house energy consumption per home

Min set	10.29	Deviation	6.844		
Max set	29.75	**House low consumption <**	13.46		
Average	20.31	**House high consumption >**	27.15		

	Monthly house energy consumption per home				Normalized values			
Day	Home 1	Home 2	Home 3	Home 4	Home 1	Home 2	Home 3	Home 4
1	10.93	23.3	29.75	16.88	0.21	0.68	0.92	0.44
2	10.29	24.68	29.36	16.13	0.19	0.73	0.91	0.41
3	10.87	24.35	29.03	17.38	0.21	0.72	0.90	0.46
4	10.87	23.93	28.4	17.17	0.21	0.70	0.87	0.45
5	10.33	24.29	29.08	16.26	0.19	0.72	0.90	0.41
6	11.7	23.5	29.29	17.71	0.24	0.69	0.91	0.47
7	11.1	24.32	28.57	17.03	0.22	0.72	0.88	0.44
8	11.56	23.42	29.67	16.91	0.24	0.69	0.92	0.44
9	11.41	23.58	28.89	17.83	0.23	0.69	0.89	0.47
10	11.61	23.94	28.18	17.38	0.24	0.70	0.87	0.46
11	10.91	23.87	258	16.92	0.21	0.70	0.92	0.44
12	11.2	23.94	29.49	17.03	0.22	0.70	0.91	0.44
13	10.67	23.15	29.33	16.66	0.20	0.67	0.91	0.43
14	11.27	23.63	29	17.19	0.23	0.69	0.90	0.45
15	11.67	24	29.32	17.24	0.24	0.71	0.91	0.45
16	11.57	24.23	28.82	16.6	0.24	0.72	0.89	0.43
17	11.27	24.17	28.94	16.56	0.23	0.71	0.89	0.43
18	11.34	23.52	29.65	17.04	0.23	0.69	0.92	0.44
19	10.99	23.79	28.83	17.06	0.22	0.70	0.89	0.44
20	10.37	23.46	29.31	17.24	0.19	0.69	0.91	0.45
21	11.63	24.24	28.75	17.31	0.24	0.72	0.89	0.45
22	11.52	23.88	29.6	16.78	0.24	0.70	0.92	0.43
23	11.44	24.43	29.46	17.27	0.23	0.72	0.91	0.45
24	11.36	24.29	28.41	16.97	0.23	0.72	0.87	0.44
25	11.14	23.94	29.4	16.42	0.22	0.70	0.91	0.42
26	10.95	24.05	29.01	17.39	0.21	0.71	0.90	0.46
27	10.87	24.25	28.96	17.24	0.21	0.72	0.89	0.45
28	11.66	24.38	28.99	16.31	0.24	0.72	0.90	0.42
29	11.21	24.86	28.48	17.49	0.22	0.74	0.88	0.46
30	10.76	23.87	28.95	17.15	0.21	0.70	0.89	0.45

Table 6 Type of environmental home

Monthly type of environmental home					Normalized values			
Day	Home 1	Home 2	Home 3	Home 4	Home 1	Home 2	Home 3	Home 4
1	2.19	9.32	17.85	6.75	0.22	0.54	0.91	0.43
2	2.06	9.87	17.62	6.45	0.22	0.56	0.90	0.41
3	2.17	9.74	17.42	6.95	0.22	0.56	0.89	0.43
4	2.17	9.57	17.04	6.87	0.22	0.55	0.88	0.43
5	2.07	9.72	17.45	6.50	0.22	0.56	0.89	0.41
6	2.34	9.40	17.57	7.08	0.23	0.54	0.90	0.44
7	2.22	9.73	17.14	6.81	0.23	0.56	0.88	0.43
8	2.31	9.37	17.80	6.76	0.23	0.54	0.91	0.43
9	2.28	9.43	17.33	7.13	0.23	0.54	0.89	0.44
10	2.32	9.58	16.91	6.95	0.23	0.55	0.87	0.43
11	2.18	9.55	17.75	6.77	0.22	0.55	0.91	0.43
12	2.24	9.58	17.69	6.81	0.23	0.55	0.91	0.43
13	2.13	9.26	17.60	6.66	0.22	0.54	0.90	0.42
14	2.25	9.45	17.40	6.88	0.23	0.54	0.89	0.43
15	2.33	9.60	17.59	6.90	0.23	0.55	0.90	0.43
16	2.31	9.69	17.29	6.64	0.23	0.55	0.89	0.42
17	2.25	9.67	17.36	6.62	0.23	0.55	0.89	0.42
18	2.27	9.41	17.79	6.82	0.23	0.54	0.91	0.43
19	2.20	9.52	17.30	6.82	0.23	0.55	0.89	0.43
20	2.07	9.38	17.59	6.90	0.22	0.54	0.90	0.43
21	2.33	9.70	17.25	6.92	0.23	0.55	0.89	0.43
22	2.30	9.55	17.76	6.71	0.23	0.55	0.91	0.42
23	2.29	9.77	17.68	6.91	0.23	0.56	0.90	0.43
24	2.27	9.72	17.05	6.79	0.23	0.56	0.88	0.43
25	2.23	9.58	17.64	6.57	0.23	0.55	0.90	0.42
26	2.19	9.62	17.41	6.96	0.23	0.55	0.89	0.43
27	2.17	9.70	17.38	6.90	0.22	0.55	0.89	0.43
28	2.33	9.75	17.39	6.52	0.23	0.56	0.89	0.42
29	2.24	9.94	17.09	7.00	0.23	0.57	0.88	0.44
30	2.15	9.55	17.37	6.86	0.22	0.55	0.89	0.43

3.2   Input 2: Type of Environmental Home

Table 6 shows the type of environmental home values per home and their normalized values.

3.3   Output: Gamified Motivation (Local Point of View)

Table 7 displays the type of gamified motivation values per home.

Table 7 The gamified motivation for each home

| Day | Gamified motivation by home | | | | |
	Home 1	Home 2	Home 3	Home 4	Mean
1	0.17	0.81	0.90	0.57	0.61
2	0.16	0.83	0.90	0.52	0.60
3	0.17	0.83	0.90	0.59	0.62
4	0.17	0.83	0.90	0.55	0.61
5	0.16	0.83	0.90	0.52	0.60
6	0.19	0.82	0.90	0.61	0.63
7	0.18	0.83	0.90	0.57	0.62
8	0.19	0.82	0.90	0.57	0.62
9	0.19	0.82	0.90	0.61	0.63
10	0.19	0.83	0.90	0.59	0.63
11	0.17	0.83	0.90	0.57	0.62
12	0.18	0.83	0.90	0.57	0.62
13	0.17	0.81	0.90	0.55	0.61
14	0.19	0.82	0.90	0.58	0.62
15	0.19	0.83	0.90	0.55	0.62
16	0.19	0.83	0.90	0.55	0.62
17	0.19	0.83	0.90	0.55	0.61
18	0.19	0.82	0.90	0.57	0.62
19	0.18	0.83	0.90	0.57	0.62
20	0.16	0.82	0.90	0.57	0.61
21	0.19	0.83	0.90	0.55	0.62
22	0.19	0.83	0.90	0.55	0.62
23	0.19	0.83	0.90	0.58	0.62
24	0.19	0.83	0.90	0.57	0.62
25	0.18	0.83	0.90	0.54	0.61
26	0.18	0.83	0.90	0.59	0.62
27	0.17	0.83	0.90	0.55	0.61
28	0.19	0.83	0.90	0.54	0.61
29	0.18	0.84	0.90	0.60	0.63
30	0.17	0.83	0.90	0.55	0.61

Figure 9 presents the ANFIS system for the global community point of view. Figure 9a shows the relationship between each home and its interaction with the other dwellings regarding its level of energy consumption and type of environmental home. Figure 9b displays the ANFIS system structure, the rules, and the surfaces of the community interaction.

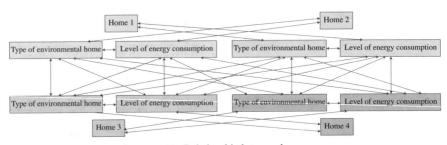

(a) Relationship between homes.

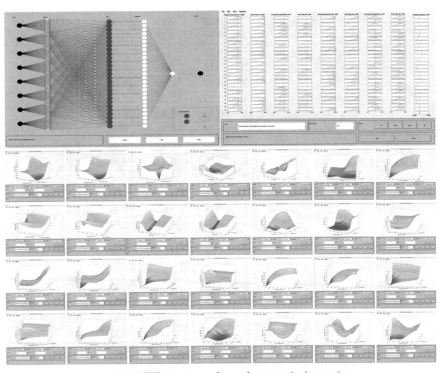

(b) ANFIS structure, rules, and community interaction

Fig. 9 ANFIS system for the global point of view (set of homes). (**a**) Relationship between homes. (**b**) ANFIS structure, rules, and community interaction

4 Results

From the local point of view, a correlation between the input and output can be seen. From the global point of view, a relationship between the data and the mean output is shown. Figure 10 displays these correlations; for the local location of view, home 1, 2 and 4 have a strong relationship; home 3 shows no correlation due to output values of 0.9, representing a constant value. However, either the fuzzy system or the ANFIS

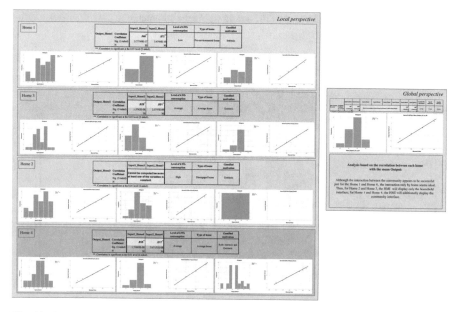

Fig. 10 Correlations between input and output for each home (local point of view) and the community (global point of view)

system demonstrates that home 3 is the home that consumes more electricity than the other houses and is cataloged as a disengaged home. This home should display in the interface extrinsic gamified motivation.

The global point of view presents a strong correlation between home 1 and 4, and the mean output values because home 2 and 3, in a local point of view, require high to very high extrinsic gamified motivation. Therefore, both houses need extrinsic motivation to interact with the community and promote energy reduction; the ANFIS system depicts this interaction between each pair of homes.

Thereby, Figure 11 shows a radar map of the level of energy consumption, type of home, and gamified motivation:

- Home 1: Energy consumption = Low; Type of home = Pro-environmental home; and Motivation: Intrinsic.
- Home 2: Energy consumption = Average; Type of home = Disengaged-environmental home; and Motivation: Extrinsic.
- Home 3: Energy consumption = High; Type of home = Disengaged-environmental home; and Motivation: Extrinsic.
- Home 4: Energy consumption = Average; Type of home = Average home; and Motivation: Intrinsic and Extrinsic (Both).

Thus, considering the gamification elements regarding energy applications and the type of motivation:

Radar map of the homes within the community

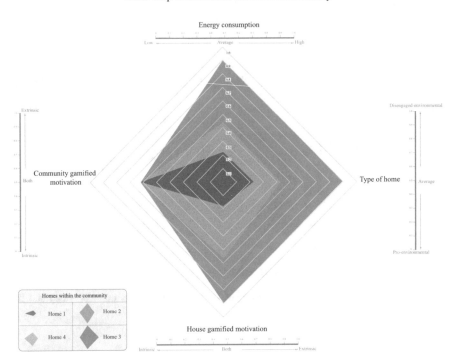

Fig. 11 Level of energy consumption, type of home, and gamified motivation for each home

- Intrinsic motivation: energy community, collaboration, control over peers, social comparison, competition; additional elements from the Octalysis framework are mentorship, community progress.
- Extrinsic motivation: offers, coupons, bill discounts, challenges, levels, dashboards, statistics, degree of control, additional elements to consider are points, badges, progress bar, and leaderboard.
- Therefore, an application with both motivation types should consider gamification elements from the extrinsic and intrinsic motivation.

Figure 12 displays the type of HMI for all home types. Figure 12a is the interface for home 1; this home is considered a pro-environmental home with less consumption. This interface emphasizes the community side by adding the community news, ability to comments and discuss, and compete to reduce energy consumption. Figure 12b is for house 3, the disengaged- environmental home, and the home that consumes more energy. This interface is focused on showing the rewards elements: coupons, prizes and bill discounts; although extrinsic motivation is not interested in challenges, it is included to subtly promote social interaction. HMI changes weekly savings to weekly expenses as a method to push the user to reduce consumption if they are visualizing a loss instead of a win. Figure 12c shows

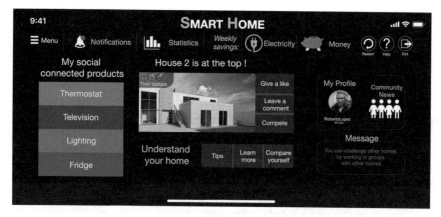

(a)   Human-Machine Interface for Home 1.

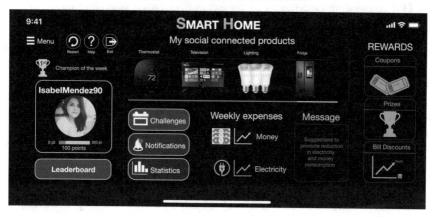

(b)   Human-Machine Interface for Home 3.

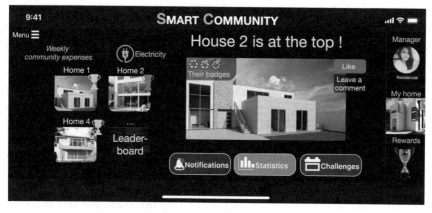

(c)   Human-Machine Interface for Home 2 and Home 4.

Fig. 12 Human machine interfaces (HMIs) for each type of home from a local point of view. (**a**) Human-machine interface for home 1. (**b**) Human-machine interface for home 3. (**c**) Human-machine interface for home 2 and home 4

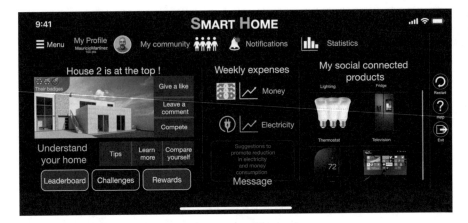

Fig. 13 Human-machine interface for the community from a global point of view

the interface for home 2 and 4, the average home, as this type of home can be motivated either by extrinsic or intrinsic triggers; this first iteration displays both motivational insights to track which of these elements interest the end-user. Finally, Fig. 13 shows the HMI for Home 1 and Home 4 at a global point of view, in smart community integration. Home 2 and Home 3 do not have a tailored global interface. According to the correlation presented from Fig. 10, they may not be interested in interacting with other homes, which is also strongly related to extrinsic motivation.

5 HMI to Improve the Quality of Life of Older People Using the Proposed Structure

Householders from Home type 2 and Home type 4 represent a type of elderly occupant. People who are older can be viewed as individuals who have a wealth of experience and knowledge, along with desires and interests, but also losses and limitations [42]. The aging process consists of biological changes including sensory, physical, and cognitive deterioration as well as social changes, e.g., social isolation and/or loss of loved ones, and potentially psychosocial variations to confidence, purpose, or value [20, 28]. Table 8 depicts the percentage of the elderly population that lives alone in Mexico, the United States, and around the world, and the 10 most common causes of death in each country and worldwide. Understanding the most common causes of death in each country, a tailored HMI can tackle specific needs [17, 41, 51].

Losing autonomy is a challenge for many as they age, often resulting in changes to living situations and environments. Social inclusion aims to provide a channel for social participation and engagement via local services, relationships, civic activities, and financial resources [46]. It is well known that healthy social relationships, and

Table 8 Percentage of older people that live alone and common diseases

Country	Mexico	United States	World
Live alone (% in 2018)	11% [17]	27% [51]	16% [51]
Most common diseases in 2017 [41]	Cardiovascular	Cancer	Cardiovascular
	Cancer	Cardiovascular	Cancer
	Kidney	Digestive	Respiratory
	Digestive	Respiratory	Digestive
	Liver	Liver	Liver
	Respiratory	Drug disorder	Tuberculosis
	Homicide	Kidney	Lower respiratory infection
	Lower respiratory infection	Lower respiratory infection	Kidney
	Road accidents	Suicide	Road accidents
	Alcohol disorder	Road accidents	Diarrheal

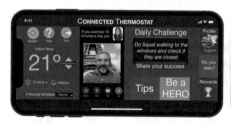 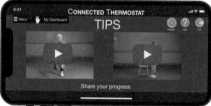

Fig. 14 Tailored HMI presented in [30] for an elderly user. This interface is designed to promote social interaction and physical activity seen at a level 1 social connected product of the local point of view

feelings of belonging and connectedness, reduce stress and promote health and well-being. Nowadays, many older adults use technology within their social context, but psychosocial aspects, such as negative or positive evaluation and opinions of technological solutions, influence use. Gamification is a useful technique for enriching enjoyment, encouraging healthcare, and promoting social participation among the elderly [25]. As rapid advancements in technology and medicine increase our life spans, there is a pronounced and timely need to design novel personalized solutions for older adults that enhance healthcare, cultivate independence, and facilitate social inclusion.

Previous research focused on the elderly using gamified interfaces include the following:

- In [30], a novel tailored gamified HMI is proposed for helping older people (Fig. 14). This interface considers the personality trait of the end-user to choose gamificiation elements for physical activity guidance.

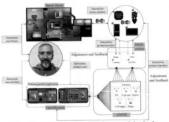

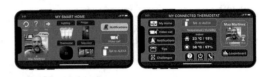

(a)   Gamified structure in an elderly home.   (b)   Tailored example of an HMI proposal for user type:
                                                              a *bit happy* older individual.

Fig. 15 Gamified structure and tailored HMI for end-users from a local point of view [31]. (**a**)
Gamified structure in an elderly home. (**b**) Tailored example of an HMI proposal for user type: a
bit happy older individual

- In [31], the inclusion of Alexa and cameras is proposed to track end-users to
  monitor daily mood and status toward enriching quality of life by encouraging
  physical activity and social participation. Physical characteristics are identified
  through the use of the smart home's multi-sensor system. Algorithms for face and
  voice detection run on the ANFIS system to select and recommend personalized
  gamification elements that operate on user type-specific HMIs. Figure 15a
  displays the gamified structure within the local point of view in a home, where
  Alexa and a camera track the user's mood, and Fig. 15b displays the tailored
  HMI.

  Both proposals aim to change how we use products such that we may leverage
  household appliances to increase social engagement and participation. Using multi-
  sensor systems and data fusion techniques, we may leverage sensors and smart
  household appliances to detect, analyze, and predict end-user behavior, patterns,
  trends, and propose personalized applications that align well with users.

  A limitation of the proposed approach is that individuals who are older as well as
  their caregivers and family members must adopt and accept automated monitoring
  in the house. Further, the type of mobile device available to the end-user may
  be limited or noncompatible due to socioeconomic levels. It is also required that
  end-users use voice assistants, such as Alexa, as an initial channel of interaction.
  Another possible limitation is face detection and emotion recognition. Emotions are
  complex and multilayered, and therefore susceptible to misclassification in certain
  circumstances, especially in the wild and in situations of limited training data. But
  technology is becoming more ubiquitous and machine learning models are evolving
  and developing robustness as data collection efforts ramp up.

  With this local perspective and by tackling end-user needs, it is feasible to
  interact with the community through continuous feedback where end-users needs
  are satisfied, and the business sector is either in the community or the city.
  Supportive and fundamental technologies can improve the satisfaction of the individual, community, and city needs. Table 9 shows the characteristics of supportive

Table 9 Supportive and fundamental technologies and their interaction at smart homes, smart community, and smart city

Supportive technologies	Customer journey, 3D printing, energy technology, gamification, voice assistants, health technology, geospatial technology, clean technology, collaborative technology, advanced materials	
Fundamental technologies	Human-computer interaction, artificial intelligence, internet of things, cloud computing, nanotechnology, mobile internet, automation, big data, robots	
Smart home	**Smart community**	**Smart city**
Healthcare: socially connected products track end-user biometrics to detect or track heart attacks, pneumonia, falls, seizures, anxiety attacks, psychosis, respiratory diseases, hearing loss, insulin status, and dementia. These products display medicament schedules, missing pills, and/or fall frequency Environment: during natural disasters, such as earthquakes, detect if all users are safe, e.g., outside the home. Avoid fires by identifying lit candles, or provide weather sensing to promote social interaction and physical activities Groceries: detect missing food or food shortages Household appliances: detect and foresee missing supplies Face-to-face virtual interaction: promote social relationships with other homes, and when possible, promote public interaction at parks	Healthcare: receive from a house its requirements, for instance, assistance with eldery occupants. Schedule medical appointments. If an accident occurs, send an ambulance to the house Environment: provide weather forecasts to inform end-users to support daily planning, such as going outside or staying in. During a pandemic, provide information on how many infected people are near the end-user Groceries: provisioning food to the home Transport: monitoring parking spaces and transportation; managing traffic; and ensuring public transportation is accessible. Establish connection with groceries to supply food to the home	The interactions between communities allow the smart city to track citizens' behavior, understand the trends, and provide accurate feedback, security, and information to the populace Participatory sensing [33]: The end-user through a smartphone becomes a sensor that shares and extracts information to monitor the environment, transportation, mobility, and energy waste

techniques and necessary technologies, and examples of interactions at the three levels: smart home, smart community, and smart city.

6 From Citizen to Smart City: A Future Vision

The *IESE Cities in Motion Index* report [5] gives a clear picture of the elements required to have a transition toward a smart city. The future of smart cities tends to integrate not only the technological aspects of life but also how they combine with and develop the rest of the indicators. Therefore, converging into a city that sees participation from all inhabitants may reduce stress from traffic, legal problems, crime and suicide rates. This may seem Utopian, however with the right planning, partnerships, and public's help, the integration of technology to achieve this ideal is a matter of time.

With the global pandemic COVID-19, at least five areas that artificial intelligence could have contributed to within a smart city were identified [22]:

- Detecting, tracking, and predicting outbreaks using big data.
- Use of face recognition and infrared-based technologies to improve public safety and security.
- Surveillance, sterilization, and supply delivery via drones and autonomous robots.
- Innovations in virus understanding, diagnostics, and treatments.
- Novel tele-communication devices and platforms to promote togetherness and connectedness during times when physical contact must be limited for safety.

Thus, in times of social distancing, the role of the HMIs takes a suitable place as they serve as a social connector between the end-user and the entire community or smart city. It is a new paradigm where end-users partake in a new type of social interaction, leveraging the internet of things, social media, and e-commerce to make a new life.

6.1 Smart City Vision in a COVID-19 Context

Figure 16 depicts a third-layer structure to achieve a smart city. A new concept considered in this roadmap is the COVID-19 global pandemic. With technology and network communications, it is feasible to continue living in a new normal and with new methods of communication where HMIs take the central role as a social connector and interactor between the end-user and the community and smart city. The three-layer topology considers the following:

- The first layer is the individual segment. The home takes advantage of the socially connected products and devices to interact with the house. Some applications

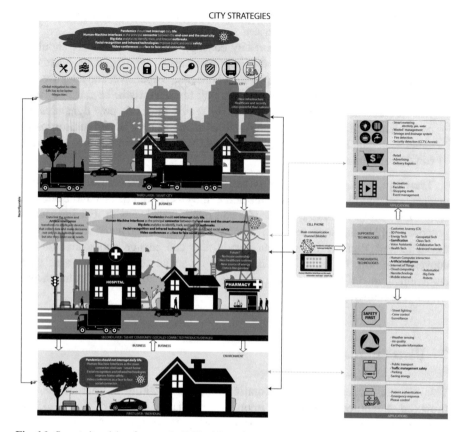

Fig. 16 Smart city vision from an individual layer into a connected smart city

consider healthcare, transportation, environment, and safety in interactions with the smart community and the smart city. HMIs connect with the home to provide new forms of social interaction and foresee if a family member is becoming ill, for instance, with cameras and communication via Alexa by detecting if the user is having fever and presenting COVID-19 symptoms. The smart fridge can identify, based on a dietary list, any food shortages, and contact the market to request provisions.

- The second layer is the smart community. This layer imagines new healthcare systems, new sources of energy, no home ownership, and data is like gasoline in the future. The data link the system, and artificial intelligence transforms devices that collect data and make decisions not only in a personal sense but also from the perspective of social needs. This layer considers applications for utilities, commerce, and entertainment. The HMIs and big data analytics bring new information to identify, track, and forecast outbreaks. The surveillance cameras and infrared technologies can detect users with erratic behavior or with fever to improve public and social safety. Video conferences allow new manners of business; for instance, physicians assist infected users and avoid physical contact to help prevent the spread of viruses.

- The third layer deepens the smart city concept. It considers that life should be better, with new developments and improvements to infrastructure, healthcare, and security. Cities should be powerful, connected, responsive, and adaptive. The safest and most reliable and convenient way to interact will be through HMIs, video conferencing, conventional calls, or mails; however, new dynamics will be implemented for social and physical interactions, e.g., access to information about a specific location and how many nearby people are infected so that a user can take precaution.

Therefore, considering the elderly sector, by taking advantage of HMIs, smart devices, and household products in the home, the elderly can receive more attention from their family, interact with friends, and monitor their health. For instance, as proposed in [31], the home can track an end-user's mood, and avoid social isolation through interaction. In this way, an elderly user can engage with Alexa through conversation. On the other hand, implementing social connectors such as video conferences in the HMIs could encourage the elderly to be more in touch with friends and family.

7 Discussion

This chapter presented socially connected products within a smart home, and proposed a tailored interface to improve the quality of life of users and the community by promoting a reduction in energy consumption. A Sugeno Fuzzy Logic decision system was used to classify the type of home based on energy consumption level and type of environmental home to propose a gamified structure that runs in a customized HMI. The proposed interface is oriented based on the preferred motivation. Although the level of energy consumption was classified based on the 2015 Residential Energy Consumption Survey public database [10], the fuzzy decision system is designed to organize the level of energy consumption from the household appliances.

This classification uses the following scale: low consumption, average consumption, and high consumption. The average value range comes from the database, by using the standard deviation; the higher consumption comes from the addition of the average value plus the standard deviation. Whereas the lower consumption comes from the subtraction of the average value minus the standard deviation. The type of energy home is classified as either a pro-environmental home, average home, or disengaged-environmental home. The type of home is related to the level of energy consumption of the house. Finally, the gamified motivation is classified in three varieties: intrinsic motivation (Low, Medium, High, and Very High); extrinsic motivation (Low, Medium, High, and Very High); or both motivation types. This interaction is included within the local point of view (see Fig. 1).

Once the decision system classifies the type of home and provides a personalized gamification interface, the multi-sensor system may be utilized inside the smart home setting to detect the level of energy consumption and the environmental type of the home to promote social interaction and energy reduction to improve the quality of life in the community. This interaction is included within the global point of view (see Fig. 1). Therefore, the ANFIS system is designed to propose the type of gamification motivation based on community behavior and a tailored community gamified interface.

Hence, a Human Machine Interface for each type of home is proposed and considers three levels:

- For a single social product, e.g., a connected thermostat. Several approaches to this type of social product have been published in [30, 39].
- For the smart home, which is the set of social products within the home. In [29, 31], saving energy in smart homes was empowered using gamification techniques.
- And lastly, for the smart community. Although there is no limitation, this interface should be included and considered based on the correlation and interaction between homes and the gamified community motivation.

This general proposal is limited in that the home should have a level of automatization and connectivity to provide real-time monitoring and feedback, as well as enable user profile creation to provide personalized interfaces. Moreover, once the community interaction is classified, if there are homes that a community structure will not allow to reduce energy consumption, then perhaps other interactions may be explored. For example, interaction between pairs of homes or groups of three homes may be proposed to offer more types of community awareness and engagement to improve quality of life.

Considering Nielsen's heuristics within the interface may increase the impact for and engagement of the end-user. These heuristics take into account [35]: the visibility of a system's current status; whether the real world matches the system; users' freedom and control; standards and consistency; error prevention; recognition (as opposed to recall); efficiency of use as well as flexibility; minimalist and aesthetic design; error recovery; and user support.

This proposal looks for a change in how connected/social products are used and how a community could interact to enhance social inclusion. It aims to produce new forms of social interaction between users and their homes. This first approach considers only the interaction between homes and the household products within the smart home; nevertheless, with further research, this interaction could include the transportation and commercial sector by taking advantage of the associated communications and promoting more connected community interaction. With a multi-sensor system, we may leverage connected smart home appliances to develop a profile of a house, and propose tailored applications triggered by intrinsic and/or extrinsic motivations that best fit the type of home.

8 Conclusion

In this chapter, a multi-sensor system for improving the quality of life by reducing energy consumption was proposed. A gamification structure triggered by outcome motivations within an HMI for a community was presented based on each home's characteristics. This strategy considers each home's interaction by profiling the level of energy consumption and type of environmental home within a fuzzy logic decision system. Then the interaction between homes to set the community was proposed through an ANFIS system that provides which gamified motivation is required to engage the home in having a reduction in energy consumption and improvement of quality of life in the community. The proposed approach aims to develop a profile of the home and improve our understanding of the type of home and the interaction of the houses in the community toward an accurate application that improves quality of life while promoting energy reduction. This HMI introduces an opportunity to create an ecosystem enabling connected products and homes to interact with the community to help residents feel included.

An example of the relevance of HMIs is the COVID-19 pandemic. HMIs tackle social distancing by taking advantage of social products and connectors such as video conferences, calls, blogs, and social media. Thus, individuals interact with others without concerns of infection; for instance, this interaction works for social relationships, work, healthcare, schools, and religious groups. As Fig. 16 indicates, HMIs work as a critical connector between each smart home, smart community, and smart city with the end-user, where the user provides information and consumption and behavior patterns to each level, improving their quality of life and fostering social synergy with other users.

Acknowledgments This research project is supported by Tecnologico de Monterrey and CITRIS under the collaboration ITESM-CITRIS Smart thermostat, deep learning, and gamification project (https://citris-uc.org/2019-itesm-seed-funding/). The authors also thank Arizona State University and the National Science Foundation for their funding support under Grant No. 1828010.

References

1. Albertarelli, S., Fraternali, P., Herrera, S., Melenhorst, M., Novak, J., Pasini, C., Rizzoli, A.-E., Rottondi, C.: A survey on the design of gamified systems for energy and water sustainability. Games. **9**, 38 (2018). https://doi.org/10.3390/g9030038
2. Aldrich, F.K.: Smart homes: past, present and future. In: Harper, R. (ed.) Inside the smart home, pp. 17–39. Springer, London (2003)
3. AlSkaif, T., Lampropoulos, I., van den Broek, M., van Sark, W.: Gamification-based framework for engagement of residential customers in energy applications. Energy Res. Soc. Sci. **44**, 187–195 (2018). https://doi.org/10.1016/j.erss.2018.04.043
4. Bartle, R.: Hearts, clubs, diamonds, spades: players who suit MUDs, 28 (1996). https://www.researchgate.net/publication/247190693_Hearts_clubs_diamonds_spades_Players_who_suit_MUDs

5. Berrone, P., Ricart, J.E., Duch, A., Carrasco, C.: IESE cities in motion index 2019. Servicio de Publicaciones de la Universidad de Navarra, Navarra (2019)
6. Bhati, A., Hansen, M., Chan, C.M.: Energy conservation through smart homes in a smart city: a lesson for Singapore households. Energy Policy. **104**, 230–239 (2017). https://doi.org/10.1016/j.enpol.2017.01.032
7. Chou, Y.: Actionable gamification beyond points, badges, and leaderboards. CreateSpace Independent Publishing Platform, Scotts Valley (2015)
8. Csoknyai, T., Legardeur, J., Akle, A.A., Horváth, M.: Analysis of energy consumption profiles in residential buildings and impact assessment of a serious game on occupants' behavior. Energ. Buildings. **196**, 1–20 (2019). https://doi.org/10.1016/j.enbuild.2019.05.009
9. Deterding, S., Dixon, D., Khaled, R., Nacke, L.: From game design elements to gamefulness: defining "gamification", Presented at the MindTrek 11: Proceedings of the 15th International Academic MindTrek Conference: Envisioning Future Media Environments (2011), https://doi.org/10.1145/2181037.2181040
10. EIA: Residential Energy Consumption Survey (RECS) – Data – U.S. Energy Information Administration (EIA). https://www.eia.gov/consumption/residential/data/2015/index.php?view=microdata
11. EIA: Total Energy Annual Data – U.S. Energy Information Administration (EIA). https://www.eia.gov/totalenergy/data/annual/index.php
12. Eltoweissy, M., Azab, M., Olariu, S., Gracanin, D.: A new paradigm for a marketplace of services: smart communities in the IoT era. In: 2019 international conference on innovation and intelligence for informatics, computing, and technologies (3ICT), pp. 1–6. IEEE, Sakhier (2019)
13. Hargreaves, T., Wilson, C.: Smart homes and their users. Springer, Cham (2017)
14. Harper, R.: Inside the smart home: ideas, possibilities and methods. In: Harper, R. (ed.) Inside the smart home, pp. 1–13. Springer, London (2003)
15. Huotari, K., Hamari, J.: Defining gamification: a service marketing perspective. In: Proceeding of the 16th international academic MindTrek conference on – MindTrek '12, p. 17. ACM Press, Tampere (2012)
16. IBM's Smarter Cities Challenge: Copenhagen report. IBM Corporate Citizenship & Corporate Affairs, Copenhagen (2013)
17. INEGI: Estadísticas a Propósito del Día Internacional de Las Personas de Edad (1o de Octubre)
18. Jang, J.-R.: ANFIS: adaptive-network-based fuzzy inference system. IEEE. Trans. Syst. Man Cybern. **23**, 665–685 (1993). https://doi.org/10.1109/21.256541
19. Kappen DL (2015) Adaptive engagement of older adults' fitness through gamification. http://dl.acm.org/citation.cfm?doid=2793107.2810276
20. Kostopoulos, P., Kyritsis, A.I., Ricard, V., Deriaz, M., Konstantas, D.: Enhance daily live and health of elderly people. Procedia Comput. Sci. **130**, 967–972 (2018). https://doi.org/10.1016/j.procs.2018.04.097
21. Li, X., Lu, R., Liang, X., Shen, X., Chen, J., Lin, X.: Smart community: an internet of things application. IEEE Commun. Mag. **49**, 68–75 (2011). https://doi.org/10.1109/MCOM.2011.6069711
22. Lii Inn, T.: Smart city technologies take on Covid-19. Penang Institute. https://penanginstitute.org/publications/issues/smart-city-technologies-take-on-covid-19/
23. Llinas, J., Waltz, E.: Multisensor data fusion. Artech House, Boston (1990)
24. Łucka, D.: How to build a community. New urbanism and its critics. Urban. Dev. Issues. **59**, 17–26 (2018). https://doi.org/10.2478/udi-2018-0025
25. Malwade, S., Abdul, S.S., Uddin, M., Nursetyo, A.A., Fernandez-Luque, L., Zhu X (Katie), Cilliers L, Wong C-P, Bamidis P, Li Y-C (Jack): Mobile and wearable technologies in healthcare for the ageing population. Comput. Methods Prog. Biomed. **161**, 233–237 (2018). https://doi.org/10.1016/j.cmpb.2018.04.026
26. Marczewski, A.: Even ninja monkeys like to play: gamification, game thinking and motivational design. CreateSpace Independent Publishing Platform, Scotts Valley (2015)

27. Marikyan, D., Papagiannidis, S., Alamanos, E.: A systematic review of the smart home literature: a user perspective. Technol. Forecast. Soc. Chang. **138**, 139–154 (2019). https://doi.org/10.1016/j.techfore.2018.08.015

28. Meiselman, H.L. (ed.): Emotion measurement. Elsevier, Woodhead Publishing, Amsterdam (2016)

29. Méndez, J.I., Ponce, P., Mata, O., Meier, A., Peffer, T., Molina, A., Aguilar, M.: Empower saving energy into smart homes using a gamification structure by social products. In: 2020 IEEE international conference on consumer electronics (ICCE), pp. 1–7. IEEE, Las Vegas (2020)

30. Méndez, J.I., Ponce, P., Meier, A., Peffer, T., Mata, O., Molina, A.: Framework for promoting social interaction and physical activity in elderly people using gamification and fuzzy logic strategy. In: 2019 IEEE global conference on signal and information processing (GlobalSIP), pp. 1–5. IEEE, Ottawa (2019)

31. Méndez, J.I., Mata, O., Ponce, P., Meier, A., Peffer, T., Molina, A.: Multi-sensor system, gamification, and artificial intelligence for benefit elderly people. In: Ponce, H., Martínez-Villaseñor, L., Brieva, J., Moya-Albor, E. (eds.) Challenges and trends in multimodal fall detection for healthcare, pp. 207–235. Springer, Cham (2020)

32. Méndez, J.I., Ponce, P., Meier, A., Peffer, T., Mata, O., Molina, A.: S4 product design framework: a gamification strategy based on type 1 and 2 fuzzy logic. In: Smart multimedia: methodologies and algorithms, San Diego, California, USA, p. 15 (2019)

33. Middya, A.I., Roy, S., Dutta, J., Das, R.: JUSense: a unified framework for participatory-based urban sensing system. Mobile Netw. Appl. (2020). https://doi.org/10.1007/s11036-020-01539-x

34. Miranda, J., Pérez-Rodríguez, R., Borja, V., Wright, P.K., Molina, A.: Sensing, smart and sustainable product development (S3 product) reference framework. Int. J. Prod. Res. **57**, 1–22 (2017). https://doi.org/10.1080/00207543.2017.1401237

35. Nielsen, J.: 10 heuristics for user interface design: article by Jakob Nielsen. https://www.nngroup.com/articles/ten-usability-heuristics/

36. Peham, M., Breitfuss, G., Michalczuk, R.: The "ecoGator" app: gamification for enhanced energy efficiency in Europe. In: Proceedings of the second international conference on technological ecosystems for enhancing multiculturality – TEEM '14, pp. 179–183. ACM Press, Salamanca (2014)

37. Ponce Cruz, P., Ramírez-Figueroa, F.D.: Intelligent control systems with LabVIEW. Springer, London; New York (2010)

38. Ponce, P., Peffer, T., Molina, A.: Framework for communicating with consumers using an expectation interface in smart thermostats. Energ. Buildings. **145**, 44–56 (2017). https://doi.org/10.1016/j.enbuild.2017.03.065

39. Ponce, P., Meier, A., Mendez, J., Peffer, T., Molina, A., Mata, O.: Tailored gamification and serious game framework based on fuzzy logic for saving energy in smart thermostats. J. Clean. Prod., 121167 (2020). https://doi.org/10.1016/j.jclepro.2020.121167

40. Ponce, P., Meier, A., Miranda, J., Molina, A., Peffer, T.: The next generation of social products based on sensing, smart and sustainable (S3) features: a smart thermostat as case study. In: 9th IFAC conference on manufacturing modelling, management and control, p. 6 (2019)

41. Ritchie, H., Roser, M.: Causes of death. Our World in Data (2018) https://ourworldindata.org/causes-of-death, last accessed 2020/07/07

42. Sayago, S. (ed.): Perspectives on human-computer interaction research with older people. Springer, Cham (2019)

43. Schiele, K.: Utilizing gamification to promote sustainable practices. In: Marques, J. (ed.) Handbook of engaged sustainability, pp. 427–444. Springer, Cham (2018)

44. Skouby, K.E., Lynggaard, P.: Smart home and smart city solutions enabled by 5G, IoT, AAI and CoT services. In: 2014 international conference on contemporary computing and informatics (IC3I), pp. 874–878. IEEE, Mysore (2014)

45. Tondello, G.F., Wehbe, R.R., Diamond, L., Busch, M., Marczewski, A., Nacke, L.E.: The gamification user types Hexad scale. In: Proceedings of the 2016 annual symposium on computer-human interaction in play – CHI PLAY '16, pp. 229–243. ACM Press, Austin (2016)
46. Victor, C.R., Scambler, S., Bond, J.: The social world of older people: understanding loneliness and social isolation in later life. Open University Press, Maidenhead (2009)
47. Waltz, E.: Data fusion for C3I: a tutorial. In: Command, control, communications intelligence (C3I) handbook. EW Communications, Palo Alto (1986)
48. Wang, X.: The optimization of smart community model based on advanced network information technology. In: 2020 IEEE 4th information technology, networking, electronic and automation control conference (ITNEC), pp. 2579–2583. IEEE, Chongqing (2020)
49. London smart city: tackling challenges with 20 initiatives. HERE Mobility. https://mobility.here.com/learn/smart-city-initiatives/london-smart-city-tackling-challenges-20-initiatives
50. My coverage of lobby of the social gaming summit. http://www.bretterrill.com/2008/06/my-coverage-of-lobby-of-social-gaming.html
51. Older people are more likely to live alone in the U.S. than elsewhere in the world. Pew Research Center. https://www.pewresearch.org/fact-tank/2020/03/10/older-people-are-more-likely-to-live-alone-in-the-u-s-than-elsewhere-in-the-world/
52. Oslo brings the future home with its multifaceted "smart city" programs. https://www.digitaltrends.com/home/oslo-norway-smart-city-technology/

Enhancing Situational Awareness and Kinesthetic Assistance for Clinicians via Augmented-Reality and Haptic Shared-Control Technologies

Jay Carriere, Lingbo Cheng, and Mahdi Tavakoli

Abstract Intraoperative situational awareness is critical for clinicians when performing complex surgeries and therapies. Augmented-reality (AR) and haptic virtual fixtures (VF) technologies can be used to increase situational awareness while still keeping the surgeon-in-the-loop. These two technologies can be used independently or together to provide various levels of assistance. 3D AR technologies provide enhanced visual feedback for the clinician, for instance, giving them the ability to "see" surgical instruments inside of tissue. Robotic assistant devices with haptic VF provide physical resistance or assistance in real-time for the clinician. Haptic VF systems can be used to enforce "no-fly zones" with varying degrees of resistance to allow the clinician to avoid damaging sensitive tissue. The assistance provided by haptic VF systems can reduce the strain on a clinician when performing a lengthy surgery, can move the surgical tool to compensate for changes in patient pose, and can increase the precision with which a clinician can perform various surgical tasks.

Keywords Medical robotics · Augmented reality · Virtual fixtures · Haptics · Assistive technologies

The original version of this chapter was revised: The author's name has now been updated to be Mahdi Tavakoli in the chapter opening page. The correction to this chapter is available at https://doi.org/10.1007/978-3-030-70716-3_11

J. Carriere (✉) · M. Tavakoli
Department of Electrical and Computer Engineering, University of Alberta, Edmonton, AB, Canada
e-mail: jtcarrie@ualberta.ca; mahdi.tavakoli@ualberta.ca

L. Cheng
College of Control Science and Engineering, Zhejiang University, Hangzhou, Zhejiang, China
e-mail: lingbo1@zju.edu.cn

1 Intraoperative Situational Awareness

Having sufficient intraoperative situational awareness is vital for physicians when performing complex procedures and therapies. Intraoperative situational awareness refers to the cognitive ability to understand where surgical tools are within the body, to determine how to manipulate the surgical tools to a desired location (or to perform a desired action), and to identify any nearby anatomical structures that should be avoided during the surgery or therapy [1]. In general, increasing a surgeon's intraoperative situational awareness will lead to an increased or successful clinical outcome of the procedure (or therapy) while reducing risks or side-effects. Using the *Perception, Planning, and Action* loop model from robotics control theory, we can think also think of intraoperative situational awareness as consisting of: *Perception* where the surgeon must be able to sense the location of surgical tools relative to anatomical areas of interest; *Planning* where the surgeon needs to know how to move the surgical tools to a desired location. Mentally, the surgeon must continuously perform these *perception* and *planning* steps while manually performing the surgery (undertaking the *action*). This chapter will discuss the following two types of assistive technologies to increase intraoperative situational awareness, *Visual Guidance* and *Haptic Guidance*.

1.1 Visual Guidance

Visual Guidance systems display a live view of the surgical tool location and relevant anatomy. These systems enhance the vision of the surgeon, presenting them with salient information from the surgical plan and allowing them to more robustly localize surgical tools inside of tissue.

For visual guidance during surgery, the clinician can be provided with visual information on a traditional 2D TV or monitor-based display system. However, more intuitive and immersive visual feedback can be provided through an augmented reality (AR) display based on optical see-through systems. In an optical see-through AR display, computer-generated images are overlaid directly on top of the operating area and patient anatomy. They are updated in real-time to match the surgeon's viewpoint [2–4]. Section 3 provides an overview of visual guidance and AR systems and their application to surgical procedures.

1.2 Haptic Guidance

Haptic Guidance systems provide physical force-feedback and assistance to the clinician during the surgery. In these systems, the force feedback is provided by a robot end-effector holding the surgical tool (or the end-effector itself is a surgical tool) to the clinician or from a surgical console (in a system like the da Vinci surgical robot).

For haptic guidance, a compliant robot controller is designed to use active constraints/virtual fixtures to provide the assistive and resistive force to the clinician. These virtual fixtures (VF) can be used to enforce rigid "no-fly" zones during the surgery, provide resistance near sensitive anatomical areas, or can provide assistance to the surgeon by helping to move the surgical tool to a desired position/location (with respect to the surgical plan) or follow anatomical motion [5]. Utilizing VF within the robot control loop allows for intuitive hands-on human/robot collaboration while still providing substantial force assistance/resistance to the clinician in a safe and stable manner [6]. Section 4 will discuss the use of virtual fixtures for haptic guidance in surgery.

1.3 Applications of Visual and Haptic Guidance in Surgery

As motivation for the visual and haptic guidance technologies discussed in this chapter, Sect. 2 will provide some background information on two surgical procedures used in the treatment and diagnosis of cancer, *percutaneous biopsy* and *mandible reconstruction*. Percutaneous (needle-based) biopsies are popular for extracting suspect tissue as part of confirming a cancer diagnosis. These needle-based biopsies are commonly performed as they are cost-effective, minimally invasive, low risk, and fast. One complication of needle-based biopsies is that the procedure's diagnostic efficacy and accuracy depend on the accuracy with which the biopsy needle is inserted into the target tissue. Mandible reconstruction is done to surgically repair or replace portions of the lower jaw bone, which have been damaged due to cancerous growths. A donor bone, typically a portion of the fibula from the patient, is used for reconstructing the jaw bone. The fibula portion is then cut into a number of precise segments. These segments are cut to different sizes and with different angles so that when they are assembled together, much like a 3D jigsaw puzzle, they will match the shape and curvature of the existing jaw bone. The success of the mandible reconstruction depends on the accuracy with which the fibula segments are cut.

This chapter will also provide an overview of practical visual and haptic guidance assistive systems to increase intraoperative awareness for biopsy and lower mandible reconstruction in Sect. 5, from our previously published works in [7] and [8] respectively.

2 Background

Oncology, dealing with the diagnosis and treatment of cancers, is a particularly complex field of medicine where diagnostic accuracy and treatment efficacy are paramount. Given the substantial number of different types of cancers, with varying degrees of severity (even within the same type of cancer), most surgical oncology procedures are either pre-planned using medical image guidance (preoperative imaging) and/or utilize real-time medical image feedback (intraoperative imaging) during the procedure [9]. This chapter will discuss assistive technologies that can be used to increase intraoperative situational awareness for clinicians during surgical oncology procedures, which capitalize on this available medical image planning/feedback. These assistive technologies help reduce the cognitive load on physicians by providing them with enhanced (visual and physical) *perception* to more accurately and effectively follow a desired surgical plan.

The surgical assistant systems described within this chapter will be discussed using two different surgical oncology procedures, biopsy and mandible reconstruction (fibula osteotomy), to provide practical examples of their utility. The assistance systems are designed to provide information (guidance) based on preoperative and intraoperative medical images used for these procedures. In general, there are numerous medical imaging modalities that can be used to detect cancerous cells, develop surgical plans, and monitor surgical progress [9]. For biopsy or percutaneous procedure guidance, the most commonly used imaging modalities are x-ray (CT or Mammogram), ultrasound (US), MRI, and optical imaging [10]. In the planning of the fibula osteotomy portion of mandibular reconstruction surgery, to be discussed below, X-ray (standard 2D and CT) images are the primary imaging modality [11–13]. Therefore, both the visual and haptic guidance technologies can theoretically provide similar benefits to other image-guided semi-autonomous surgical systems.

2.1 Biopsy

Percutaneous, or core needle, biopsy is a common procedure to collect tissue samples from suspected cancerous tissue within the body. In percutaneous biopsy, a biopsy needle is inserted through the skin and guided into the tissue to be sampled. Once the biopsy needle has been correctly positioned a small sample of tissue is extracted using a cutting head on the tip of the needle. Core needle biopsies are generally preferred over surgical biopsies as they are faster, easier to perform, have minimal cosmetic effect, and are less invasive for the patient [14, 15]. For accurate diagnosis, the correct placement of the biopsy needle tip is critical and often intraoperative US, MRI, and x-ray (mammogram) images are used to help guide the clinician during needle insertion [14].

A number of retrospective studies have shown that, even with image guidance, roughly 2.2–3.5% of core needle biopsies result in false negatives [16, 17]. The primary reason for these false negative tests is the result of improperly placing the needle with respect to the desired target tissue. The placement inaccuracy is primarily caused by poor visualization and localization of the needle tip and target tissue in the intraoperative images [16, 18]. While MRI is an ideal imaging modality for accurate localization of the needle with superior soft-tissue contrast capability, MRI imaging is time consuming, expensive, and not universally available. Therefore, US imaging is the preferred imaging modality for most core needle biopsy procedures, and has been shown to result in more accurate needle placement than

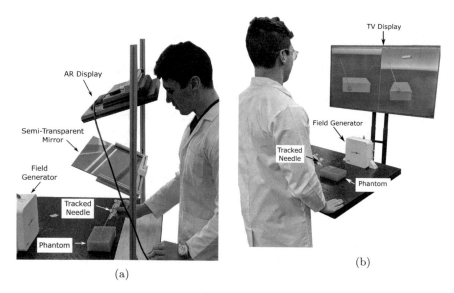

Fig. 1 The two different display methods, AR and monitor-based, used for visual guidance during biopsy experiments. Both displays show current needle position, desired needle trajectory, and target phantom tumour. (**a**) Augmented-reality display used for visual guidance during the biopsy experiments. (**b**) 2D Monitor-based display used for visual guidance during the biopsy experiments, showing a front and side view of the surgical scene

x-ray mammography [16]. There are limitations to US image guidance, in that current clinical US machines tend to be low resolution, noisy, and only provide moderate soft tissue contrast.

Percutaneous biopsy, therefore, provides an ideal example of a procedure that can be assisted through the use of enhanced visual guidance. A brief summary of the experimental setup for visual guidance, from [7], will be presented in Sect. 5 where the amount of assistance provided by visual guidance technologies in both the 2D monitor-based display and the AR display modalities was compared; shown in Fig. 1b and a respectively.

2.2 Mandible Reconstruction

A mandibulectomy may be performed if a tumor threatens or invades the mandible (lower jaw bone) of a patient. If the tumour is small, or well confined to a specific area, the tumour and a minimal portion of the impacted jaw bone will be removed (marginal mandibulectomy). For more aggressive or widespread cancers, where a marginal mandibulectomy would be ineffective, it is necessary to remove the entire mandible and the tumor tissue surrounding it in a procedure known as segmental mandibulectomy.

After segmental mandibulectomy, the lower jaw bone must be surgically recreated through a procedure known as mandibular reconstruction. There has been a great deal of interest and significant progress in mandibular reconstruction over the last 50 years [19–21]. An autograft bone coming from the patient, and surrounding soft/vascular tissue, is used to recreate the mandible. Fibula free-flap reconstruction, utilizing a portion of the fibula and calf tissue, is the most widely used autograft source [11–13]. After removal, the fibula has to be cut down into a number of precisely shaped pieces (fibula osteotomy) that are bonded together to recreate the shape and curve of the removed jaw bone. Using CT and x-ray images, virtual surgical planning is used to develop the cutting plan for fibula osteotomy to maximize the esthetic and functional outcomes of the reconstructed mandible. Fibula osteotomy is a highly challenging surgical procedure, where there may be compound angles between the desired cutting planes on either side of each cut fibula piece. Any deviation from the virtual plan and the shapes of the fibula pieces after cutting will impact the resulting esthetic and functional outcomes of the reconstructed mandible, and can increase the risk of rejection and severe side-effects [11–13].

Due to these risks, in conventional mandibular reconstruction, fabrication and use of patient-specific cutting guides/templates is used to minimize the deviation between the surgical plan and the resultant cut fibula segments. These templates, along with rapid prototyped models of the patient's jaw and fibula bones, has led to significant improvements in mandible reconstruction [22–25]. The fabricated cutting guide/templates significantly improve the accuracy with which fibula free flap osteotomy can be done [26, 27], however, they have some significant limitations. Due to precision, strength, and sterility requirements for the cutting guide/templates, they are expensive, time-consuming to produce, and extremely difficult to modify after fabrication.

As a more flexible and dynamic alternative to the fabricated cutting guide/templates, an alternative is to use a (non-robotic) image-guided navigation system when cutting the fibula based on the initial surgical plan [28]. In these systems, the surgeon is guided by the pre-planned cutting planes/locations, which are projected onto the skeletal anatomy. While these image-guided systems provide clinical benefits by allowing more freedom during preoperative planning and allow for modifying the plan intraoperatively, it is extremely difficult for a surgeon to match the position and orientation of the projected cutting planes with the required precision, as shown in Fig. 2. To compensate for this, surgical robotic and image-guided robotic systems have been developed for fibula extraction and cutting. These systems have shown significant advances in terms of planning flexibility, time and cost savings, and cutting precision with respect to the conventional template or non-robotic image-guided approaches [29–31].

Fig. 2 (**a**) Desired fibula
segments from the front view.
(**b**) Measured results of fibula
segments implemented by
using guidance with AR and
VF from the front view, units
are in mm

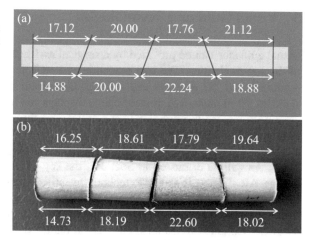

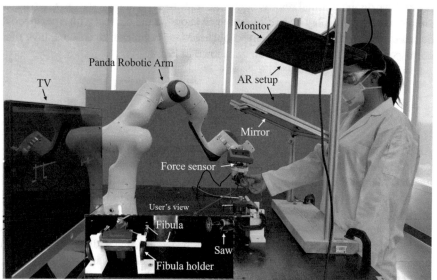

Fig. 3 Experimental setup for fibula osteotomies: robot, force sensor, saw, simulated fibula bone, fibula holder, TV screen, and AR setup

Given the existing research on image-guided robotic and non-robotic systems for fibula osteotomy, it is clear that the precision and accuracy required during fibula osteotomy provides an ideal surgical procedure with which to evaluate visual guidance and haptic guidance assistant systems. A brief description of the experimental setup used in [8] for visual and haptic guidance are given in Sect. 5, and are shown in Fig. 3.

3   Visual Guidance Technologies

Visual guidance can be provided by a surgical assistance system through a number
of display modalities. The two modalities we will discuss within this chapter are
monitor-based 2D displays and AR displays. Here it is important to note that
standard 2D monitor, TV, or smartphone displays can be used as components when
creating video-see-through (VST) and optical-see-through (OST) AR displays. The
distinction between what we refer to as a 2D display and AR display is based on
the Virtuality Continuum, which was proposed by Milgram and Kishino [32]; see
Fig. 4. As will be discussed in Sect. 3.1, the key difference between a 2D display
and an AR display is that AR technology utilize perspective, scaling, and pose
information to display virtual objects such that they appear to co-exist with (or are
overlaid on top of) real-world objects from the observer's viewpoint. Within the
Virtuality Continuum in Fig. 4, augmented reality is shown as being more akin to
the real-world than virtual reality. When we refer to 2D displays, we are referring to
simple rendering/display technologies which show virtual objects with a perspective
or scale independent from real-world objects. Our definition of 2D displays then
corresponds to the virtual environment shown in Fig. 4.

3.1   Augmented Reality Display

AR is defined as a technology that projects (or overlays) virtual objects onto real-
world objects. The key feature of AR displays is that there is a continuously
updated mapping between the viewpoint of the observer, real-world locations and
objects, and the locations of virtual objects. This mapping allows for the motion
of virtual objects to seamlessly match those of real-world objects with respect to
the observer's viewpoint. The use of AR technologies during surgical interventions
has been and continues to be an active area of research [2–4]. Advances in medical
image and 3D graphic processing technologies have allowed for AR systems to
be adapted to a growing number of surgical applications, including general open
surgeries [2], laparoscopic oncology surgeries [33], and orthopedic surgeries [4].
The real-time 3D rendered graphics, and image overlaying, used in immersive
AR displays can be implemented using any number of available general-purpose

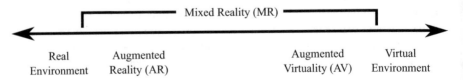

Fig. 4 The Virtuality Continuum introduced by Milgram and Kishino [32] to categorize different
mixed reality environments

3D graphics rendering libraries/toolkits, such as Unity (Unity Technologies, San Francisco, CA, USA), or with specialized toolkits for medical image display and analysis such as 3D Slicer [34].

Depending on the application area, there are a number of possible ways that AR displays can work to project virtual objects onto real-world objects. For instance, video-see-through displays are a common AR display method where virtual objects are superimposed on top of real-world objects captured in a live video stream. This projection style is commonly used for AR videogames, for example, Pokemon Go (Niantic Inc., San Francisco, CA, USA), as it can be easily implemented using the built-in camera and screen in smartphones and tablets. This style of AR display has also been used for prototype and research medical AR systems, with some using smartphones or tablets, or to overlay virtual objects onto a video stream captured by an endoscopic or laparoscopic camera during surgery [3, 33].

The AR display used in this work is an optical-see-through system, where the user can see the simulated surgical scene through a semi-transparent (half-silvered) mirror [7, 8, 35, 36]. The rendered images for the AR display are output to a monitor, which are then reflected on the half-silvered mirror to blend with the user's view of the surgical scene. This allows any salient surgical tool or anatomical information to be placed correctly on top of real-world reference objects in the surgical scene when presented to the user, giving them an x-ray-like ability to see things inside of tissue (or any other real-world object). The mirror and monitor are mounted at an appropriate distance above the surgical workspace to ensure an adequate amount of free workspace for the user to manipulate surgical tools, when performing the simulated surgical procedure. One major advantage of optical-see-through displays, like this one, is that they offer an additional safety factor over video-see-through AR displays. Even if the screen or display device fails, it is still transparent and therefore, will not abruptly obstruct the view of a clinician during surgery.

The half-silvered mirror AR display can be mounted either rigidly or with a swivel joint, such that it can be rotated out of the way, in front of the surgical scene. While head-mounted optical-see-through devices, such as the Microsoft HoloLens and HoloLens2 (Microsoft, Redmond, WA), are commercially available, they have been found to be generally unsuitable for use within surgical settings due to cost, complexity, weight, and optical limitations, making it difficult to focus on both real-world and virtual content simultaneously [37, 38]. The semi-transparent mirror optical-see-through AR display is both low-cost and does not suffer from the same optical limitations as a head-mounted optical-see-through [7, 8, 36]; see Fig. 1a.

With a single monitor being reflected by the semi-transparent mirror, the AR display is able to provide a single-view camera/viewpoint perspective. To provide an immersive display for the user, the user's head is tracked in 3D, using a Kinect v2 depth camera, and the position of the rendering camera in Unity (see Fig. 5) is updated to follow the user's head in 3D. Being as the system provides only a single-view camera rendering, the 3D position of the user's two eyes are tracked and the desired position for the Unity camera is calculated to be centered between them (roughly corresponding to the bridge of the user's nose). With this live head tracking, the Unity camera view of the surgical scene matches the user's view and perspective,

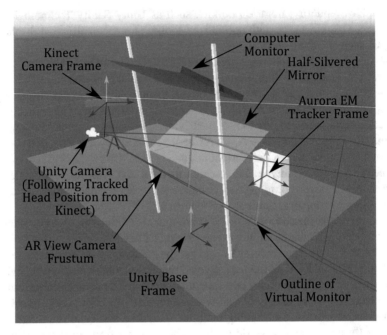

Fig. 5 For the AR display system, a scale-accurate copy of the physical setup was modelled within Unity for the biopsy and fibula osteotomy experiments. The position of the Unity camera is updated in real-time to follow the user's head motion to ensure that the overlaid projection of objects rendered from the virtual-world surgical scene matches their real-world counterparts

which not only allows the virtual objects to be overlaid correctly but also provides parallax (depth-cue) information. The effect of these parallax depth-cues is that as users move their head around they are able to see different sides of the virtual objects (which are mapped appropriately to match the user's viewing angle). Due to how the human visual system processes and retains visual information, these depth cues are stored and processed such that the user perceives a rich 3D environment which is a phenomena known as motion parallax [39]. With the head-tracking and depth-cue information, the AR display is able to provide immersive AR information, overlaid onto the surgical scene, in a low-cost and highly-configurable platform.

When looking at the surgical scene, the user sees a reflection of the 2D monitor in the semi-transparent mirror. The reflected monitor, referred to as the "virtual monitor", appears to be hovering in space between the back-side of the mirror and the surgical scene; see Fig. 6. The location of the virtual monitor is dependent on the relative distances and angles between the physical monitor and the mirror. By measuring these angles and offsets, using landmarks on the AR setup, the location of the corners of the virtual monitor can be calculated. By using a generalized perspective projection [40], the view frustum of the Unity camera can be constrained to correspond exactly with the corners of the virtual monitor (as if the user is looking through a virtual window); a full explanation of the projection calibration

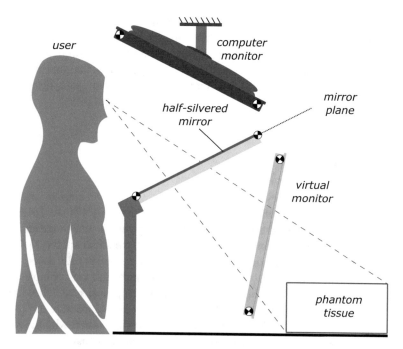

Fig. 6 Diagram of the single-camera AR setup for the biopsy experiment. The "virtual-monitor" is the reflected image of the physical monitor in the semi-transparent mirror

is given in [7]. The parameters of the perspective projection matrix are designed such that the AR images are automatically flipped (during rendering), to provide a correct view when reflected in the mirror; ensuring the rendered virtual objects match the position, scale, and orientation of real-world objects from the user's viewpoint. Figure 5 shows the corners of the virtual monitor, and the constrained view frustum of the Unity camera, as a result of the generalized perspective projection calculations.

3.2 Monitor-Based 2D Display

For 2D visual guidance during surgery, the system displays two 2D images, top and front views of the surgical scene and shows the current pose of the surgical tool, the biopsy needle or saw. As with the AR display system, the virtual surgical scene was modelled and rendered using Unity. The 2D display provides salient surgical guidance information through projections of the desired biopsy target or the fibula cutting planes in both views. Thus, this image-guided surgery task provides visual guidance comparable to conventional surgical tool tracking, wherein a live image of the surgical tool is overlaid on top of CT or x-ray patient images. For visualization, a standard computer monitor was placed near physical simulated surgical setups and showed real-time surgical performance by displaying desired and actual tool (saw or biopsy needle) positions and orientations. During the simulated surgical procedures using the 2D-only visual guidance assistance in [7] and [8], the goal was for the operator to orient the surgical tool to match the desired tool pose shown on the display.

4 Haptic Guidance

The level of assistance provided during surgery by a robotic surgical system can be defined in terms of six discrete levels of automation [41, 42]. At *Level 0*, the first level of automation, the robotic or surgical system is under the clinician's direct control and no assistance is provided (i.e. fully manual surgery). At *Level 5*, the highest level of automation, the robotic surgical system is fully automatic and requires no input or control from the clinician. Given the inherent complexity and safety issues associated with high levels of automation, most research within the literature is focused on providing unobtrusive surgical assistance with the *surgeon-in-the-loop*, where the robotic system is working in collaboration with the surgeon while they are performing most aspects (or all) of the surgery manually.

Haptic guidance force-feedback during surgery can be provided to a clinician, or a user controlling a robot, through a force-feedback capable control console in a dual-robot teleoperated system, or directly to the clinician holding on to a surgical tool which is connected to the end-effector of a single-robot collaborative system. In either single-robot or dual-robot teleoperated systems, haptic fixtures can be used to model and implement resistive and assistive force fields in free space [5]. For human-robot cooperation, virtual fixtures provide an excellent balance between full autonomy and direct human control [6]. Haptic guidance during the fibula osteotomy surgical simulation was provided by a single Panda collaborative robot; see Fig. 3. An admittance controller was used to render the effect of the haptic fixtures while ensuring the robotic system remained compliant. Within the level of automation frameworks outlined in [41, 42], the admittance control and virtual fixture technologies for increasing situational awareness are part of *Level 1* of automation, providing enhanced perception and/or guidance to the surgeon.

4.1 Admittance Control

Admittance control is a common control methodology used to allow for hands-on direct co-manipulation of a surgical tool attached to the end-effector of a robotic system [43]. The admittance controller was utilized to allow for the operator to collaborate with the surgical robot assistant smoothly and to minimize the operator's hand tremor and the vibration caused by the surgical saw [44–50].

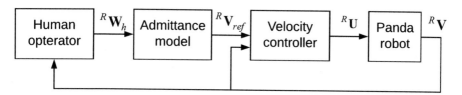

Fig. 7 Admittance controller for the robot

The admittance controller ensures that the surgical robot is compliant while still providing appreciable haptic guidance to the user.

The controller design is outlined in Fig. 7. Here, $^R\mathbf{W}_h$ is the interaction force-torque (wrench) between the robot end-effector and the operator, which is measured directly through a 6-DOF force sensor, as expressed in the frame $\{R\}$. The pre-programmed admittance model receives inputs, $^R\mathbf{W}_h$, and generates reference Cartesian (both translational and angular) velocity for the robot, $^R\mathbf{V}_{ref}$, to track. As the saw is mounted on the robot end-effector, we use the position and orientation of the robot end-effector to indicate the position and orientation of the saw blade for the sake of brevity. A velocity controller is used for the robot and outputs control signals, $^R\mathbf{U}$, to the robot. The actual Cartesian velocity of the robot end-effector is denoted as $^R\mathbf{V}$.

The desired admittance model in this study is designed as

$$\mathbf{M}\,^R\mathbf{V}_{ref} + \mathbf{C}\,^R\mathbf{V}_{ref} = k_f\,^R\mathbf{W}_h \tag{1}$$

where $\mathbf{C}$ and $\mathbf{M}$ are the virtual damping and inertia (6-by-6 diagonal) matrices of the admittance model given in [8]. In order to avoid restoring forces in free-space, the stiffness term is set to be zero matrix. Also, k_f is a force scaling factor.

5 Experimental Setup for Demonstration Assistive Systems

The experimental setups (shown in Figs. 1a, b, and 2) for the demonstration assistive systems, in [7, 8], contain some equipment in common. The virtual surgical objects and scenes for 2D and AR displays used in both setups for visual guidance were rendered using the Unity Engine (Version 2019.2.21 Unity Technologies, San Francisco, CA, USA). The calculations of the AR display projective parameters and experimental data analysis were done in MATLAB/Simulink R2019a (The MathWorks Inc, Natwick, MA, USA).

5.1 Experimental Percutaneous Biopsy Setup

For the percutaneous biopsy task, phantom tumours were fabricated and embedded into a rectangular opaque tissue phantom. Super soft plastisol (M-F Manufacturing Company, Fort Worth, Texas, USA), which is similar in characteristics to biological tissue, was used to create the tumour and phantom tissue. The plastisol phantom tumours, located inside the tissue phantom, have the same material properties as the surrounding tissue and are sized to approximate tumors seen clinically. Using the same plastisol for the phantom tissue and tumour replicates the characteristics of a non-palpable tumour. To track the location of the biopsy needles in real-time an electromagnetic tracker, the NDI Aurora V2 System (NDI Medical, Waterloo, Ontario, Canada), was used. The biopsy needle and tissue phantom were instrumented with 6-DOF sensors (NDI Item ID 610029) to track the position and orientation of the needles and tumour. The needle tracking information was used to update the position of the biopsy needle for both the 2D and AR display modality experiments.

5.2 Experimental Fibula Osteotomy Setup

For haptic guidance in the fibula osteotomy study, a Panda Robotic Arm (Franka Emika GmbH, Munich, Germany) equipped with an Axia80-M20 force/torque sensor (ATI Industrial Automation, Inc., Apex, NC, USA) was used as the surgical robot (Fig. 2). A rotary saw (Dremel 4300-5/40, Toluca, Mexico) was attached to the robot end-effector to act as a proxy for a surgical bone saw used in fibula osteotomy. The feasibility of the proposed methods is verified through proof-of-concept experimentation by performing fibula osteotomies on several simulated fibula bones which are wood dowels with a diameter of half an inch. Although the stiffnesses of the wood dowel and the fibula bone are slightly different, both are rigid objects, and both are designed to effectively cut through them. Therefore the difference in material properties has a trivial and negligible effect on the experimental results. The admittance controller for the virtual fixtures was implemented using MATLAB/Simulink R2019a, on a PC running Ubuntu 16.04 LTS, containing an Intel Core i5-8400 running at 4.00 GHz (Intel Corporation, Santa Clara, CA, USA).

References

1. Nomikos, I.N.: "Situational awareness in surgery. Hellenic Journal of Surgery **90**, no. 6, pp. 282–284, 2018. [Online]. Available: https://doi.org/10.1007/s13126-018-0490-y
2. Fida, B., Cutolo, F., di Franco, G., Ferrari, M., Ferrari, V.: Augmented reality in open surgery. Updates Surg. **70**(3), 389–400 (2018) [Online]. Available: https://doi.org/10.1007/s13304-018-0567-8

3. Eckert, M., Volmerg, J.S., Friedrich, C.M.: Augmented reality in medicine: systematic and bibliographic review. JMIR Mhealth Uhealth **7**(4), e10967 (2019). [Online]. Available: http://mhealth.jmir.org/2019/4/e10967/

4. Jud, L., Fotouhi, J., Andronic, O., Aichmair, A., Osgood, G., Navab, N., Farshad, M.: Applicability of augmented reality in orthopedic surgery - a systematic review. BMC Musculoskelet. Disord. **21**(1), 103 (2020). [Online]. Available: https://doi.org/10.1186/s12891-020-3110-2

5. Bowyer, S.A., Davies, B.L., Rodriguez y Baena, F.: Active constraints/virtual fixtures: A survey. IEEE Trans. Robot. **30**(1), 138–157 (2014)

6. Abbott, J.J., Marayong, P., Okamura, A.M.: Haptic virtual fixtures for robot-assisted manipulation. In: Thrun, S., Brooks, R., Durrant-Whyte, H. (eds.) Robotics Research, pp. 49–64 Springer Berlin Heidelberg, Berlin, Heidelberg (2007)

7. Asgar-Deen, D., Carriere, J., Wiebe, E., Peiris, L., Duha, A., Tavakoli, M.: Augmented reality guided needle biopsy of soft tissue: A pilot study. Front. Robot. AI **7**, 72 (2020). [Online]. Available: https://www.frontiersin.org/article/10.3389/frobt.2020.00072

8. Cheng, L., Carriere, J., Piwowarczyk, J., Alto, D., Zemiti, N., de Boutray, M., Tavakoli, M.: Admittance-controlled robotic assistant for fibula osteotomies in mandible reconstruction surgery. Adv. Intell. Syst. **3**, 2000158 (2020)

9. Frangioni, J.V.: New technologies for human cancer imaging. J. Clin. Oncol. **26**(24), 4012 (2008)

10. Rossa, C., Tavakoli, M.: Issues in closed-loop needle steering. Control Eng. Pract. **62**, 55–69 (2017). [Online]. Available: http://www.sciencedirect.com/science/article/pii/S0967066117300606

11. Hidalgo, D.A.: Fibula free flap: A new method of mandible reconstruction. Plastic Reconstr. Surg. 84(1), 1989 [Online]. Available: https://journals.lww.com/plasreconsurg/Fulltext/1989/07000/Fibula_Free_Flap__A_New_Method_of_Mandible.14.aspx

12. Hidalgo, D.A., Pusic, A.L.: Free-flap mandibular reconstruction: a 10-year follow-up study. Plastic Reconstr. Surg. **110**, 438–49; discussion 450–1 (2002)

13. Chang, E.I., Jenkins, M.P., Patel, S.A., Topham, N.S.: Long-term operative outcomes of preoperative computed tomography-guided virtual surgical planning for osteocutaneous free flap mandible reconstruction. Plastic Reconstr. Surg. **137**, 619–623 (2016)

14. Liberman, L.: Percutaneous imaging-guided core breast biopsy: state of the art at the millennium. Am. J. Roentgenol. **174**(5), 1191–1199 (2000)

15. Parker, S.H., Burbank, F., Jackman, R.J., Aucreman, C.J., Cardenosa, G., Cink, T.M., Coscia Jr, J.L., Eklund, G., Evans 3rd, W., Garver, P.R.: Percutaneous large-core breast biopsy: a multi-institutional study. Radiology **193**(2), 359–364 (1994)

16. Boba, M., Kołtun, U., Bobek-Billewicz, B., Chmielik, E., Eksner, B., Olejnik, T.: False-negative results of breast core needle biopsies–retrospective analysis of 988 biopsies. Polish J. Radiol. **76**(1), 25 (2011)

17. Liberman, L., Dershaw, D.D., Glassman, J.R., Abramson, A.F., Morris, E.A., LaTrenta, L.R., Rosen, P.P.: Analysis of cancers not diagnosed at stereotactic core breast biopsy. Radiology **203**(1), 151–157 (1997)

18. Youk, J.H., Kim, E.-K., Kim, M.J., Lee, J.Y., Oh, K.K.: Missed breast cancers at us-guided core needle biopsy: how to reduce them. Radiographics **27**(1), 79–94 (2007)

19. Castermans, A., van Garsse, A., Vanwijck, R.: Primary reconstruction of the mandible after resection for oral cancer. Acta Chir. Bel. **76**, 203–208 (1977)

20. Defries, H.O.: Reconstruction of the mandible: Use of combined homologous mandible and autologous bone. Otolaryngol. Head Neck Surg. **89**(4), 694–697 (1981), pMID: 6793984. [Online]. Available: https://doi.org/10.1177/019459988108900433

21. Lowlicht, R.A., Delacure, M.D., Sasaki, C.T.: Allogeneic (homograft) reconstruction of the mandible. Laryngoscope **100**, 837–843 (1990)

22. Liu, Y.-f., Xu, L.-w., Zhu, H.-y., Liu, S.S.-Y.: Technical procedures for template-guided surgery for mandibular reconstruction based on digital design and manufacturing. Biomed. Eng. Online **13**, 63 (2014)

23. Matros, E., Santamaria, E., Cordeiro, P.G.: Standardized templates for shaping the fibula free flap in mandible reconstruction. J. Reconstr. Microsurg. **29**, 619–622 (2013)
24. Rodby, K.A., Turin, S., Jacobs, R.J., Cruz, J.F., Hassid, V.J., Kolokythas, A., Antony, A.K.: Advances in oncologic head and neck reconstruction: systematic review and future considerations of virtual surgical planning and computer aided design/computer aided modeling. J. Plast. Reconstr. Aesthet. Surg. JPRAS **67**, 1171–1185 (2014)
25. Sieira Gil, R., Roig, A.M., Obispo, C.A., Morla, A., Pagès, C.M., Perez, J.L.: Surgical planning and microvascular reconstruction of the mandible with a fibular flap using computer-aided design, rapid prototype modelling, and precontoured titanium reconstruction plates: a prospective study. Br. J. Oral Maxillofac. Surg. **53**, 49–53 (2015)
26. Logan, H., Wolfaardt, J., Boulanger, P., Hodgetts, B., Seikaly, H.: Exploratory benchtop study evaluating the use of surgical design and simulation in fibula free flap mandibular reconstruction. J. Otolaryngol. Head Neck Surg. Le Journal d'oto-rhino-laryngologie et de chirurgie cervico-faciale **42**, 42 (2013)
27. Papadopoulos-Nydam, G., Wolfaardt, J., Seikaly, H., O'Connell, D., Harris, J., Osswald, M., Nayar, S., Rieger, J.: Comparison of speech and resonance outcomes across three methods of treatment for maxillary defects. Int. J. Maxillofac. Prosthetics **1**, 2–8 (2017)
28. Rozen, W.M., Ting, J.W.C., Leung, M., Wu, T., Ying, D., Leong, J.: Advancing image-guided surgery in microvascular mandibular reconstruction: combining bony and vascular imaging with computed tomography-guided stereolithographic bone modeling. Plast. Reconstr. Surg. **130**, 227e–229e (2012)
29. Chao, A.H., Weimer, K., Raczkowsky, J., Zhang, Y., Kunze, M., Cody, D., Selber, J.C., Hanasono, M.M., Skoracki, R.J.: Pre-programmed robotic osteotomies for fibula free flap mandible reconstruction: A preclinical investigation. Microsurgery **36**, 246–249 (2016)
30. Kong, X., Duan, X., Wang, Y.: An integrated system for planning, navigation and robotic assistance for mandible reconstruction surgery. Intell. Serv. Robot. **9**(2), 113–121 (2016). [Online]. Available: https://doi.org/10.1007/s11370-015-0189-7
31. Zhu, J.-H., Deng, J., Liu, X.-J., Wang, J., Guo, Y.-X., Guo, C.-B.: Prospects of robot-assisted mandibular reconstruction with fibula flap: Comparison with a computer-assisted navigation system and freehand technique. J. Reconstr. Microsurg. **32**, 661–669 (2016)
32. Milgram, P., Kishino, F.: A taxonomy of mixed reality visual displays. IEICE Trans. Inf. Syst. **77**(12), 1321–1329 (1994)
33. Nicolau, S., Soler, L., Mutter, D., Marescaux, J.: Augmented reality in laparoscopic surgical oncology. Surg. Oncol. **20**(3), 189–201 (2011), special Issue: Education for Cancer Surgeons. [Online]. Available: http://www.sciencedirect.com/science/article/pii/S0960740411000521
34. Kikinis, R., Pieper, S.D., Vosburgh, K.G.: 3D Slicer: a platform for subject-specific image analysis, visualization, and clinical support. In: Intraoperative Imaging and Image-Guided Therapy, pp. 277–289. Springer New York, New York (2014). [Online]. Available: https://doi.org/10.1007/978-1-4614-7657-3_19
35. Bimber, O.: Interactive rendering for projection-based augmented reality displays, Ph.D. dissertation, University of Technology Darmstadt, 9 2002
36. Rossa, C., Keri, M.I., Tavakoli, M.: Brachytherapy needle steering guidance using image overlay. In: Habib, M. (ed.) Handbook of Research on Biomimetics and Biomedical Robotics, pp. 191–204. IGI Global, Hershey, PA (2018). [Online]. Available: http://services.igi-global.com/resolvedoi/resolve.aspx?doi=10.4018/978-1-5225-2993-4.ch008
37. Ferrari, V., Carbone, M., Condino, S., Cutolo, F.: Are augmented reality headsets in surgery a dead end? Expert Rev. Med. Devices **16**(12), 999–1001 (2019), pMID: 31725347. [Online]. Available: https://doi.org/10.1080/17434440.2019.1693891
38. Condino, S., Carbone, M., Piazza, R., Ferrari, M., Ferrari, V.: Perceptual limits of optical see-through visors for augmented reality guidance of manual tasks. IEEE Trans. Biomed. Eng. **67**(2), 411–419 (2020)
39. Howard, I.: Depth from motion parallax. In: Perceiving in Depth: Volume 3 Other Mechanisms of Depth Perception. Oxford University Press, Oxford (2012), ch. 28
40. Kooima, R.: Generalized perspective projection. J. Sch. Electron. Eng. Comput. Sci, 6 (2009)

41. Attanasio, A., Scaglioni, B., De Momi, E., Fiorini, P., Valdastri, P.: Autonomy in surgical robotics. Ann. Rev. Control Robot. Auton. Syst. **4**(1), null (2021). [Online]. Available: https://doi.org/10.1146/annurev-control-062420-090543

42. Yang, G.-Z., Cambias, J., Cleary, K., Daimler, E., Drake, J., Dupont, P.E., Hata, N., Kazanzides, P., Martel, S., Patel, R.V., Santos, V.J., Taylor, R.H.: Medical robotics—regulatory, ethical, and legal considerations for increasing levels of autonomy. Sci. Robot. **2**(4) (2017). [Online]. Available: https://robotics.sciencemag.org/content/2/4/eaam8638

43. Hogan, N.: Impedance control: An approach to manipulation: Part I–theory. J. Dyn. Syst. Meas. Control **107**(1), 1–7 (1985). [Online]. Available: https://doi.org/10.1115/1.3140702

44. Carriere, J., Fong, J., Meyer, T., Sloboda, R., Husain, S., Usmani, N., Tavakoli, M.: An admittance-controlled robotic assistant for semi-autonomous breast ultrasound scanning. In: 2019 International Symposium on Medical Robotics (ISMR), pp. 1–7 (2019, April)

45. Cheng, L., Tavakoli, M.: Ultrasound image guidance and robot impedance control for beating-heart surgery. Control Eng. Pract. **81**, 9–17 (2018). [Online]. Available: http://www.sciencedirect.com/science/article/pii/S096706611830460X

46. Cheng, L., Tavakoli, M.: Switched-impedance control of surgical robots in teleoperated beating-heart surgery. J. Med. Robot. Res. **03**(03n04), 1841003 (2018). [Online]. Available: https://doi.org/10.1142/S2424905X18410039

47. Cheng, L., Sharifi, M., Tavakoli, M.: Towards robot-assisted anchor deployment in beating-heart mitral valve surgery. Int. J. Med. Robot. Comput. Assisted Surg. **14**(3), e1900 (2018), e1900 RCS-17-0094.R2. [Online]. Available: https://onlinelibrary.wiley.com/doi/abs/10.1002/rcs.1900

48. Sharifi, M., Salarieh, H., Behzadipour, S., Tavakoli, M.: Impedance control of non-linear multi-dof teleoperation systems with time delay: absolute stability. IET Control Theory Appl. **12**(12), 1722–1729 (2018)

49. Sharifi, M., Salarieh, H., Behzadipour, S., Tavakoli, M.: Beating-heart robotic surgery using bilateral impedance control: Theory and experiments. Biomed. Signal Process. Control **45**, 256–266 (2018). [Online]. Available: http://www.sciencedirect.com/science/article/pii/S174680941830123X

50. Piwowarczyk, J., Carriere, J., Adams, K., Tavakoli, M.: An admittance-controlled force-scaling dexterous assistive robotic system. J. Med. Robot. Res. **05**(01n02), 2041002 (2020)

Correction to: Enhancing Situational Awareness and Kinesthetic Assistance for Clinicians via Augmented-Reality and Haptic Shared-Control Technologies

Jay Carriere, Lingbo Cheng, and Mahdi Tavakoli

Correction to:
Chapter 10 in: T. McDaniel, X. Liu (eds.),
Multimedia for Accessible Human Computer Interfaces,
https://doi.org/10.1007/978-3-030-70716-3_10

"Owing to an error on the part of the editor and corresponding chapter author, the author's name in the chapter opening page of chapter 'Enhancing Situational Awareness and Kinesthetic Assistance for Clinicians via Augmented-Reality and Haptic Shared-Control Technologies' was presented wrongly. The author's name has now been updated to be Mahdi Tavakoli in the chapter opening page, table of contents, and wherever applicable throughout the book."

The updated online version of this chapter can be found at
https://doi.org/10.1007/978-3-030-70716-3_10

Printed in the United States
by Baker & Taylor Publisher Services